T0200461

KIRK'S
BASIC SURGICAL
TECHNIQUES

Eighth Edition

KIRK'S BASIC SURGICAL TECHNIQUES

Fiona Myint, FRCS

Consultant Vascular Surgeon
Royal Free Hospital

Professor of Surgical Education
University College London
London, UK

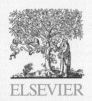

ELSEVIER

© 2025, Elsevier Limited. All rights are reserved, including those for text and data mining, AI training, and similar technologies.

First edition 1973
Second edition 1978
Third edition 1989
Fourth edition 1994
Fifth edition 2002
Sixth edition 2010
Seventh edition 2018

The right of Fiona Myint to be identified as author of this work has been asserted by her in accordance with the Copyright, Designs and Patents Act 1988.

No part of this publication may be reproduced or transmitted in any form or by any means, electronic or mechanical, including photocopying, recording, or any information storage and retrieval system, without permission in writing from the publisher. Details on how to seek permission, further information about the Publisher's permissions policies and our arrangements with organizations such as the Copyright Clearance Center and the Copyright Licensing Agency, can be found at our website: www.elsevier.com/permissions.www.elsevier.com/permissions.

This book and the individual contributions contained in it are protected under copyright by the Publisher (other than as may be noted herein).

Notices

Practitioners and researchers must always rely on their own experience and knowledge in evaluating and using any information, methods, compounds or experiments described herein. Because of rapid advances in the medical sciences, in particular, independent verification of diagnoses and drug dosages should be made. To the fullest extent of the law, no responsibility is assumed by Elsevier, authors, editors or contributors for any injury and/or damage to persons or property as a matter of products liability, negligence or otherwise, or from any use or operation of any methods, products, instructions, or ideas contained in the material herein.

ISBN: 978-0-4431-1367-3
      978-0-4431-1442-7

Senior Content Strategist: Alex Mortimer
Content Project Manager: Supriya Barua Kumar
Design: Miles Hitchen
Marketing Manager: Deborah J. Watkins

Working together
to grow libraries in
developing countries

www.elsevier.com • www.bookaid.org

Printed in India

Last digit is the print number: 9 8 7 6 5 4 3 2 1

For Reo

'Success is no accident. It is hard work, perseverance, learning, studying, sacrifice and most of all, love of what you are doing or learning to do'.

– Pelé

RAYMOND MAURICE (JERRY) KIRK

Jerry Kirk was born and brought up in Nottingham. While he was still at school the Second World War began, and after a brief interim as a bank clerk he served as an ordinary seaman in the famous cruiser *HMS Ajax* during Operation Torch—the first combined American-British landings in North Africa. Commissioned in charge of a minesweeper in the Mediterranean Sea, he swept no mines, but the ship, renamed 'Calypso', was famously converted by the oceanographer Jacques Cousteau. After demobilization, and financed by an ex-service grant, Jerry attended Medical School at Kings College London and Charing Cross Hospital. He became an anatomy lecturer at Kings College London and went on to work for Professor Ian Aird at the Royal Postgraduate Medical School, Hammersmith Hospital. He held registrar posts at Charing Cross Hospital and subsequently the Royal Free Hospital, where he became a consultant general surgeon in 1964 and remained for the rest of his career.

He was an elected member of the Council of the Royal College of Surgeons of England, and devised the original basic surgical skills (BSS) course, as well as the first minimal access course, alongside Professor Sir Alfred Cuschieri. As director of the Overseas Doctors Training Scheme he was proud to see trainees return home with greater confidence and competence to deal with the surgical challenges in their homelands.

Jerry Kirk was privileged to work with a series of wonderful teachers, colleagues, students and patients. Notable among these were Professor Ian Aird, a scintillatingly brilliant intellect, and Norman Tanner, who from modest beginnings became internationally celebrated as a pioneer of standardized, safe gastric surgery, resulting in outstanding long-term outcomes. A third giant was the eminent oesophageal surgeon Hiroshi Akiyama of Tokyo, who could have been a twin brother of Tanner in character, both matching each other in talent, commitment, honesty and teaching by example. All three left Jerry recognizing the privilege of being a teacher.

He was a former president of the Surgical Section of the Royal Society of Medicine, the Medical Society of London and the Hunterian Society. He held honorary fellowships of the Association of Surgeons of Poland and the College of Surgeons of Sri Lanka and was a fellow of the Royal Society of Medicine. After retiring from clinical surgical practice in 1989, Jerry was appointed an honorary consulting surgeon at the Royal Free Hospital and Honorary Professor of Surgery at University College London teaching anatomy, basic surgical skills and essential clinical insights. He had a second career teaching aspiring surgeons for more than 25 years.

He was past editor-in-chief of the *Annals of the Royal College of Surgeons* and wrote and edited numerous books for surgeons in training, including *Basic Surgical Techniques*, *Clinical Surgery in General* and *General Surgical Operations*.

Preface

The first edition of *Kirk's Basic Surgical Techniques* was published in 1973. Since that time Professor Jerry Kirk updated and revised his classic work five times, reducing and refining the text into a more synoptic publication. He intended it to be a reference and learning text for trainee surgeons learning the foundations of their surgical craft. I was one of those surgical trainees who carried a well-thumbed third edition in my now defunct white coat. Thus, I was most honoured when he personally asked me to update the previous, seventh, edition, in particular as it was his personal favourite of all of his publications. Sadly, Professor Kirk is no longer with us, but I hope this further update of his little book will give both a flavour of his direct and personal teaching method and a source of reference for aspiring and practising trainee surgeons.

The book is intentionally written in the second person. This was Professor Kirk's style, providing personal instruction by addressing the reader directly. It is not intended to be an operative surgery book, and any reference to specific operations is to put into context the basic techniques used. If you are reading this book as a trainee surgeon, I wish you every success in your surgical career.

Fiona Myint
London, 2024

Acknowledgements

This book is still Kirk's book. Many of the words and illustrations are his. I am, as he was, grateful to all of those who supported him in writing and refining the book over the years. I am also very grateful my colleagues who have supported me for the last two editions. In particular, I wish to acknowledge the advice and sense checking provided by Mr Tim Lane, Mr Rovan D'Souza, Mr Akash Patel and Mr Ibidumo Igah.

Fiona Myint
London, 2024

Contents

Chapter | 1 |

Handling yourself

The personal qualities you bring to medicine are the same as those that drive all clinicians. We are all primarily physicians, endeavouring to apply the same knowledge and judgement that our medical colleagues apply to diagnosing and treating patients.

1. As a surgeon, the extra, practical aptitude you must acquire beyond clinical competence is operating skill – the ability to manipulate living human tissue with intimate knowledge of its characteristics in health and disease while endeavouring to preserve its physical and functional qualities. In the medieval period surgeons, unlike physicians, did not study at a university but were ranked as craftsmen, learning as apprentices from masters. As in other trades, surgeons use tools or instruments to facilitate controlling their materials but recognise that they are intermediates between their hands and the object of their skill. Your awareness of this should impress on you the need to use every practical task you perform as a means of improving the skills required in surgery all day, every day; not just in the operating theatre.

2. Individual components of operative skill can be listed but do not define the way in which they are put together to create a successful surgeon. Few of us are fully equipped mentally and physically, but by putting in the extra effort to overcome our weaknesses we hope to compensate for them. In contrast, some fortunate enough to be born with natural aptitudes fail to put in the extra effort.

3. From reading this chapter, identify in yourself some of the qualities you need to utilise and develop in order to become a skilful surgeon. You can recognise the presence or lack of them in your everyday life and initiate your training even before you step into the operating theatre. Continue this process when you watch operations, become an assistant, and are eventually allowed to perform part or all of an operation.

4. It is not necessary to see someone operating to identify the presence or absence of desirable

qualities. Watch others performing everyday tasks such as carving a joint of meat, peeling fruit, and eating a meal; is the food on the plate still orderly, or does it look like a battlefield? Note someone who habitually drops objects and swears at them muttering, 'Bad luck. That happens every time'. Why do experts not suffer such misfortunes? They recognise the likelihood and incorporate precautionary measures into their routines.

5. Some accomplish everyday tasks calmly, safely, and in an orderly manner, maintaining uncluttered surroundings. Others are casual, messy, rough, clumsy with their hands, the equipment, or the object they are handling, and do not seem to anticipate an imminent fault or accident that is evident to the onlookers. They may be outstanding at their vocation, but you would feel anxious if they claimed to be surgeons or intended to pursue such a career.

Key points

- **'Get it right first time'** incorporates the recognition that faults occur and that they must be anticipated and avoided.
- Do not hope for the best. If an error is likely, build into your routine a check or corrective.
- Correcting errors is more time consuming than avoiding them.

ATTITUDES – THE FIVE 'Cs'

1. *Common sense* encompasses being aware at all times of what is going on around you and reacting to it in a logical and rational manner. It is eroded if you are distracted or lose your composure and temper. Thus, your anticipation of impending danger is blunted, as is your ability to react sensibly and perform effectively. If you encounter a difficulty, do not rush wildly into 'doing something'. Respond to changed circumstances; errors often result from dogged and blind continuation with the intended procedure.

2. *Competence.* Make it a habit in your everyday life to carry out your duties in a relaxed atmosphere of expertise and calm. List your intentions in descending order of priority and ensure you are able to carry them out proficiently and professionally. Take each step in its correct order, complete it, check it and continue with the next one but react to new input and respond to it if necessary.

3. *Commitment.* Keep in mind your prime purpose. Unless circumstances change, concentrate on this and do not be deflected from it without good reason. Be willing to defer or cancel other duties in order to fulfil the most important one. Except in an emergency, complete every task.

4. *Compassion.* How privileged you are to be a physician, able to treat patients who are in pain, or anxious. Now you wish to add to your skills and offer another means of treatment. Operating on people can be dramatically successful and potentially disastrous. Expect to have occasional sleepless nights from anxiety and guilt as you retrospectively consider your recent actions.

5. *Communication.* You are in a professional relationship with your patients, their relatives and your colleagues. Technical skill in the operating theatre is not sufficient on its own to make you a successful surgeon. It is a vital add-on, but it is one component among many others. You must communicate and be open to communication; in other words, be willing to listen as well as to talk.

Key point

- You will carry these attitudes that you strive to develop, from your everyday life to the operating theatre.

PHYSICAL ATTRIBUTES

Hands

1. There is no ideal surgeon's hand. The shape of your hand has little or no bearing on your manipulative skill. However, identify the peculiarities of your own hands and fingers in order to exploit the benefits and make the best use of them. For example, the terminal phalanx, nail shape and extent of nail bed towards the tips of your fingers affect your preference for fingertip pressure or pulp pressure.

2. Your hands are important assessors of tissues. Their sensitivity is affected by wearing gloves. When clinical circumstances require you to

wear gloves, consciously note the changes. Make sure you wear the correct sise of gloves and wear them correctly. Do not allow the glove fingertips to project beyond yours. Rather, pull the glove fingers on fully, if necessary creating concertina'd wrinkles near the base of your fingers.

3. There are many outstanding left-handed surgeons, so this is no disability, even though many instruments are designed for right-handed people. Some instruments are also available for left-handed surgeons.

Stability

1. Surgeons do not usually have extraordinarily steady hands. Our ability to perform finely controlled movements diminishes as we age.

2. If you hold long-handled instruments at arm's length, the tips magnify the tremor and anxiety exaggerates this. Do not feel embarrassed. The further the distance from a firm base to the point of action, the less steady are your hands.

3. Stand upright with feet apart, arms and fingers outstretched. You will detect a slight tremor at your outspread fingertips. Now press your elbows into your sides and you should find your hands are steadier. Sit, or brace your hips against a fixture to become even steadier. Rest your elbows on a table; also rest the heel of your hand or your little finger on the table (Fig. 1.1).

Key point

- Keep a firm base as close as possible to the point of action.

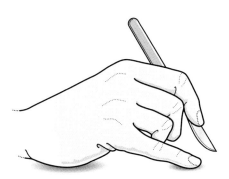

Fig. 1.1 Your wrist and little finger rest on the base, forming a steadying bridge while you hold the scalpel to make a precise incision.

4. If you cannot use a base close to the active fingers, use the other hand to steady the dominant hand by grasping the wrist. If you need to reach to make an action (for example, when you are cutting ligatures as an assistant), use the fingers of the inactive hand on which to rest the scissors (Fig. 1.2). If no other base exists, place the 'heels' of your hands together when carrying out a manoeuvre such as the nowadays rare need to thread a needle (Fig. 1.3), or when untying an inadvertent knot in your thread.

5. If you need to carry out a smooth movement, try practising it in the air first, as a golfer does before making a stroke.

WHAT IS SKILL?

---

1. The Old Norse word 'skil' signified distinction (from *skilja* = to separate, discriminate). In everyday use, it commonly signifies expertise and dexterity in performing a practical procedure as opposed to a facility in a theoretical or abstract accomplishment.

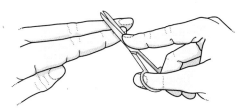

Fig. 1.2 Steadying an instrument by resting it on the fingers of the other hand.

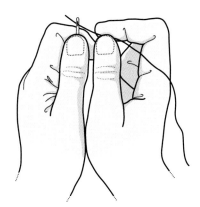

Fig. 1.3 Press your wrists together while threading a needle.

2. As an example, a tennis beginner must learn to control the racket to strike a ball. Initially, the player must concentrate on the dominant hand controlling the racket head. As the presence of the racket becomes a familiar extension of the hand, the concentration can be transferred increasingly to the ball, which becomes the prime focus as its flight is observed and predicted. The racket head is relegated to subsidiary focus[1] and seems to move naturally so that the sweet spot impacts the ball.

3. This ability to 'download' the means of accomplishing something, so freeing the performer to focus attention on the prime object of the procedure, is a skill. It is a fundamental achievement that has to be acquired by assiduous, intelligent practice. It frees the player to see the game as a whole, able to plan, anticipate and be correctly positioned for the next shot.

4. It is remarkable that having acquired a skill and then trying to add further ones, the first skill is initially lost. When you learn to drive a car, having learned to control the accelerator and brake, if you now look at the other traffic, as you wish to signal your desire to move off and steer into the road, your control of the accelerator and brake pedals often regresses. Likewise, as a child, you probably spent hours learning the alphabet, but now it is incorporated into your language skills without reference to these basic building blocks.

5. When you have acquired a skill, however simple, you will find that if you concentrate on it, you become clumsy. If you are familiar with a QWERTY keyboard on a computer or typewriter, ask yourself if you can continue the line of letters after the 'Y' or list the next line. Why do you have difficulty? Your fingers go to them automatically because you have relegated them to a subsidiary awareness. Your focal awareness is directed at what you are writing.

6. You will appreciate that if you attempt to hurry, you are moving your primary focus from the accomplishment of the skilful performance to the individual movements, and you make mistakes. Take the example once again of the keyboard. Try typing at speed. Your focal awareness shifts to the keys, not the content, and you make mistakes.

7. In order to acquire a skill, you must practise it assiduously until you can perform it repeatedly and reliably. Just going through movements does not demonstrate a skill. You need to perform it perfectly, every time.

Key points

- Having acquired a skill, always perform it at a natural pace.
- Hand speed and work speed are not parallel – they may even be opposed.
- Indeed, it often takes longer to repeat and correct a rushed and imperfect act than to perform it deliberately and correctly in the first place.

8. Watch and copy experts. Of course, they cannot bestow skill. Differentiate between trainers and masters. A trainer or coach can tell you what to do, assess you and identify ways for you to improve but does not necessarily have the personal skill to do so at a high level. A craft master (L *magister*) is one who is an expert at *performing* the craft and can show you. Watch and remember how they achieve their success. Trainers may not be masters and masters may not be good trainers.

EXERCISES VERSUS PRACTICE

1. Since you need to carry out the task repeatedly to acquire skill, differentiate between exercise and practice. It is a distinction recognised more by instrumental musicians and those pursuing a career in sports than by surgeons.

2. *Exercise.* If you wish to become accomplished at a particular procedure you have been shown, you may repeat it until it becomes second nature, and you can carry it out without the need to concentrate on the component actions. Each repetition is the same as the previous one. For example, young violinists use the Suzuki method of teaching.

3. *Practice.* You may instead perform the manoeuvre, identify a difficulty or a means of facilitating it and adjust the next trial to judge its success in eliminating the difficulty; this will make the procedure feel easier, better controlled and more natural. Continue until you cannot improve it further; only then should you convert it into an exercise.[2]

4. Ask for feedback from trainers and colleagues. Undertake work-based assessments as a formative process throughout training and do not leave their use until the end as purely summative assessments. The more feedback you

receive, the more you have to reflect upon and base your development upon.

5. Remain willing to modify it again if you find a better routine. One of the benefits of watching others is that it gives you the opportunity to see new approaches to difficult manoeuvres. Musical instrumentalists often ask experts to 'finger in' passages which they find difficult.

6. This intelligent practice augments the natural process of skills learning in which as we repeat a manoeuvre we develop a confidence in the probability of the next result and adjust the 'feed-forward' motor signals. During the performance, sensorimotor signals provide 'feedback' adjustments to create the optimum result. This is a form of Bayesian integration.[3]

HAPTICS

1. Do not be distracted by this word (G *haptein* = to fasten). It becomes increasingly important as we introduce methods of 'handling' tissues by instruments that reduce or remove our ability to feel them, assess their surface, texture and temperature, and appreciate the force we are applying to them and their resistance to that force. It is the science of touch (possibly related to L *tangere* = to touch), creating an interface mainly between us and technological apparatus and instruments.[4]

2. During clinical examination of our patients we recognise and identify many structures by touch, assessing the surface, texture and temperature. We employ our kinaesthetic sense (G *kinein* = to move + *aisthesis* = perception) to explore them for homogeneity, strength, friability, flexibility and attachments. We may receive force feedback from resistance or vibrations. We rely heavily on our knowledge of the texture of structures and when we wear gloves, even thin surgical gloves, our appreciation of touch is impaired.

3. When you interpose an instrument between your hand and the target structure, your tactile input is drastically reduced. Rigid instruments such as dissecting forceps transmit more than soft or flexible ones; when you pass a soft urinary catheter into the bladder, you need to move it extremely delicately to appreciate the progress through the urethra. The more complex the link between the hand and the target structure, the greater the loss of touch.

4. You will find, as you embark on your surgical career, that much of your training will be using instruments. Do not be misled into feeling that skill in manipulating them alone confers surgical skill. However, many surgical procedures are now performed without the operator touching the tissues. In order to reduce exposure, minimal-access procedures have been widely developed. When using instruments, whether handheld or mechanically or electronically linked, the sense of touch is reduced or lost. You may have the opportunity to experience on a simulator the use of minimal-access instruments, often with relatively long handles. In laparoscopic surgery, you need to move your hand in the opposite direction to the intended tip movement, a pivoting movement about a fulcrum. In robotic surgery the hand and target tissue are decoupled, being driven through electronic systems, and you move your hand in the same direction as the intended tip movement. Much research is directed at providing force feedback to the operator to help in the estimation of the tissues held within graspers.

5. *Force and torque.* In other occupations, artificially produced haptic feedback systems are in use to provide operators with – as yet limited – sensation of feel and measure of applied force and torque (L *torquere* = to twist). These are being introduced into surgical applications. When you watch an expert tighten a ligature, it is impossible to know, and accurately replicate, the tension. Again, in the case of handheld or electronically controlled robotic instruments, appreciation of the force transmitted is reduced or not sensed. It is now possible to measure the force exerted through some instruments.[5] An important finding is that novices tend to exert up to 130% more force or torque than is required by experts to perform the same procedure. You do not need elaborate equipment to recognise the potential damage you can inadvertently create by pinching tissues with instruments. If the handles of hinged forceps are twice as long as the blades, your squeezing force is doubled at the tips. You may exert very high compression per unit area through fine forceps with tip surfaces as fine as 2–3 mm^2. Use too much force and, when you release your pressure, the crushed tissue soon looks normal, but it will die or – at best – be partially replaced with a scar. When you look at some old wounds, you see scarred

lines crossing the healed wound; they result from sutures tied too tightly.

6. Whenever you encounter resistance of any type, make it a habit to apply the minimum force to overcome it. Often this means changing your approach or method or removing an obstacle that adds to the difficulty. When you watch or assist an expert surgeon you will be surprised how little force is used. Magically, the tissues seem to behave well out of respect for the surgeon. It is not magic. It is the result of intimate familiarity in guiding the tissues to conform to the operator's wishes. This is the essence of craftsmanship.

Key points

- Make it a habit in everyday activities, to achieve manipulations with minimal force.
- Consider trying several methods and choose the gentlest.

TRANSFERABLE SKILLS

1. Even before you enter the operating theatre you can start to develop or improve the manipulative facility and sensitivity that you will require as a surgeon. Adapt every possible normal routine to hone your skills. Watch skilled workers in other vocations and you will see common traits, some of which you can incorporate into your training. It is a joy to see someone carefully assessing a problem, unhurriedly preparing the materials and tools, doing the preparatory work to facilitate the task, and now seemingly effortlessly carrying out the needed procedure, reassembling, testing and approving the result. This is a demonstration of seamless assessment, decision, preparation, accomplishment and final assessment without haste or the need to correct imperfections.

2. The French surgeon Alexis Carrel (1873–1944) developed his suturing technique after watching an expert embroiderer in Lyon. He practised by inserting up to 500 stitches in a cigarette paper without once tearing it, becoming a founder of vascular surgery, for which he received the Nobel Prize in 1912. The British surgeon Lord Moynihan (1865–1936), who was famously skilled, was reported to carry a piece of string with which he practised tying knots whenever he had a spare moment.

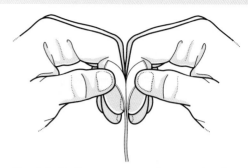

Fig. 1.4 Peeling apart two adherent strips. Trap the strips between the thumbs and index fingers. As you supinate your wrists, you separate the strips but maintain contact between your index fingers and then your middle fingers. This keeps the length of strips being distracted to a minimum. Do not separate your hands but repeatedly change your grip.

3. For example, when you peel fruit or open a sealed envelope, you can practise separating tissues without damaging them, while keeping them in the correct plane. You achieve this by keeping the distance between the adherent surfaces and the distracting force to a minimum. Every time you open a sealed envelope, raise an edge of the flap and extend the parting. Grasp each edge between the thumb and index finger. While keeping your index fingers pressed together, evert your hands so that the edges are separated. Limit the extent of the cleaving tension by compressing the still sealed section just ahead of the split between your middle fingers (Fig. 1.4). You are remarkably sensitive to incipient tearing. Unless you readjust your grip every few millimetres, your hands move apart, the extent of paper at risk is lengthened and you may not detect a tear starting anywhere along it.

4. Use your ingenuity to find other practice opportunities. Try to perform every action gently, neatly and with minimum disturbance.

Speed

The examples of focal awareness demonstrate the importance of allowing your hard-won skill to be applied naturally. Do not compromise the benefits of this by hurrying.

Sequence (L *sequi* = to follow)

If you need to take apart, adjust or repair any structure or equipment, determine to attempt doing so without misplacing or dropping any part and carry out the dismantling and reassembly in the correct sequence. The value of the habit will be evident when you watch or participate in a surgical operation. There is a well-tried procedural order.

SKILLS COURSES

1. In the past trainee surgeons watched, assisted and then operated on patients. Indeed, there was an adage, 'See one, do one, teach one'. It is preferable for you to be shown in a course, away from the potentially tense atmosphere of an operating theatre, how to perform the procedures and carry them out under supervision and guidance. Take every opportunity to attend such courses.

2. Practice operations on live but anaesthetised animals is an ethical dilemma and is strictly limited except for microsurgery. Dead animal tissue has been used for many years, but simulated tissues are increasing in use. The available models may look like real body parts, but it is not yet possible to create simulations with the complex, varied structure and consistency that you will encounter in surgical practice. Make the most of these opportunities to reach the highest level of skill that you can with these models, remembering that the ultimate purpose of these courses is to teach you to operate on living tissue.

3. You must become familiar with handling surgical instruments – courses offer you this facility. You initially need to concentrate your attention on controlling them, rather than controlling what is at the other end of them. As you become more familiar, they become natural extensions of your hands, and when you come to operate on living tissues, you can focus your concentration on the tissues rather than on the instruments, with which you are now proficient (see below).

4. Laparoscopic surgical courses are particularly valuable because you need to become familiar with the opposite effects of hand movements on instrument tip movement through the pivoted access port (see Ch. 13).

5. Virtual reality and augmented reality instruments and courses based on them provide you with the opportunity to learn how to control complex instruments that further remove you from the target tissues. At present, they mainly offer exercises that you control under visual guidance. They offer the promise

Key points

- Skills courses offer excellent introductions to operative procedures. They are adjuncts, not replacements, for becoming skilled at operating on living tissues.
- Skills courses do not transfer skills to you; they should reveal to you what skills you need to acquire through active practice.

of greater haptic and force/torque feedback, but this is still rather crude (see above).

6. *Create your own simulations.* Courses offer you limited experience in carrying out operations. You need to create opportunities for practising the routines and become familiar with them. Use your ingenuity to create an arrangement that allows you to repeatedly follow through part or all of an operation. When you are offered the opportunity to carry out the same procedure in the operating theatre, you will have the confidence to perform it competently. In the future, the surgeon, who is responsible to the patient, will be more willing to delegate a procedure to you if you have already demonstrated during a simulation that you can perform it safely.

THOUGHT PROCESSES

Kahneman describes two thought systems: system 1 is a fast, subconscious automatic system, and system 2 is a slow, conscious system. When we begin to learn surgery, system 2 is at the forefront as we try and remember the sequence of the procedure and what we have been taught. As we become more proficient, some of what we do uses system 1, for instance automatically tying a knot when we have placed a suture. The more that the processes come into system 1, the more proficient we become. However, we can also learn bad habits. It is therefore important to learn correctly from the start in order to avoid forming any unconscious bad habits.

RATIONAL ASSESSMENT OF INFORMATION

1. Part of your complex development as a competent surgeon is how you discriminate

the information you receive. You will be simultaneously trying to improve as a physician-scientist, a practical craftsman, learning current accepted practice, yet being aware that this may be rapidly changing.

2. Be willing to follow the practice of your teachers. This often means that you have to change your methods as you pass through the rotating appointments. It is important that you do not become too rigid early in your career. Sometimes an unfamiliar method proves, with practice, to be an improvement on your current one. Ultimately, your own practice will be a conglomeration of the best that you have learned from trainers and experiences.

3. Your trainers may claim that their success depends upon some possibly unique change in their technique or material, but they seem to get similar results to others who do not perform in the same manner. You will learn that it is not the method or the material that is the component of success, but rather the care with which it is incorporated into the procedure. Your teacher is too modest in attributing success to one change; success is the result of outstanding commitment to skill and competence.

4. Improvements in techniques, instruments and materials constantly appear. Welcome them but assess them critically. Those who introduce them often unconsciously or consciously select the patients, and by committing to it greater effort and enthusiasm, obtain improved outcomes. Improvement in performance may also result from increased attention to it. This is often called the 'Hawthorne effect', named after a noted rise in productivity at a factory in Hawthorne near Chicago when the workers became aware that they were being assessed. It is only when uncommitted researchers detect improvement that you should embrace the claimed improvement.

COMMUNICATION

Throughout your surgical career, you will communicate with patients, their relatives and colleagues from your own department and others. Be aware of the effect that your communication has on others. As a surgeon, you hold a position of respect and authority for many around you, and it sometimes helps to imagine yourself in

their shoes when you communicate with them. This applies to verbal, non-verbal and written communication. Remember that lack of communication can also convey messages to others.

Do not bring your external worries and sorrows to work with you.

If you are physically or mentally unwell, consider taking a break to recover. You are human too.

BURNOUT

1. Surgery is a rewarding and fulfilling career. However, as with all aspects of life, there are good days and bad days. Caring for one's patients is an honour and a privilege. Occasionally the onus of caring can lead to anxiety and emotional exhaustion. If continuously repeated or prolonged, this can lead to burnout. This is more likely to occur if you have high ideals and high expectations of yourself and your performance, or if you are in a higher-risk or higher-acuity specialty.

2. Look out for the signs. Are you in a constant low mood at work? Are you being uncharacteristically grumpy either at work or at home? It is important that you look after yourself as well as your patients. Share your concerns with a trusted colleague, family member or mentor. Don't be afraid to take a step back, even if only for a short period of time.

PROCEDURAL PRACTICE

There are a number of general principles that you will always follow:

- Conduct yourself with professionalism at all times (it is worth reflecting on what this means)
- Ensure good communication
- Ensure good handwashing and infection control procedures
- Wear appropriate personal protective clothing (apron, gown, gloves, double glove, face mask)
- Handle all tissues with care and respect
- Consider the whole patient and not just the small area on which you are working
- Remember that you are a doctor as well as a surgeon
- Do not practise beyond your capabilities
- Have insight into your own capabilities

- Do not be afraid to ask for advice and help
- Learn and practise constantly
- Ask for feedback and accept and act on it if necessary
- Reflect on your own performance
- Be responsible for your own actions

You should aim to be the best possible surgeon that you can be. Of course, this is open to reflection; you may model yourself on one of your surgical heroes (or heroines). However, throughout your surgical career, you will observe many good qualities in senior and junior colleagues. Learn from these and practise those with which you can develop yourself for the better.

> **Key point**
>
> - You are a better carer for your family and your patients if you are in a good physical and psychological place yourself.

REFERENCES

1. Polanyi M. *Personal knowledge of J Kirk.* London: Routledge & Kegan Paul; 1973.
2. Cross KD. Role of practice in perpetual-motor learning. *Am J Phys Med.* 1967;46:487–510.
3. Kording KP, Wolpert DM. Bayesian integration in sensorimotor learning. *Nature.* 2004;427(6971): 244–247.
4. Robles-de-La-Torre G. Principles of haptic perception in virtual environments. In: Grunwald M, Ed. *Human haptic perception.* Basel, Switzerland: Birkhäuser Verlag; 2008: 363–379.
5. Kirk RM. Surgical skills and lessons from other vocations. *Ann R Coll Surg Engl.* 2006;88:95–98.

FURTHER READING

Kahneman D. *Thinking, fast and slow.* New York: Penguin; 2012.
Kirk RM. Teaching the craft of operative surgery. *Ann R Coll Surg Engl.* 1996;78:25–28.
Kirk RM. Surgical excellence–threats and opportunities. *Ann R Coll Surg Engl.* 1998;80: 256–259.
Rosen J, MacFarlane M, Richards C, et al. Surgeon-tool force/torque signatures: evaluation of surgical skills in minimally invasive surgery. *Proceedings of Medicine Meets Virtual Reality,* *MMVR* – 7. San Francisco, CA: IOS Press; 1999. http://bionics.soe.ucsc.edu/publications/ CP_03.pdf Online. Available: June 26, 2009.
Rothenberger DA. Physician burnout and wellbeing: a systematic review and framework for action. *Dis Colon Rectum.* 2017;60(6): 567–576.
Thomas WEG. Teaching and assessing surgical competence. *Ann R Coll Surg Engl.* 2006;88: 429–432.

Chapter | 2 |

Handling instruments

Key points

- Do not delude yourself into thinking you are an expert because you can handle instruments.
- Your expertise is measured ultimately by how you deal with the tissues and the result of your surgery.
- Once you are familiar with handling the instruments, you can concentrate on performing the operation well.
- Learn the names of instruments and their usage so that you do not have to stop to think about what you want. Likewise, if you don't ask for a specific instrument by name, you may be given something similar, but which you do not want, which is inefficient.
- *You are ultimately responsible for the swab, needle and instrument count*.
- Make sure you retrieve them all before closing. If a swab, needle or instrument cannot be accounted for, organise a plain X-ray over the operative field before asking the anaesthetist to wake the patient up to ensure it has not been left in the wound.

Learn to handle and become familiar with standard instruments, since they are surgical extensions of your hands. Practise handling instruments that are employed in open surgery to carry out functions that you would expect to carry out in surgical procedures. Acquaint yourself with minimal-access instruments using simple simulations (see Ch. 13), and for both these and endoscopes, attend courses and practise on any available simulation and virtual reality kit.

SCALPEL

The scalpel (from the Latin *scalpere* = to cut) is the traditional instrument of surgeons. The majority of scalpel blades in use are disposable whilst some whole scalpels are totally disposable.

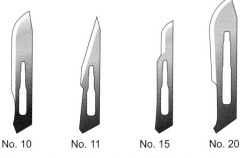

No. 10 No. 11 No. 15 No. 20

Fig. 2.1 Commonly used scalpel blades. Note that the no. 20 blade requires a larger handle.

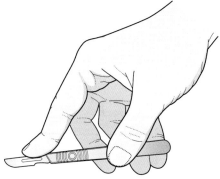

Fig. 2.2 Hold the scalpel to make a long smooth incision. Draw the belly of the knife, not the point, from your nondominant to your dominant side. If you are cutting along a sagittal plane, cut from far to near.

If you use a scalpel with a disposable blade, fit and remove the blade while holding it clear of the sharp edge with a haemostat, not with fingers. If it slips, you will avoid sustaining a cut. Take care not to flick the blade across the room. Likewise, when removing a scalpel blade from the handle, aim the point of the blade downwards, preferably at a sharps receiver. Some sharps-retaining devices have a scalpel blade remover that grips the blade and allows you to lever it off the handle.

Your choice of blade will depend upon the procedure that you are going to undertake with it. A small incision is made with a 15-blade, which has a small belly. For a moderate-sized incision, you would choose a 10-blade, and for a large or long incision a 20-blade. A stab-type incision is made with an 11-blade which has a pointed tip. In this case, the point of the blade is used (Fig. 2.1).

1. Use a scalpel to make deliberate cuts into tissues, dividing them with the minimum trauma in order to cut skin or separate tissues. Stay in the same line of the cut to avoid multiple adjacent incisions or jagged edges.
2. Draw the belly of the blade across the target rather than exerting excessive pressure that may result in an uncontrolled cut. Use controlled pressure to determine the depth of the cut. Be careful to use the belly and not the tip for incisions as you will have better control of depth. Sometimes steadying your hand by resting your little (fifth) finger on an adjacent steady surface can help for fine incisions.
3. For cutting skin and similar structures, hold the knife in a manner similar to that for holding a table knife (Fig. 2.2). Keep the knife horizontal, suspended below your pronated hand,

held between your thumb and middle finger. Place your index finger on the back of the knife at the base of the blade, to control the pressure exerted on it. Wrap your ring and little fingers around the handle to reinforce your steadying grip, so that the end of the handle rests against the hypothenar eminence.
4. When you need to produce a small puncture, a short, precise incision or cut a fine structure, hold the knife like a pen (see Fig. 1.1) and use the tip rather than the belly. An 11-blade is useful for stab incisions.
5. As a rule, you cut in the sagittal plane (from the Latin *sagitta* = arrow; the path of an arrow directly away from you), from far to near, and in the transverse plane from nondominant to dominant side. If you need to cut from the dominant to the nondominant side, consider going to the other side of the operating table, using your nondominant hand, or using scissors.
6. Do not misuse the scalpel by attempting to cut metal or bone or try to lever the knife during a cutting manoeuvre. Do not continue to use a blunt scalpel, since once the sharp edge is lost, you need to apply excessive pressure, the incision is uneven, and the tissues are traumatised.
7. Never make a casual incision without first assessing the exact situation; some are irretrievable. Before making a critical incision, plan it and, if necessary, first draw an intended line on the skin with a marker pen, though be aware that a marker pen may leave a tattoo mark. If an important structure is endangered, interpose a protective instrument such as a

retractor. When you are about to cut a linear structure in the depths, you may be able to place a grooved dissector beneath it, to protect deeper tissues.

8. A special scalpel exists, called a bistoury, conjectured to be named after Pistorium (modern Pistoja) in Tuscany where they were made. It has a long thin curved blade, blunt ended for side cutting, sharp tipped for end cutting through a small opening. They are not commonly used as it is better to cut under direct vision.

9. Invariably keep and pass sharp instruments in kidney dishes to avoid the risks of acquiring, or passing on, infection including viral diseases. Never hand a scalpel directly to another person.

OTHER 'SCALPELS'

In the modern age of infection control and 'sharps free' operating, scalpel alternatives are widely used. The diathermy can be set to 'cutting' and using the point of the diathermy blade can cut tissues with ease. In setting the diathermy to 'coagulation' you can still use this to cut through tissues but will also establish haemostasis at the same time. There are devices that you can utilise which both diathermy coagulate and then cut the now avascular section at the flick of a switch.

SCISSORS

The cutting action of scissors (from the Late Latin *cisorium* = a cutting instrument, from *caedere* = to cut) results from the moving edge contact between the blades, which are given a slight set towards each other. If you hold them up to the light, edge on, you should see light between the blades except at the joint and at one point of contact which moves towards the tips as you close the blades. If the blades spring apart the cutting action is replaced by a chewing effect and this results if delicate scissors are used to cut tough tissues.

Scissors are made for right-handed users and the lateral pressure of the right-handed thumb tends to result in the blades being pressed together. When held in the left hand the pressure of the thumb tends to lever the blades apart. If you are left-handed, you may wish to acquire some left-handed scissors.

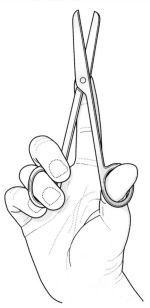

Fig. 2.3 Insert only half the distal phalanx of your thumb and all the distal phalanx of your ring finger through the rings of scissors. Wrap your middle and little fingers around the ring finger. Place your index finger on the hinge.

Most surgical scissors have round tips but for special purposes pointed blades may be used. The blades may be straight, curved or angled.

1. With your hand in midpronation, hold scissors by inserting only part of the first phalanx of the thumb through one ring (called a 'bow' by the manufacturers); this controls the moving blade. Insert only the first phalanx of the ring finger into the other ring and wrap the middle and little fingers around the handle to steady it; this will be the fixed blade (Fig. 2.3). Place the tip of your index finger on the hinge. In this way you are able to steady the scissors in more than one plane.

2. If you are left-handed, using right-handed scissors to make a crucial cut, insert the whole terminal phalanx of your thumb through its ring so you can flex it at the interphalangeal joint and draw the ring to your left to increase the binding force between the blades.

3. As a rule, your hand is most comfortable in the midprone position but if you are cutting down a deep hole try fully supinating your hand so that you have a clearer view of the structures at the tip. The knuckles of a hand in pronation may obstruct your view. For the majority of scissor work, the curve of the

scissors will be in a direction that is almost in continuity with the curve of your partially flexed wrist.

4. Choose the correct scissors for the task. McIndoe scissors are commonly used for soft tissue dissection (named after the eminent plastic surgeon Archibald McIndoe born in 1900). Mayo's are excellent rounded-tipped all-purpose scissors (from the celebrated Clinic of the brothers William, born 1861, Charles, born 1865, both died 1939, came well-designed scissors and needle-holder). Use lighter scissors for very light work only. Remember that it is more difficult to make curved scissors' blades accurately engage along their whole length. In general, use straight scissors for cutting in straight lines and curved scissors where there is a curvature to your cut. If you are cutting down a hole prefer long-handled scissors so that the rings remain outside the hole. The longer the scissors, the more likely is any tremor magnified, so be willing to rest the hinge on the fingers of your nondominant hand (see Fig. 1.2).

5. It is fortunate that scalpels and scissors cut in opposite directions. Scissors cut in the sagittal plane from near to far but when you need to cut from far to near, it may be practical to use a scalpel. In the transverse plane, scissors cut most conveniently from the dominant towards the nondominant side. When you need to cut in the transverse plane from your nondominant side towards your dominant side, consider moving to the other side of the operating table or using a scalpel. If you are reasonably ambidextrous change the scissors to your nondominant hand; alternatively swing the scissors around in your dominant hand, so they point towards your elbow (Fig. 2.4).

6. You may also use scissors for blunt soft tissue dissection. Nudge the tips of the closed scissors into the plane that you are developing and gently prise the blades of the scissors apart in the line of that plane. Withdraw the scissors to the extent that you have opened them and close them again before repeating the same movement. Be careful not to close the tips of the scissors before you can see that they are clear of the tissues to avoid inadvertent sharp dissection.

7. Scissors can be 'palmed' freeing up the index, second finger and thumb to continue operating. To do this the scissor is rotated anticlockwise around your ring finger until it is grasped against the palm by the ring and little finger, with the blades pointing towards your elbow. The scissor can then be rapidly brought back into use by effecting the reverse action, rotating clockwise around your ring finger until your thumb is in position to loop the free ring of the scissor.

> **Key point**
>
> - Invariably keep and pass sharp instruments in kidney dishes to avoid the risks of acquiring or passing on infection, including viral diseases.

DISSECTING FORCEPS (THUMB FORCEPS)

It is not clear whether the word is derived from *ferriceps* (from the Latin *ferrum* = iron + *capere* = to take) or from *formus* (from the Latin = hot + *capere*). They grip when compressed between the thumb and fingers. When released the blades separate because they are made of springy steel. Dissecting forceps form an excellent multipurpose instrument. The commonest types are toothed and nontoothed but various shaped tips are available, such as rings for grasping soft viscera. Vascular and cardiac surgeons favour a DeBakey forcep (named after the esteemed US cardiovascular surgeon Michael DeBakey, 1908–2008) which offers a firm grip with minimal crush and no piercing of the tissue. Delicate forceps have a post on the inside of one blade that engages with a hole in the other blade, to ensure that the tips meet accurately. If you compress the forceps tightly the sharp post will protrude through the opposite blade and potentially pierce your glove or your skin; a sure sign that you are crushing the tissue between the blade

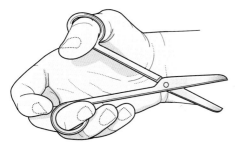

Fig. 2.4 Cut from left to right while holding the scissors in your right hand.

tips. Dissecting forceps may be extremely delicate for use during microsurgery or large and strong for grasping tough tissues.

Toothed forceps have at least one tooth on one tip, interdigitating with two teeth on the opposing tip. The intention is that the teeth puncture the surface of the tissue, tethering it and preventing it from slipping, rather than holding it by strong compression, which may be more damaging. Skin is tolerant of punctures but is severely injured by crushing, so toothed forceps are usually employed to grasp it. Very tough slippery tissues such as fascia, fibrocartilage and bone are best grasped with toothed forceps.

Nontoothed forceps exert their grip through serrations on the opposing surfaces. Use them when manipulating blood vessels, bowel and small ducts, since punctures of these cause leakage. Provided the closed tips are used to act as counter pressure and manipulate tissue rather than to grip it, they are suitable for use on skin, but skin hooks are preferable (see Ch. 6).

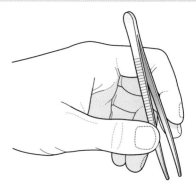

Fig. 2.5 Grip dissecting forceps like a pen but usually in your nondominant hand since you usually hold a scalpel or scissors in your dominant hand while dissecting.

> **Key points**
>
> - The pressure exerted per unit area when fine-tipped forceps are forcibly closed is extremely high.
> - Tissues crushed by this force will appear normal soon afterwards, but will die.
> - Whenever possible use the closed tips to stabilise or distort tissues and create counter pressure.

1. As a rule, hold dissecting forceps like a pen in your nondominant hand since you usually have another instrument in your dominant hand (Fig. 2.5). They do not usually have a locking mechanism because they are intended to provide only a temporary grip.
2. You can palm forceps (Fig. 2.6), retaining them with your ring and little fingers, to free the index and middle fingers, and thumb, while tying knots.
3. The closed blades of round-nosed nontoothed forceps make an excellent dissecting tool to open up a longitudinal tissue plane. Gently insert them in the desired plane as a wedge and allow their springiness to open up and create a space between the blades along which you can identify and selectively divide the overlying tissue (see Ch. 9). This method is valuable when displaying a longitudinal structure such as a blood vessel, nerve or tendon.

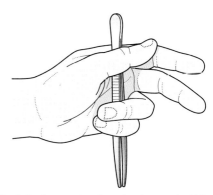

Fig. 2.6 If you palm dissecting forceps, hold them with your ring and little fingers, freeing your important fingers to hold other instruments or tissues or to tie knots.

ARTERY FORCEPS (HAEMOSTATIC FORCEPS, HAEMOSTATS)

Haemostatic forceps (from the Greek *haema* = blood + *stasis* = stoppage) were devised by the great French surgeon Ambroise Paré (1510–1590) with scissors and were then improved by the addition of a ratchet so they could be locked, by Sir Thomas Spencer Wells (1818–1897) after whom one of the larger sizes is named. Note that the tips alone meet when they are lightly closed; the proximal parts of the blades are slightly separated. The basic design is so versatile that it has been adapted from fine 'mosquito' forceps to heavy, toothed grasping forceps. Some haemostats are straight, but most are curved. In cardiovascular surgery, small, snug rubber or plastic covers are often applied to the tips of small haemostats to clip the suture out of the field of surgery without fracturing it. These are referred to as 'shods' because they are like little shoes on the tips of the instrument.

1. Insert the first phalanx only of your thumb and of your ring finger into the rings of the opened forceps, with your index finger on the hinge. When the handles are compressed, the ratchets lock. To release them you need to compress them lightly to overcome the slight overhang of the ratchet, separate the handles in a plane at right angles to the hinge action, and open the handles. Practise the action so that you can skilfully and controllably apply and remove them automatically.

2. As an assistant learn to use your nondominant hand because you usually have scissors in your dominant hand, ready to cut the ligature. An alternative method of opening and closing the artery forceps using your nondominant hand is to hold one ring of the forcep between the index finger and thumb while the other rests between the palps of the third and fourth finger and the dorsal aspect of the terminal phalanx of the fifth finger. If you push towards the thenar eminence with the third and fourth finger and then ulnarward, the ratchet can be opened and closed. This allows you to clip with your nondominant hand and cut with your dominant hand with economy of movement.

3. Because these forceps can be applied and left in place, always ensure the shafts are sufficiently long so that the handles remain outside the wound. Short-handled forceps left in the wound are easily forgotten, so always check the number at the end of the procedure.

4. Apply artery forceps to bleeding vessels with your hand supinated, the convexity of curved forceps facing down (Fig. 2.7). Grasp vessels so the tips of the forceps protrude; this retains the subsequently applied ligature, preventing it from slipping over the tip and trapping the forceps in the tied ligature. If this happens, when the forceps are removed, they will pull off the ligature. A single click of the ratchet may suffice.

5. Avoid picking up extraneous tissue. If you apply a ligature around it and the vessel, the attachment will anchor the ligature and allow the vessel, as it retracts, to withdraw from it and rebleed.

6. If you are the assistant, you will be expected to remove the forceps when the vessel is

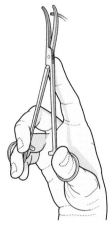

Fig. 2.7 When applying curved haemostatic forceps to capture bleeding vessels, prefer to have your hand supinated, and with curved forceps, have the convexity down, and ensure the tips just project beyond the vessel.

ligated. Aim to remove the haemostat with your non-scissor-holding hand, so that you can swiftly cut the thread with your scissor-holding hand in a time-efficient way, without having to put the haemostat down and then pick up the scissors. The surgeon will either expect you to lift the handle of the forceps to allow the end of the ligature to be passed from hand to hand on your side of the vessel or will stretch the ligature between two hands on your side of the vessel while you reach over it to grasp the handles of the forceps. As the first half-hitch is formed and tightened, you should, when requested, release and remove the haemostat in a controlled manner. If you leave the forceps, they may prevent the first half-hitch from being tightened. Grasp the far ring between your index finger and thumb; this is to be the static ring. Insert part of the first phalanx of the ring finger in the other ring and steady it by pressure from outside the ring, with the little finger (Fig. 2.8). Gently compress the rings together to release the overlap of the ratchet, lever the handles in opposite directions at right angles to the joint and gently open the forceps without pulling them off. When the final half-hitch has been tightened the surgeon will hold up the ends of the ligature while you cut them, using the scissors held in the right hand. When an important vessel is being tied you may be asked to slacken the forceps while a first ligature is being tied and tightened; then re-clamp

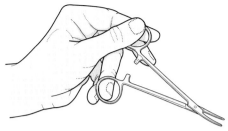

Fig. 2.8 Learn to remove artery forceps with your nondominant hand in a controlled manner, without allowing them to spring off. As an assistant you normally hold your scissors in your dominant hand, ready to cut the ends of the ligature to the correct length.

the forceps while a second ligature is tied and tightened, before removing the forceps; this is sometimes referred to as an 'ease and squeeze'. Where there is a thicker bit of tissue or a vascular bundle being tied, a transfixion stitch may be used. The first surgeon will place a stitch through the tissue and tie a half-hitch on one side before taking the thread around the whole circumference of the tissue and tying a knot. In this case, you will hold up the forceps and not release it until after the first half-hitch has been placed around the whole circumference.

7. Haemostats are also useful in dissection. The blunt tips make good blunt dissection instruments in the same manner as you would blunt dissect with scissors. The advantage of using a haemostat is there is not inadvertent sharp dissection when closing the instrument. Additionally, haemostats are often used to grip small swabs variously called pledgets, 'peanuts' or Lahey dabs, which are used almost like a fingertip for gentle blunt dissection (see Ch. 9).

TISSUE FORCEPS

These rely on their grip on the shape and apposing surfaces of their blades in contact with the tissues to grasp but not damage them. Some encircle the tissues, some have large ring blades through which the tissues bulge, or rough surfaces, or teeth (Fig. 2.9). For instance, a Babcock is commonly used for holding the bowel, a Duval for holding the gallbladder and an Alliss for holding skin edges or fascia.

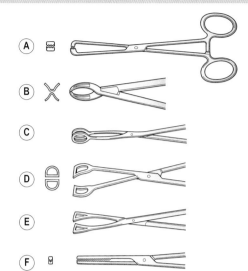

Fig. 2.9 Tissue-holding forceps. (A) Allis. (B) Lane's. (C) Ring. (D) Babcock's. (E) Duval. (F) Kocher's.

1. Use them in circumstances when traction sutures or a sharp hook may cut out, when the tissues are too slippery to be held with smooth retractors, and when the direction of traction needs to be varied. Do not use metal forceps when gravity, tapes, packing, or extending the incision could be less damaging.
2. If you need to apply strong traction of tough tissues, use forceps with a powerful grip rather than inadequate forceps that are likely to pull off, tearing the tissues and straining the forceps. When the tissues are fragile, use delicate forceps, apply them carefully, do not drag on them and remove them as soon as possible. Several lightweight forceps may give a better grip and do less damage than a single pair of heavy forceps.

NEEDLE-HOLDERS

In the past, we frequently held needles in our hands. The risk of sustaining or transmitting infection, especially viral and prion diseases, has made the practice unsustainable. There is a great variety of needle-holders (Fig. 2.10). They grip the needle with specially designed jaws. Most of them are straight and are designed to be rotated in their long axis with a pronation/supination action of the hand to drive the needle through the tissues in a curved path. Mayo's is the simplest

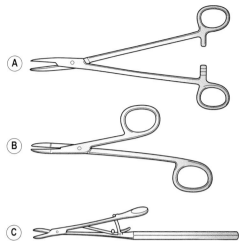

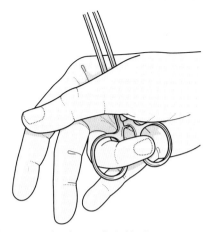

Fig. 2.10 Needle-holders. (A) Mayo's. (B) Gillies' incorporating scissors. (C) One type of ophthalmic needle-holder.

Fig. 2.11 Palm the needle-holder by removing your thumb from its ring and rotating the instrument on your ring finger so that it lies in the interspace between the thumb and the second metacarpal. This slightly restricts movement of the thumb.

model, used in many modifications, similar in design to haemostatic forceps, with ratchet closure, and controlled in the same manner. Sir Harold Gillies (1882–1960), the New Zealand-born father of British plastic surgery, invented a nonlocking combined needle-holder and scissors. Ophthalmic surgeons use a small holder for the fine stitching required.

1. Do not allow needles to come into contact with your skin but always hold them with a needle-holder, manoeuvring them within the needle-holder using dissecting forceps. Most needles are now curved but use the needle-holder to drive all types of needles through the tissues.

2. Grip the curved needle between the jaws of the needle-holder. The needle makes a right angle with the holder. Have the needle point facing towards your nondominant side and pointing upwards when your hand is in the midprone position because you more easily drive the needle through by starting with your hand fully pronated, progressively supinating. This is a natural action whether you are inserting stitches from far to near or from dominant to nondominant side. It is important that you follow the curve of the needle as you push it through the tissues or else you will traumatise the surrounding tissue. Furthermore, if you are in tough tissue you could inadvertently straighten the curved needle which will further traumatise the tissue and may break.

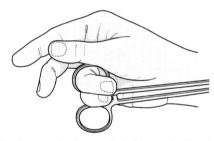

Fig. 2.12 Palm the needle-holder so that it points towards your elbow and flex your little finger to lie between the rings, leaving your thumb and main fingers free.

3. If you are stitching in the depths of a wound, use a long-handled needle-holder, otherwise your hand is inside the entrance, blocking your view.

4. When you are inserting and tying stitches, or need to carry out some other short action, it is very convenient to palm the needle-holder. Remove your thumb from one ring, retaining your ring finger in the other. Swing the shaft of the needle-holder into the first interspace between the thumb and second metacarpal (Fig. 2.11) or swing it until it points back towards your elbow and flex your little finger into the space between the rings to retain it (Fig. 2.12). Do not retain the needle in the holder if you intend to palm it.

5. Occasionally you need to stitch alternately from right to left and then left to right, or far to near then near to far. To avoid the need to

Fig. 2.13 To reverse the direction of the needle, rotate it in the needle-holder, through 180°. This manoeuvre has been popularised by Mr W. E. G. Thomas of Sheffield.

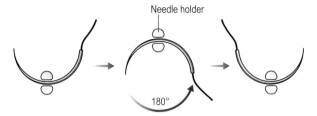

Needle holder

180°

remove and replace the needle, merely turn it in the needle-holder, then turn the needle-holder through 180° in its long axis and gain a fresh grip (Fig. 2.13).

6. It is good practice to hand the used needle back to the scrub nurse with the point of the needle held in the needle-holder and pointing towards the shaft of the needle-holder.

Laparoscopic and robotic needle-holders

1. Needle-holders for use in open surgery generally have ringed handles for thumb and finger and come in a variety of sizes and lengths to suit particular needs and/or procedures. Despite the variety of different needle-holders available, they all conform to a generally universal design pattern.

2. Laparoscopic needle-holders however, whilst serving the same purpose, necessarily have significant design differences. They consist of a long shaft of approximately 30 cm in length and with handles placed in a straight axial alignment with the surgeon's wrist which ultimately provides for a more natural motion on suturing. The jaws are generally operated by a spring-loaded palm grip which opens and closes the jaw accordingly. A ratcheted locking mechanism secures the needle. The flat jaws of a standard needle-holder will keep the needle in the position in which it was originally grasped.

3. By contrast self-righting needle-holders force the grasped needle into a fixed position (either 45° or 90° to the shaft). The effect is achieved either by using corresponding convex and concave jaws designed to precisely fit the curve of the needle or by the use of interlocking protrusions on upper and lower jaws.

4. Robotic needle-holders represent a whole further level of advancement in design. The robotic arms are linked to specialised *Endowrist* instruments which allow seven degrees of freedom (or axes of movement) as compared to the four degrees available in laparoscopy.

In addition to the increase in the axes of movement, there is the additional 90° of articulation allowing the instruments to work with a function equivalent to the human wrist. The increased dexterity allows for more accurate suturing in minimally invasive surgery.

RETRACTORS

These are extremely useful when you wish to display and carry out a procedure on a deeply placed organ. Some are hand held and some are self-retaining (Fig. 2.14). For major abdominal operations, a large metal ring or modular ring may be placed to encircle the wound, to which can be attached various retractors. A retractor may

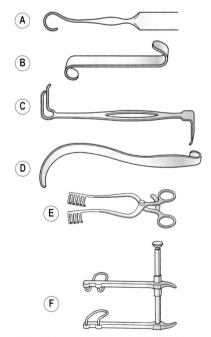

Fig. 2.14 Retractors. (A) Hook. (B) Malleable copper. (C) Czerny. (D) Deaver. (E) Self-retaining. (F) Gosset self-retaining.

be attached to a frame placed over the patient, to lift the lower sternum, improving access to the upper abdomen.

1. Use them carefully so you do not damage structures inadvertently. Ensure that the assistant who is retracting for you uses minimal traction and relaxes it whenever it is unnecessary.
2. If you are retracting with a hand-held retractor, in general, pull in the direction of the handle with a slight lifting action. Always be aware of the tissue that you are retracting and use the appropriate level of force. For instance, do not pull too hard on the viscera, for risk of causing significant soft tissue damage. Placing a damp swab on the viscera and placing the retractor over it will reduce the trauma of the bare metal.
3. Exploit a change of approach: retraction by a hand placed over a pack is less damaging than a metal retractor. Sometimes a change of position of the patient or part allows gravity to produce the required effect.
4. There are now some self-retaining retractors available that have lights incorporated into them, enabling illumination of the operative field when operating in deep tissues.

CLAMPS

A wide variety of clamps fulfil the differing needs of grasping, joining and compressing structures (Fig. 2.15), and the mechanisms for fixing them vary from spring handles to ratchets, locking hinges and screws. As opposed to haemostatic forceps that are intended to clamp blood vessels that will be permanently sealed, vascular clamps such as bulldog clips, deBakey clamps and Potts artery clamps are designed to occlude them temporarily without damaging them.

1. In order to prevent leakage of contaminating contents from the bowel, control oozing from the cut edges; to steady the ends while carrying out an anastomosis, many surgeons apply noncrushing clamps near the ends, including the vessels in the mesentery. In some models, the clamps on each side of the anastomosis can be fixed together. Other surgeons condemn the use of bowel clamps. Make up your own mind. If you do apply them across the mesentery, make sure you apply them very lightly, or just firmly enough to occlude the arteries. Do not merely occlude the veins while leaving

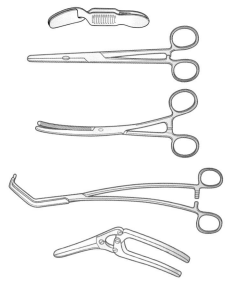

Fig. 2.15 Clamps. From above there are four noncrushing clamps: bulldog, Potts arterial, intestinal, and Satinsky types; these allow part of the vessel to be isolated without totally obstructing the lumen. Below is a crushing, lever-action, intestinal clamp.

the arteries patent. If you do so, the bowel and the occluded veins in the mesentery will become congested, may rupture and bleed into the mesentery, and be difficult to identify.

2. When you resect the bowel you may place two crushing clamps side by side at each point of division and cut between them. In this way, the cut ends are sealed. If you then intend to join the bowel ends do not fail to excise the crushed, sealed strip to expose the lumen. Stapling devices (*vide infra*) may preclude the need for crushing clamps.
3. A noncrushing bowel clamp can be most useful to place across the splenic hilum and temporarily control bleeding in a ruptured spleen.
4. In vascular surgery, select the clamp that is enough to temporarily occlude blood flow. However, using too large or too tight a clamp may damage the blood vessels. For delicate vessels, such as the axillary artery or the profunda femoris artery, sometimes a vessel loop is preferable to a clamp.

HAEMOSTATIC CLIPS

Metal clips fit into the jaws of special forceps and can be applied across blood vessels and ducts to

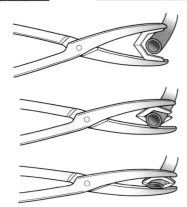

Fig. 2.16 Vascular clip. As you compress the clamp the clip first closes at the tips, preventing the enclosed structure from being squeezed out, before being compressed and occluded.

occlude them. The chevron shape ensures that as they close their tips meet first so that the tubular structure does not slip away (Fig. 2.16). Further compression occludes the lumen. Some instruments apply a series of clips from a mechanical or powered applicator. Another instrument applies two clips across a structure while cutting between them with a single action. Metallic clips are useful as radio-opaque markers to help identify their position after operation. They can be placed at intervals around a tumour in order to plan radiotherapy and to estimate subsequent shrinkage as a result of treatment. Those made from titanium allow scatter-free computerised tomography and are magnetic resonance imaging compatible. A disadvantage of clips compared with ligatures and sutures is that they catch on hands, instruments and swabs and can be pulled off. They are also more expensive. Bio-degradable clips are available as an alternative to metal clips. They are slowly absorbed.

STAPLING DEVICES

The principle of mechanical staplers in surgery is exactly the same as paper stapling machines. An inverted U-shaped staple is driven through the target tissues and then hits a shaped anvil that turns the ends (Fig. 2.17). The tissues should not be crushed because the ends are so turned as to form the shape of the letter 'B' lying on its face.

Straight staplers apply lines of staples, usually two offset parallel lines, and can be employed to seal, or seal and cut, tubular or vascular viscera

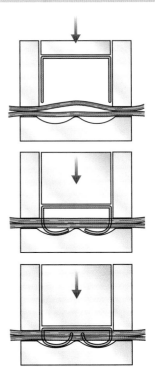

Fig. 2.17 The principles of stapling action. As you close the instrument you drive the staple points through the two layers of tissue before they impact on the anvil and are turned over to form the shape of a letter B lying on its face.

(from the Latin = flesh or soft organs), and seal major blood vessels. A linear cutter applies four parallel lines and at the same time cuts along the centre to produce a double line of staples on each side of the cut. This can be used to produce a stoma between two segments of bowel. A miniature version of this instrument can be inserted through a laparoscopy port to doubly occlude a major structure such as a large blood vessel and divide it between the staple lines.

1. To unite two hollow viscera such as intestine, insert the limb containing the staple magazine into one bowel lumen through a stab wound and the anvil bar into the other bowel lumen through a stab wound.
2. Lock the two limbs together and actuate the instrument. When you unlock and remove the two limbs there remain only the two stab wounds to close, leaving a side-to-side anastomosis (Fig. 2.18).
3. Close the stab wounds with sutures or place a straight stapler across the everted edges of each of the holes and seal them.

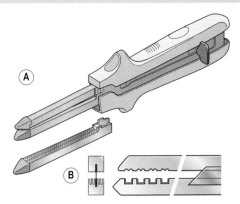

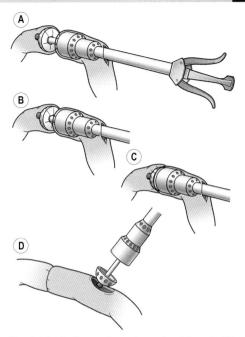

Fig. 2.18 Linear stapler. (A) There are four lines of staples in the lower jaw and four matching lines of anvils in the upper jaw. Tissues can be placed between the two jaws which are then locked together. When the instrument is activated the staples are driven through the intervening tissues and folded over against the anvils. At the same time, a knife is driven through the centre line of the staple lines, cutting the intervening tissues and separating them with each side sealed with a double line of staples. (B) A diagram shows how the staple lines are placed in the jaws with the anvil lines opposed to them. The knife will cut between the lines as shown in the end-on view.

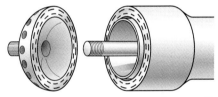

Fig. 2.19 The head of a circular stapler. Two offset concentric rings of staples sit in the magazine with ends pointing upwards. The anvil has been unscrewed and turned towards you. When the anvil is reattached and screwed down onto the magazine, and the instrument is activated, the staples are driven up through any intervening material or tissue and then bent over as they hit the anvil. A circular knife blade is also driven through, cutting off any protruding material or tissue, so the lumen is not obstructed.

4. Sometimes an additional layer of interrupted handsewn sutures can be applied to complete a 'two-layer' anastomosis. This is sometimes referred to as a 'goodnight' stitch because the surgeon sleeps better.

Circular staplers (Fig. 2.19) produce an end-to-end anastomosis. There are two concentric offset rows of staples in the magazine head. At the end of a spindle is a removable circular anvil.

1. To form an anastomosis, insert the staple head through a side hole in the bowel wall, or, for

Fig. 2.20 End-to-end anastomosis of bowel. (A) Insert the staple head into the bowel through a side incision (or through the anus for a low colorectal anastomosis), pass it through the end and into the segment to be joined on. (B) Insert purse-string sutures around both ends and tie them to draw a ring of bowel end into the gap between the magazine and anvil. (C) Close the gap between the anvil and magazine to bring the peritoneal surfaces of the inverted bowel ends into contact. Now actuate the instrument to staple the bowel ends together and cut off the internal fringes of bowel. (D) After separating the anvil from the empty magazine, gently withdraw the stapler with a twisting motion before closing the side entry hole.

example, when performing a low colorectal anastomosis, insert it through the anus. Fix the anvil on the end of the spindle and introduce it into the other end of bowel (Fig. 2.20). Insert a purse-string suture around each bowel end and tighten and tie them. This draws one end over the staple magazine end, the other over the anvil head.

2. Screw down the anvil to trap the two inverted bowel ends between the staple heads, without crushing them. Now activate the instrument. The staple ends are thrust through both layers of inverted bowel ends, hit the anvil and are turned over. Simultaneously an inner circular knife is pushed through to cut off the excess inverted bowel ends.

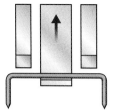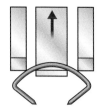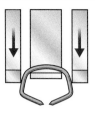

Fig. 2.21 The principle of the skin stapler. Since there is no anvil beneath, against which to turn over the staple ends, the sequence is from left to right. The central column of the stapler has a lip beneath the staple to hold it. The outer parts thrust the staple ends through the skin and as they continue, the staple ends are forced to turn in towards each other.

3. Now separate the anvil from staple head and gently withdraw the instrument with a twisting motion. Examine the trimmed ends encircling the central spindle. They should be complete toroids –'doughnuts', confirming that the anastomosis has been perfectly carried out through the whole circumference. Check the circumference externally. If you created a side hole to insert the instrument, close it.

Skin staplers must be inserted without the presence of an anvil to turn the tips (Fig. 2.21). The central section of the U-shaped staple is held while the outer ends are pushed through the skin and then bent so that the ends meet, forming a closed ring. When applying them it is useful if you ask your assistant to evert the edges of the skin with two toothed forceps, drawing the skin edges together for each clip. Alternatively, if you are alone, you can pick up the skin just beyond the end of the wound that you are working towards with an Alliss forcep. This everts the ends and the traction allows you to apply the skin clips. They are removed by straightening the base of the 'U' to open out the ends so that the staples can be withdrawn. Special staple removers are available for this purpose. Staples can be inserted from a magazine containing a number for convenience.

> **Key points**
>
> - Staples can be invaluable when stitches are difficult to place or are time consuming in a major procedure.
> - Stitching remains the most versatile method of joining tissues.
> - As a trainee concentrate on acquiring suturing skill whenever it is convenient and safe to do so.

DISSECTION AIDS

You will, as a trainee, see a number of instruments used to aid dissection both in open and in minimal access procedures. Learn the principles of their properties and be aware of any side effects and dangers. They offer selective tissue destruction combined with haemostasis and with varied penetrating effects on nearby tissues. There is a variety of instruments from different manufacturers, each with its advantages and disadvantages, and new and updated products appear regularly.

> **Key point**
>
> - Do not attempt to use these complex and potentially dangerous instruments without proper understanding and training.

Electrosurgical dissection

Diathermy. The name should properly be applied to high-frequency electromagnetic waves as in a microwave machine. I have continued to use the term for the machine long used in surgery in which the electrodes are usually applied to the tissues, mainly to achieve haemostasis. For more recent, complex machines I have used the term electrosurgery. A high-frequency (400 kHz–10 MHz) alternating current passing through the tissues between two electrodes may produce 1000°C heat.

Monopolar diathermy localises the effect at the point of one (active) electrode. A self-adhesive dispersive electrode (often referred to as the diathermy plate) is applied to the patient outside the operating area. This should not be over an open wound, metal implant or bony area. The heating effect is greatest when using interrupted pulses of 50–100 per second, producing tissue coagulation where the electrode is touching the tissues into a semisolid mass. Fulguration or spray causes tiny sparks to jump from the electrode to the tissues allowing slightly wider coagulation and haemostasis. A continuous current of sinus wave form vaporises cell water, producing a cutting effect. A blend combines the effect allowing progressive dissection and haemostasis. For sealing bleeding over large surfaces an ionised argon gas flow can be used to complete the circuit between a monopolar diathermy electrode and the surface, spreading the effect.

Bipolar diathermy has the current passing only between the two tips of an instrument that encloses the tissues. A dispersive electrode plate is not used. This is ideal to use when your patient is awake as the current in the patient only passes between the two electrodes of the forceps. It is also preferable to use when you are using diathermy near nerves as the current does not transmit to the nerves (except if you pick up a nerve with the forceps, which you should not do).

1. Diathermy is a valuable method of occluding blood vessels before dividing them or sealing cut vessels. The combined action makes it a valuable dissector, especially during minimal access procedures; a piece of tissue can be elevated with a hook, free of other structures, sealed and gently broken (see Ch. 13). By picking up the tissue with a bipolar forceps, the current passes only between the tines of the forceps, to produce a similar effect.
2. Beware the interference effects on pacemakers. Beware of using diathermy soon after applying alcohol-based skin preparation, and in the presence of inflammable anaesthetic or bowel gas, for fear of causing an explosion. In particular, do not allow alcohol-based skin preparation to pool anywhere near the patient's skin as it will conduct the current and cause a burn. Do not leave the diathermy forceps or needle lying on the patient; keep it in its quiver when not in use.
3. Use bipolar diathermy whenever possible and stop diathermy if arrhythmia develops.
4. If the indifferent plate of monopolar diathermy does not have good skin contact, the skin may be burned. Test the connections and use short bursts whenever possible. Do not place the plate over a metal implant such as a hip replacement.
5. Capacitative coupling occurs if a metal object or instrument is near but insulated from the diathermy which induces a charge in the metal. Design changes have reduced the risk but beware also of bringing the electrode near another instrument.

> ### Key points
>
> - Do not apply diathermy for prolonged periods—the damaging heating effect spreads into previously normal tissues causing severe tissue destruction.
> - Do not apply diathermy to large tissue masses—take small pieces.
> - Prefer cutting, or combined cutting and coagulation.

LigaSure is able to seal vessels by compressing them between the jaws to obliterate the lumen, with computerised sensing of the collagen content, melting it and the elastin to create a seal. A knife can now be triggered to transect the tissue. It is claimed to be capable of sealing vessels up to 7 mm in diameter with minimal charring and with very limited spread of heat into adjacent tissues.

Ultrasonic dissection

The mechanical energy transmitted by ultrasound can be used to disrupt tissues. If there is a high water content in the cells or tissues, it is vaporised, disrupting the parenchymal cells (from the Greek *enchyma* = infusion, inpouring: from an ancient belief that the specialised cells were poured into the matrix scaffold and congealed), but sparing those with low water content such as blood vessels and ducts. At higher power levels, the vibration and resulting heat generation directly destroy cells.

Blood vessels and ducts can be sealed using ultrasonic energy provided the walls are flattened together within a clamp. The ultrasound energy produces heat to about 80°C; protein is denatured (Fig. 2.22).

The *Cavitron Ultrasonic Surgical Aspirator (CUSA)* consists of a titanium tube oscillating at 23 kHz which fragments tissue within 1–2 mm of the tip. The irrigation and suction facilities allow the fragments to be washed and sucked away. The parenchymal cells are disrupted leaving the vessels and ducts intact, so they can be sealed with ligatures, clips or other means, before being divided. This is used by dentists to clean teeth and by neurosurgeons to remove brain tumours.

The *Harmonic Scalpel*, producing 55.5 kHz, cuts using a hook dissector, or coagulates using

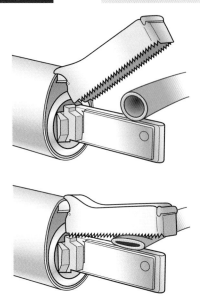

Fig. 2.22 Principle of dissection combined with haemostasis by ultrasound energy. A vessel is compressed between the active and passive jaws of the clamp to appose the endothelial linings. The heating effect causes coagulation and 'welding' of the vessel walls to seal it.

a ball coagulator. Combined cutting and haemostatic vessel sealing can be achieved using low power. The vessel is compressed to appose the walls within a clamp, one blade of which is inactive, and the other is the ultrasound emitter (Fig. 2.21). Sealing is dependent on good vessel wall coaptation, low power and allowance of sufficient time for the weld to form. Claimed advantages over electrosurgical methods are that no electric current passes through the patient and heating of surrounding tissues is minimal.

Key points

- Dissection with electrosurgery or ultrasound both produce damaging heating effects, although less so with ultrasound.
- Dissection in layered tissue that can be separated into small bites causes minimal damage but dissection into solid organs and tissues presents the danger of creating inadvertent and macroscopically undetectable damage to important structures in advance of the dissection, which will subsequently undergo necrosis.

INTRAOPERATIVE DIAGNOSTIC ULTRASOUND

Mechanical waves above a frequency of 20,000 cycles/second (20 kHz) are inaudible to humans. Using low power intensity can be valuable in intraoperative diagnosis, especially within solid tissues, such as the liver, when deeply placed structures are impalpable. It can be used during open procedures and especially during laparoscopic operations since during these procedures the operator is precluded from palpating large organs or masses.

MISCELLANEOUS METHODS

Laser dissection is widely used in various branches of surgery, employing variable wavelengths to suit the circumstances and the tissues involved. It is valuable for debulking large tumours.

Microwave dissection can be carried out using microwaves with a frequency of 2450 MHz to prevent bleeding.

Cryosurgery (from the Greek *kryos* = frost) is performed by freezing the tissues to −40°C with liquid nitrogen. Ice crystals form in the cells, disrupting them. The frozen tissue forms an ice ball which subsequently separates spontaneously from the surrounding tissues.

High-velocity water jet can be employed as a dissecting method since it selectively separates the tissues. Although it is not haemostatic, it disrupts loose parenchymal cells while leaving the blood vessels intact, which can then be dealt with by other means.

Radiofrequency tissue destruction is a valuable method of tissue destruction. An internally cooled needle delivers energy directly to the tissues to produce coagulative desiccation (from the Latin *siccus* = dry).

Chapter | **3** |

Handling threads

Threads of various materials are used extensively for ligating (binding) and suturing (sewing).

Manufacturers strive to produce threads that are strong, reliable, and produce minimal inflammatory response. In some cases the threads are coated to improve the surface characteristics. Most threads are sterilised by gamma rays and presented in sealed packets.

All foreign materials inserted into the body evoke a reaction, but some are relatively inert. Natural products tend to generate an inflammatory reaction, stimulating manufacturers to produce synthetic (from the Greek *syn* = together + *thesis* = a placing; hence, putting together) materials that are less reactive.

Threads may be absorbable, and these are virtually all synthetic, predictably assimilated by hydrolysis, and so produce minimal inflammation. Nonabsorbable threads are also nearly all synthetic including a polyamide such as nylon. The only commonly used natural thread is silk. 'Nonabsorbables' almost always undergo changes within the tissues.

THREAD CHARACTERISTICS

1. Synthetic threads are usually extruded as a viscous substance through a fine hole, hardening to create a smooth-surfaced thread. A single monofilament thread has 'memory', which tends to make it return to its original straightness unless it is restrained, and since it has a smooth surface, loosely tightened knots tend to unfasten spontaneously. If the smooth surface is damaged by, for example, being roughly handled or grasped with a metal instrument, the thread is seriously weakened. Multifilament threads, made up of fine monofilaments, are virtually always braided, rather than twisted, so that when you roll them in your fingers, they remain intact, instead of unlaying.

2. Absorbable threads may be monofilament or multifilament. Catgut is banned in many countries for fear of transmitting prion disease. Synthetic absorbable threads evoke

little reaction, and are absorbed predictably by hydrolysis, not by inflammation. Some slowly absorbed materials retain strength long enough to replace nonabsorbable threads in certain circumstances. Monofilament substances include polydioxanone (PDS), polyglyconate (Maxon) poliglecaprone (monocryl), polypropylene (Prolene) and glycomer 631 (Biosyn). Monofilaments, since they expose less surface to the body tissues, cause less reaction than do multifilaments and are preferable in the presence of infection because their smooth surfaces do not provide a nidus for microorganisms. Against this they are often difficult to handle and because they have smooth surfaces, knots do not hold so well. Multifilament threads, formerly often held together by twisting, are now almost invariably braided. They include polyglactin 910 (Vicryl), polyglycolic acid (Dexon) and lactomer 9-1 (Polysorb). These handle excellently, tie well and retain their strength for prolonged periods. Do not pull them roughly through the tissues; their surfaces are not as smooth as monofilaments, so there is a dragging and sawing effect.

3. The only commonly used natural nonabsorbable thread is braided silk, popular because of its soft pliability, and easily formed, reliable knotting. Polyesters, polypropylene and polyamides are synthetics and evoke minimal tissue reaction. Monofilament forms are strong, but because of their smoothness, they do not bind together well and require multiple knotting to create reliable knots. Multifilament forms handle well and knot well. Stainless steel is favoured in some circumstances because it causes almost no tissue reaction—but it is difficult to handle. Have your assistant guide the loops of wire to avoid snags and twists.

4. Whatever the type of thread, do not use excessive force when pulling it. You may break it, but then at least you are aware of this and can replace it. Worse, you may weaken it and it will break later. Do not drag it over sharp edges, or roughly snatch the strands together when tightening knots. Do not grasp threads with metal instruments except in sections that you will excise. In cardiovascular surgery, rubber or plastic 'shods' are paced on the tips of haemostats to use as clamps for threads placed to one side.

5. If you twist a slack thread, it forms a loop (Fig. 3.1). Threads have an almost fiendish

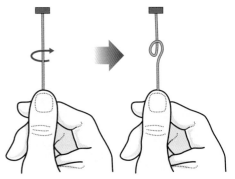

Fig. 3.1 Effect of twisting a thread. Modern monofilament and braided threads do not unlay as did twisted threads.

propensity to catch around the handles of surgical instruments or any other projection.

6. Surgeons vary in their choice of threads. As a trainee, note and use those chosen by your consultant. Make up your own mind so that at the completion of training you will have experienced a range of materials and can make a sensible choice.

7. Whenever you are handling threads arrange them so that they do not catch, remove all unnecessary instruments from the area or cover the projections with towels to protect them. If the thread becomes twisted when you are drawing it through the tissues, it may kink and cause damage, so run it through your fingers at intervals while the needle hangs freely, to allow the twists and possible snags to straighten out.

8. In laparoscopic surgery, extracorporeal knots that are effectively tied outside the patient and then tightened inside the patient are commonly used. They are mostly slip knots, and a pusher is used to snug the knot down. Examples of this are the Roeder knot and the Tayside knot.

9. A V-Loc suture is a unidirectional barbed self-locking thread with a loop at the end such that the need for knotting is almost entirely eliminated. The sutures effectively 'lock' after each pass and so evenly distribute tension along a wound or anastomosis. V-Loc suture use results in a significant reduction in suturing time (especially for laparoscopic procedures) and is reported to reduce the risk of infection and suture extrusion.

10. Other techniques for tying off structures may be threadless, including metal clips,

Table 3.1 A comparison of thread sizes															
Metric	0.1	0.2	0.3	0.4	0.5	0.7	1	1.5	2	3	3.5	4	5	6	7	8
Others	10/0	9/0	8/0	7/0	6/0	5/0	4/0	3/0	2/0	0	1	2	3 & 4	5	7

The top line shows metric sizes, which if divided by 10, give minimum thread diameter in millimetres. The bottom line ('Others') shows the equivalent BP and BPC gauges, including both nonabsorbables and synthetic absorbables.

endoloops and automatic staplers (both endoscopic and open).

Key points

- If a thread frequently catches during certain manoeuvres, incorporate into your technique a routine to avoid it happening.
- Do not wait for it to happen, to disturb your smooth progression, and then correct it.

Sizes

Thread diameter was formerly recorded as British Pharmacopoeia (BP) but is now usually quoted in metric gauge (Table 3.1).

KNOTS

As you read these accounts of knot tying, have a length of string attached to a convenient base so you can practise the movements. This does not give you skill. It demonstrates what movements of the *thread* you must create. How you create them depends on your personal preference—what feels natural. You need to practise how best you can use your fingers, or instruments, to create them in differing circumstances and from different aspects. As you do so, you create automatic movements that you can perform perfectly every time. Then, and only then, have you acquired a skill.

Key points

- Recognize that it is not sufficient to learn how to form knots. At least as important is how you tighten and bed them down while retaining the correct relationships between the threads within the knot.
- In all these descriptions, the loose ends are kept under complete control so that you do not need to look for them. They can be passed from finger to finger or finger to instrument.

1. A knot (strictly a bend or hitch since a knot is a node or knob) is an intertwining of threads for the purpose of joining them. The ends of ligatures and sutures are joined in this manner. Secure fastening results from friction between threads and this is affected by the area of contact, the thread surface, the tightness of the knot and the length of thread left projecting from the knot.
2. The *half-hitch* (also called an overhand hitch) forms the basis of most knots used in surgery. Cross two threads to form a closed loop (Fig. 3.2). Pass one end through the loop. A half-hitch may be formed by crossing one thread over or under the other, thus making two forms of half-hitch possible (Fig. 3.3). The initial crossing may be left over right (on the left) or right over left (on the right).
3. If the two ends are to be tied in a half-hitch, they must be crossed and both tightened on the opposite sides of the knot from which they started (Fig. 3.4).
4. If you tie one half-hitch left over right and on top of it tie a second half-hitch also left over right, you produce a *granny knot* (Fig. 3.5). You could also tie two half-hitches right over left, right over left. A granny knot

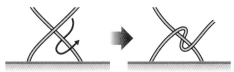

Fig. 3.2 Forming a half-hitch. Cross the threads and pass one end under the crossing to emerge on the other side.

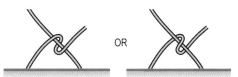

Fig. 3.3 Two types of half-hitch: starting left over right or right over left.

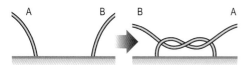

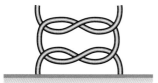

Fig. 3.4 When forming a half-hitch, the ends must be crossed and drawn in opposite directions. Note that end A starts on the left but ends on the right, and end B starts on the right and ends on the left.

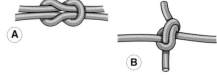

Fig. 3.7 (A) Looking down at a reef knot. The ends lie parallel to the standing threads. In panel B the ends tend to project at right angles to the standing parts—this is a granny knot.

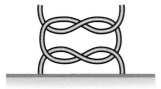

Fig. 3.5 Granny knot. Follow the path of the threads; for the first half-hitch, the left thread was passed in front of the right one, then underneath, to emerge in front on the right side. For the second half-hitch, the new left thread (the former right thread) is also passed in front of the new right thread (the former left thread) and emerges in front on the right.

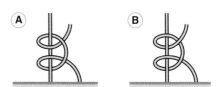

Fig. 3.8 Two varieties of slip knot. (A) The result of pulling one thread of a reef knot straight—or keeping it straight while you form hitches round it. The other thread is converted to form two half-hitches round it. (B) The result of pulling one thread of a granny knot. Note that the other thread is converted to form the well-known clove hitch round it (clove = past participle of cleave, from Old English *clifian* = to unite, adhere).

Fig. 3.6 Reef knot. The left thread was passed behind the right thread for the first half-hitch, then under it through the loop and taken to the right. The right thread emerges on the left. For the second hitch the new left thread passes in front of the new right and passes under it to emerge on the right.

has much greater holding power than a single half-hitch.

5. After tying one half-hitch, say left over right, crossing the threads so the left one is drawn to the right and the right one drawn to the left, create the second half-hitch by crossing what is now the right thread to the left over the left thread. This forms a *reef knot* (from Old Norse *rif* = fold; the knot used when folding and gathering a ship's sail to reef, or shorten it, in a strong wind; Fig. 3.6). You could pass right over left, then left over right.

6. In the granny knot the threads of the two half-hitches cross rather than run parallel as in the reef knot, shortening the length of

contact. Note the difference by looking down on the knots. In a reef knot the ends lie parallel to the standing parts; in a granny knot the ends tend to lie at right angles to the standing part (Fig. 3.7).

7. If you create the same half-hitches as for a granny and a reef knot but keep one thread taut, you produce a slip knot. In the days of square-rigged ships, sailors used the reef knot because it was not only secure but also because it could be released easily and rapidly. Pull one thread straight and it produces a *slip knot* (Fig. 3.8). The two half-hitches can be slid off the straight, standing thread. This emphasises the critical need when tightening the knots to maintain their relationship correctly.

8. After tying a reef knot, form a third half-hitch, creating a reef knot with the second half-hitch, to produce a *triple throw knot* (Fig. 3.9). This is even more reliable and is used as the standard method in surgery when security is essential.

9. The hands that control the ends must either cross each other or exchange ends. If they are crossed in the horizontal plane after the manner of crossing hands at the pianoforte (Fig. 3.10), they obscure the knot as they cross.

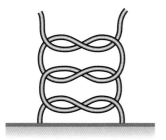

Fig. 3.9 Triple throw knot.

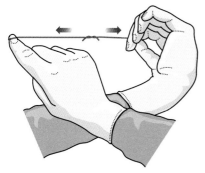

Fig. 3.10 Hands crossed in the horizontal plane obscure the field and are less in control.

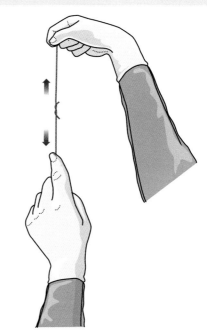

Fig. 3.11 Cross your hands in the sagittal plane.

If the hands pass each other in the sagittal plane, towards and away from the body (Fig. 3.11), the knot is not obscured at any time. You may be able to tie knots in the sagittal plane by adjusting your posture, either physically or mentally.

Two-handed knot

I believe this is the safest knot. Why? Both hands are actively involved and sense exactly the tension on the threads, which must be even, ensuring that you do not distort the knot or pull on their attachment. At all stages you are fully in control of the thread ends, and of the direction and amount of tension, matching them on each side. It is a valuable facility to use either hand to form the crossing of the threads. If you are inserting sutures, holding the needle-holder in the dominant hand and using it to draw the thread through the tissues, you capture the short thread with the nondominant hand. Right-handed surgeons hold the needle-holder with and draw through the thread with the right hand. The left hand captures the short end.

1. If the short end of thread is towards you, capture it and hold it vertically between the

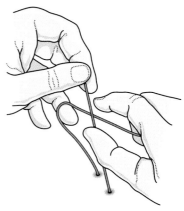

Fig. 3.12 If the short end is near you, hold it vertically by its tip, grasped between thumb and index finger of your pronated left hand. With the ring finger of your left hand, draw a loop of the long thread to the left, behind the vertically held short thread.

thumb and index finger of the pronated left hand. Grip the longer end with the fully flexed right ring and little fingers, allowing the spare thread to hang from the curled little finger, leaving the thumb, index and middle fingers free. With your left ring finger draw a loop of the long thread to the left behind the short thread (Fig. 3.12).

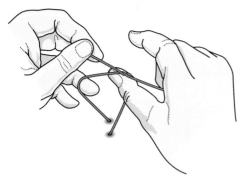

Fig. 3.13 Dorsiflex your right hand to place your extended thumb under the crossing of the threads.

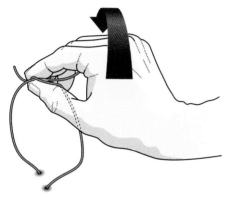

Fig. 3.14 Trap the crossing with your index finger. Now release your grasp of the short end by left thumb and index finger. Prepare to palmar-flex your right hand, carrying the short end over and back under the crossing.

2. Dorsiflex your right hand to thrust the pulp of the right thumb under the crossing of the threads, trapping the crossing between the thumb and the right index finger (Fig. 3.13). Release the grip of left index finger and thumb on the short thread to free it (Fig. 3.14).
3. Now palmar-flex your right hand, carrying the short end under the crossing of threads so that it points towards you (Fig. 3.15). Grasp the end once more between the left thumb and index finger and take it away from you as you draw the long thread in your right hand towards you, to tighten the hitch (Fig. 3.16).
4. If the short end of the thread is away from you, pick it up between the thumb and index finger of the pronated left hand.
5. Grip the longer thread with the fully flexed ring and little fingers of the right hand, letting the spare thread hang from the curled little

finger, leaving the right thumb, index and middle fingers free. Draw a loop of the long thread to the left in front of the short thread, using your left ring finger (Fig. 3.17).
6. Supinate and palmar-flex your right hand to thrust your index finger under the crossing of the threads, pointing towards yourself (Fig. 3.18). Pronate your left hand to draw the short thread pointing towards you and release it as you trap the crossing with your right thumb. Now fully pronate your right hand, carrying the short end under the loop to emerge on the other side, pointing away from you (Fig. 3.19).
7. Capture the end of the short thread again with your left index finger and thumb (Fig. 3.20) and draw it toward you as you take the long thread in your right hand away from you to tighten the hitch (Fig. 3.21).
8. If you start with the short end toward you, tie the hitch and carry straight on to tie the hitch with the short end pointing away from you. If you start with the short end pointing away from you, tie the hitch and carry straight on to tie the hitch with the short end pointing toward you.

Key points

- How tight? This is most difficult to judge from watching experts, or for them to judge you.
  - To ligate a blood vessel, just a little tighter than successful occlusion but not tight enough to risk damaging the integrity of the wall and risking separation of the stump. In an artery, not loose enough to risk pulsations rolling off the ligature.
  - Tight enough to gradually cut through in the case of ligatures intended to cause ischaemic necrosis and separation.
  - In living tissues, usually just enough to appose the tissues without blanching. Local oedema will later tighten the constriction and risk necrosis of the contained tissues with prejudiced healing.
- With delicate tissues, snug the knot down with your index finger on the knot to avoid avulsing the tissue.
- Cut the thread long enough so that it does not come undone. This may be slightly longer for a monofilament thread than for a braided thread.
- Likewise, if you are excising tissue distal to the ligature, the greater the volume of tissue that is tied, the slightly longer it is cut above the ligature to prevent it from sliding out of the knot when it retracts.

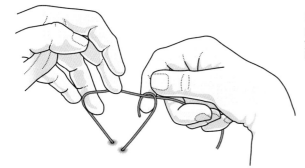

Fig. 3.15 Your right index finger now pushes the short end under and towards you as you release the loop held by your left ring finger.

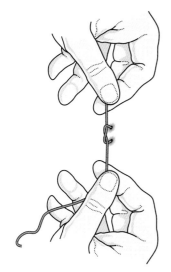

Fig. 3.16 Grasp the end of the short thread between thumb and index finger of your left hand and carry it away, while drawing the long thread towards you with your right hand, to tighten the hitch.

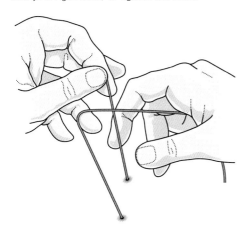

Fig. 3.17 If the short thread is away from you, hold it up between the index finger and thumb of your left hand. Draw a loop of the long thread in front of the short thread with your left ring finger.

One-handed knot tied with the left hand

This is a perfectly good knot, tied with the left hand, used effectively by surgeons while holding an instrument in the right hand. Do not try to emulate the speed and elegance of experts without recognising that although it is named 'one-handed' for forming, it is two-handed for tightening; in consequence they hold one hand still, form and tighten the hitches around it—and create a slip knot (see Fig. 3.8). Prefer slower, secure, two-handed knots unless you are confident that every hitch is not only formed but tightened perfectly every time, with crossing of the hands.

Key points

- If you are tying a ligature or suture in very delicate tissue, avoid this knot. You cannot control exactly the tension you put on the standing parts as you hook your fingers round the vertically held threads to capture one of them.
- In contrast, you can form and tighten a two-handed knot while retaining exactly even tension, or no tension at all, on the strings as you form and tighten the knot.

---

1. As with the two-handed knot, there are two types of half-hitch. When the short end is away from you, use the index finger (index-finger hitch). When the short end is close to you, use the middle finger (middle-finger hitch). The index-finger hitch and the middle-finger hitch must be tied alternately to produce a reef knot.
2. For the index-finger hitch, when the short end is away from you, pick up the short end with the thumb and middle finger of the left hand and hold it vertically. Flex the wrist so

31

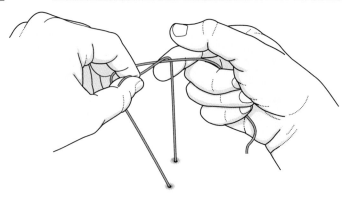

Fig. 3.18 Flex your right wrist and supinate the hand to place the extended right index finger under the crossing of the threads and pronate the left hand to draw the end of the short thread pointing towards you.

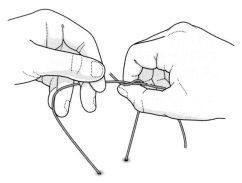

Fig. 3.19 Trap the crossing of the threads with the thumb of your fully supinated right hand as you release the short end with your left hand. Fully pronate your right hand and extend the wrist as you carry the short end under the crossing to point away from you.

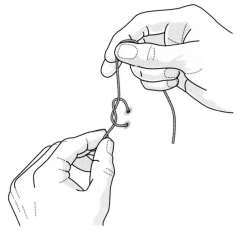

Fig. 3.21 Draw the short thread towards you and take the long thread away to tighten the half-hitch.

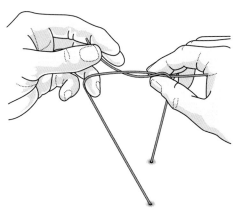

Fig. 3.20 As the short end emerges from under the crossing, pointing away from you, capture it once more with the left hand.

your left hand hangs from it, then supinate your hand and extend the index finger to create a loop of the short thread over it.

3. Pick up the long thread with your right hand and hold it vertically in front of the short thread so that it crosses the short thread in the section between the index finger and the grasp of the middle finger and thumb of your left hand (Fig. 3.22).

4. Flex the terminal interphalangeal joint of your left index finger around the long thread to reach behind the short thread (Fig. 3.23). The short thread lies against your nail on the dorsum of the finger. As you pronate your left hand, extend the tip of the left index finger, carrying the loop of short thread under the loop of long thread (Fig. 3.24).

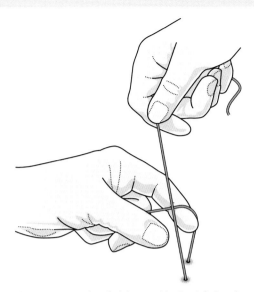

Fig. 3.22   One-handed knot with the left hand. Hold the short end between the thumb and middle finger of the pronated left hand. Supinate the left hand, swinging the left index finger to push a loop of short thread behind and beyond the long thread held vertically in the right hand. This is the index-finger half-hitch.

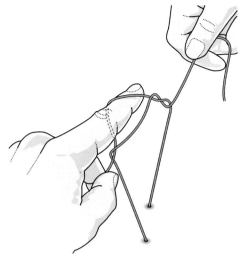

Fig. 3.24   While still holding the short end with the left thumb and middle finger, pronate your left hand, carrying the loop of short thread under the loop of long thread on the back of your index finger.

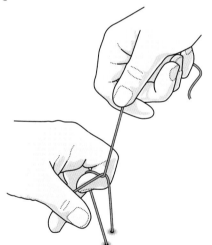

Fig. 3.23   Flex your left index finger around the vertically held long thread so that you can pull a loop of long thread up with the pulp of the index finger, while the short thread crosses the nail.

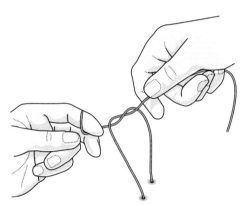

Fig. 3.25   As the loop of short thread emerges, release the left thumb and middle finger grip on the end of the short thread and use your middle finger to trap the emerging end of short thread against the index finger to be replaced by your thumb.

5. Release the middle finger contact with the thumb of the left hand to allow the end of the short thread to be carried through and use the middle finger to trap the emerging end against the index finger (Fig. 3.25).

6. Now bring the short end toward you and take the long end away from you to tighten the hitch (Fig. 3.26).

7. For the middle-finger hitch, when the short end lies near you, pick it up between the index finger and thumb of the pronated left hand and hold it vertically. Pick up the long thread with your right hand and hold it vertically.

8. Supinate your left hand as you extend the middle finger between the near short thread

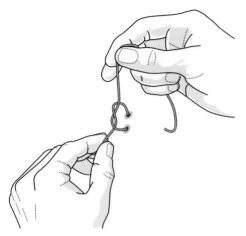

Fig. 3.26 Now draw the short end towards you and take the long end away to tighten the hitch.

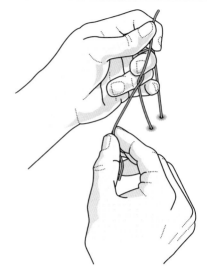

Fig. 3.28 Flex the terminal phalanx of the middle finger to pass over the long thread but behind the part of the short thread above the crossing of the threads. The nail lies in contact with the short thread.

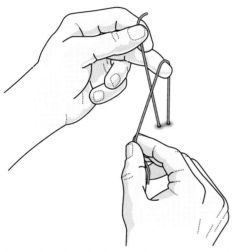

Fig. 3.27 When the short end lies near to you, pick it up between the index finger and thumb of your left hand and pick up the long thread with your right hand. Supinate your left hand and extend your middle finger behind the short thread. Draw the long thread over the extended finger from the far side, pointing towards you. This is the middle-finger half-hitch.

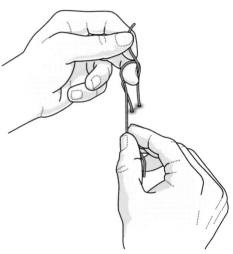

Fig. 3.29 Extend the terminal phalanx of your middle finger to carry a loop of the short thread away from you, under the long thread as you pronate your left hand.

and the far long thread and pull the long thread over it toward yourself (Fig. 3.27), crossing the short thread.

9. Flex the tip of your middle finger over the top of the horizontal section of the long thread and beneath the section of the short thread between the crossing of the threads and the grip of the left thumb and index finger; the nail of your middle finger lies in contact with the short thread (Fig. 3.28).

10. As you pronate your left hand, extend your middle finger (Fig. 3.29) to carry the end of the short thread underneath the long thread, to point away from you, as you release the grip of your index finger and thumb on the tip, and extend your ring finger to trap the end against the middle finger (Fig. 3.30).

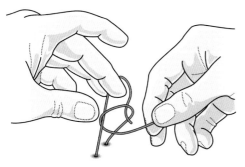

Fig. 3.30 As the loop of the short thread emerges, release the end so that it is carried through; move your left ring finger to trap the end against the middle finger.

11. Now carry the short end away from you and bring the long end toward you (Fig. 3.31) to tighten the hitch.

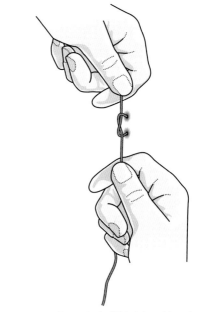

Fig. 3.31 Tighten the half-hitch by taking the short end away from you and drawing the long thread towards you.

Key point

- Note that when tying the index finger hitch, you need to pick up the short thread between thumb and middle finger, leaving the index finger free; when tying the middle-finger hitch, you need to pick up the short thread between thumb and index finger, leaving the middle finger free.

Three-finger hitch

An alternative to the middle-finger hitch might be called the three-finger hitch.

1. When the short end lies near you, pick it up between the index finger and thumb of the pronated left hand and hold it vertically.

2. Supinate your left hand while extending the medial three fingers so that the short thread lies on the little, ring and middle fingers. Take the long thread over the middle finger from the far side and across the ring and little fingers, coming towards you (Fig. 3.32).

3. Flex the terminal phalanx of the left middle finger over the top of the long thread and under the section of short thread lying between the little finger and the grip of the thumb and index finger (Fig. 3.33). You can immediately trap the short thread onto the back of the middle finger, with the pulp of your ring finger.

4. As you pronate your left hand, carry the loop of short thread under the long thread by

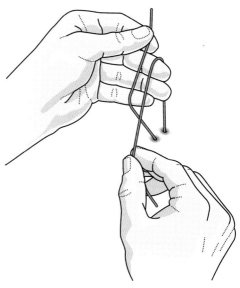

Fig. 3.32 'Three-finger hitch'. When the short thread is closer to you, pick it up with your index finger and thumb of the pronated left hand. Now supinate your left hand but instead of extending just your middle finger, extend the medial three fingers, allowing the short thread to stretch from the little finger to the index finger and thumb. Take the long thread in the right hand on the far side of the middle finger and lay it over the three medial fingers towards you.

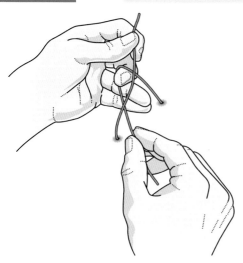

Fig. 3.33 Flex the terminal phalanx of the middle finger over the long thread and under the short thread. Prepare to extend the middle finger to draw a loop of short thread under the long thread as in Fig. 3.29.

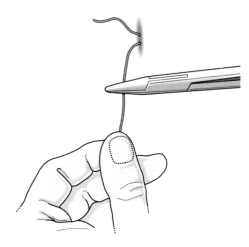

Fig. 3.34 If the short thread is farthest from you, lay the needle-holder on the long thread nearer to you.

extending the middle finger and ring fingers as in Fig. 3.29 and tighten it by taking the short thread away from you and the long thread towards you as in Fig. 3.31.

5. The advantage of using three fingers instead of the middle finger only is that it is often easier to dip the terminal phalanx of the middle finger under the longer stretch of short thread. You can achieve this without exerting tension on the thread.

Knot tied using instruments

Use instrument ties for repetitive routine knot tying as when inserting a line of interrupted skin stitches. Do not use the method indiscriminately. When tying important knots, revert to the two-handed method.

The method avoids the need to put down the needle-holder to tie two-handed knots. However instruments can be 'palmed'—held by the medial fingers while using the lateral fingers to perform manoeuvres such as knot-tying (see Chapter 2). A less justifiable reason for using instrument ties is that the method is economical of suture material, since the short end need be only long enough to be grasped by the instrument, but this tempts you to hold it taut so the long thread forms a slip knot around it.

1. If the short end is away from you and the longer thread toward you, lay the needle-holder (it

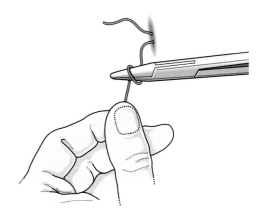

Fig. 3.35 Take a turn of thread round it.

may be a haemostat or dissecting forceps—but I shall not continue to repeat this) on the long thread (Fig. 3.34).

2. Take the long thread closest to you and pass it over the tip of the needle-holder, around it and back towards you (Fig. 3.35). While maintaining the loop, manoeuvre the needle-holder through it so you can grasp the short end (Fig. 3.36) and draw it back through the loop towards you, while taking the long thread away from you to tighten it (Fig. 3.37).

3. If the short end is near you, take the long thread away. Lay the needle-holder on top of the long thread (Fig. 3.38). Take a turn of the thread around it (Fig. 3.39), then grasp the

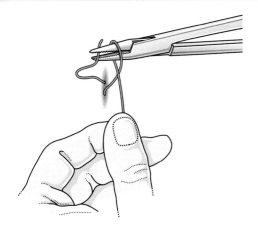

Fig. 3.36 Reach through the loop to grasp the short end.

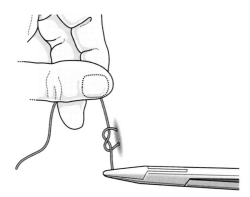

Fig. 3.37 Draw the short end through the loop towards you and take the long thread away from you to tighten the hitch.

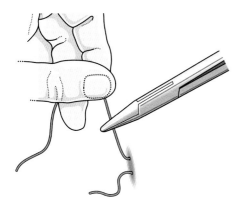

Fig. 3.38 When the short thread is towards you, lay the needle-holder on the long thread lying away from you.

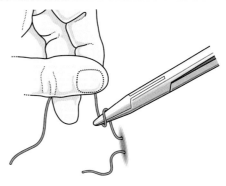

Fig. 3.39 Take a turn of the long thread around the needle-holder.

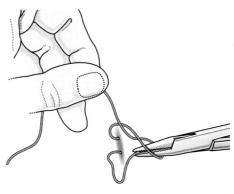

Fig. 3.40 Grasp the short end through the loop.

short end through the loop (Fig. 3.40) and draw it through.

4. Tighten the hitch by taking the short thread away from you and drawing the long thread towards you (Fig. 3.41).

Knot tying using instruments only has been brought to a fine art during minimal access surgical procedures, but this is not a basic technique (see Chapter 13). Try practising the technique.

Laying and tightening knots

Key points

- Arranging the threads to lie in the correct relationship to each other is as important as forming the knots correctly.
- A carefully tightened knot weakens the thread significantly. A roughly tightened knot weakens it critically.

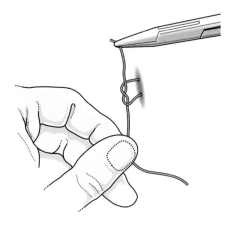

Fig. 3.41 Carry the short end through the loop and take it away from you while drawing the long thread towards you.

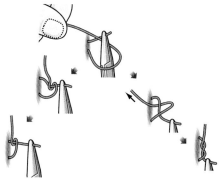

Fig. 3.42 When one end is short and you form a loop around it, draw the short end through the loop, being careful not to tauten, and thus straighten, the short end. Allow it to remain slack while you take up the slack in the large loop through which it was drawn. On the left, it is drawn out straight and a slip half-hitch results. On the right, the short end remains slack while you draw through the large loop to match it. Only then are the two ends evenly distracted to tighten a correct half-hitch.

1. Before you tighten a hitch ensure that the loops are of equal size. We automatically move our hands apart at equal speeds. If one loop is larger than the other, the shorter one tends to become tautly straight before the slack is taken up by the other (Fig. 3.42).
2. This fault occurs particularly when you attempt to tie a knot when one end is short. To avoid losing it, you tend to keep it taut.
3. Once you have secured it, slacken it off until you have drawn the longer end through to match it. Plastic surgeons often pull the thread

through when stitching, to leave a protruding end so short that when they have tied the knot they need to cut only the long thread. If you attempt to copy this technique, take the greatest care to lay and tighten the knot correctly.
4. The force and direction of pull for both threads must be equal and lie along a straight line passing through the centre of the knot. Any other force or direction displaces the knot and puts traction on the attached tissues.
5. Carefully adjust the tension of the first half-hitch.

> ### Key points
>
> - To appose tissues and encourage them to unite, do not overtighten the stitch and constrict them.
> - Remember that inflammatory oedema is inevitable following a surgical procedure; if the tissues are already constricted, they will die or the tie will cut out.
> - If your knot is too tight, if possible, cut it out and tie it again.
> - If your knot is too loose, if possible, cut it out and tie it again. If you cannot cut it out then, if possible, place a second tie and consider cutting the first one out.

6. Conversely, when you are tying a vital ligature around a major blood vessel, if the tie is too slack, it will be insecure. Tighten the second hitch fully onto the first. It is the binding effect of the threads of the two hitches that secures the knot.
7. When tying an important knot onto strong tissue, be willing to 'bed down' the hitches by gently and evenly tugging the ends apart two or three times (Fig. 3.43). Tighten the second hitch onto the first in a similar manner. Finally, tie and securely tighten a third half-hitch, forming a reef knot with the second.
8. Remove knots that are too tight or too loose and redo the suturing. If you have a row of continuous suturing that is loose, you can gently tighten each loop from the start to the loose, untied end with a nerve hook (do not use a skin hook, as this will cut your thread). If you have tied a knot at the end of a continuous suture which is too loose and cannot be cut out and restarted, you may be able to tighten the suture as follows: take a second suture and make a stitch a short distance from the loose loop. Tie the new stitch with a sound knot. With one of the free ends of the new knot, tie a further knot to the loose loop of

the continuous suture, using an instrument tie. If the loose loop is not long enough, then pass the needle of your new, tied stitch through the loop and re-tie the new stitch pulling the loop to be incorporated in the knot. These strategies should only be used when you really cannot afford to untie the original suture and start again.

Tightening under tension

Of course we should not tie under tension—but we do not always have the choice.

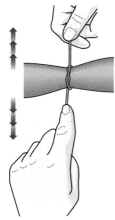

Fig. 3.43 'Bed down' the hitch on a thick structure by gently pulling the threads apart several times.

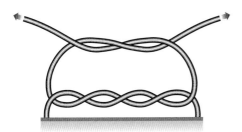

Fig. 3.44 This is a true surgeon's knot. The first half-hitch has two 'throws' or turns. The second is a standard half-hitch; I believe it should be finished off with a third half-hitch that forms a reef knot with the second half-hitch.

1. If two structures must be brought together and held there with sutures or ligatures, use your assistant's hands to draw and hold them together while you tie the knots.

2. In order to create increased contact and therefore increased friction between the threads of the first half-hitch, pass the short end twice through the closed loop. When this is pulled taut, it has less tendency to slip than a normal half-hitch. Now tie a normal second half-hitch onto it to form a *surgeon's knot* (Fig. 3.44). I believe you should always tie a third, normal half-hitch, forming a reef knot with the second normal half-hitch.

3. A knot in which the second hitch also has two turns is sometimes recommended—and incorrectly called a surgeon's knot. When tying smooth-surfaced, extruded synthetic material, a number of methods are recommended, such as a surgeon's knot with a third hitch having two 'throws' or turns, or a standard reef knot finished with a third hitch also having two throws (Fig. 3.45).

4. If you are tying a thread around a structure that cannot be compressed by your assistant, such as a bulky elastic duct, then the thread itself must be capable of constricting and holding tight while you form and tighten a second hitch onto it. Try keeping the threads taut after tying and tightening the first half-hitch while you form the second hitch and tighten it onto the first (Fig. 3.46).

5. Particularly when suturing skin, the edges tend to separate after you have brought them together with the first half-hitch, which slackens while you are forming and tightening the second half-hitch. Try rotating the threads clockwise or anticlockwise, to lock them (Fig. 3.47). They will lock only in one direction depending on which type of half-hitch you have tied. As you tighten the second hitch, they unlock to form a secure reef knot but only if you form and tighten the second hitch correctly. Just as the second hitch

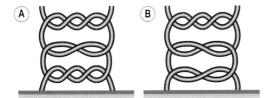

Fig. 3.45 Recommended knots for tying synthetic absorbable materials. (A) A double throw, then a single throw, followed by a double throw. (B) Tie a reef knot, then add a double throw.

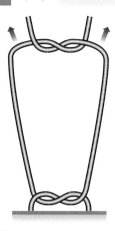

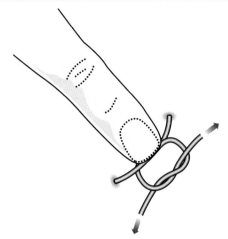

Fig. 3.46 Tying a knot under tension. After tying and tightening the first half-hitch, keep the threads taut while you form and tighten the second hitch, to stop the first hitch from slipping.

Fig. 3.48 Your assistant's finger traps the first half-hitch while you tie the second half-hitch. You must lead the tightening threads under the assistant's finger—without capturing part of the glove.

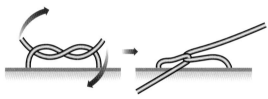

Fig. 3.47 After tying and tightening the first half-hitch, rotate the ends clockwise or anticlockwise to 'lock' the threads while you tie and tighten the second hitch onto it. You must rotate the threads correctly, and you must tie and tighten the second hitch correctly to create a reef knot.

tightens, it unlocks the trapped first hitch without giving it a chance to slacken.

6. If you deliberately keep one thread taut as you throw two half-hitches around it to form a slip knot (Fig. 3.8), you can tighten it, to be held temporarily by the friction of the threads, while you now add two correctly formed and tightened hitches to make a reef knot. This is most effective if your slip knot is the result of pulling one thread of a granny knot, rather than a reef, which is more likely to lock before you have snugged it down.

7. An effective method of preventing slippage is to ask your assistant to compress the tightened first half-hitch with a finger while you form and tighten the second hitch, leading the tightening loop under the compressing finger (Fig. 3.48). Take care that you do not capture a small piece of the assistant's surgical glove, which will tear off when the finger is removed.

8. Another valuable method is to insert one or more temporary stitches to draw separated edges together while you insert and tie the definitive stitches, and then remove the temporary stitches (Fig. 3.49). You may tie them, or merely cross the ends and have your assistant hold them taut.

9. Alternatively, you may close the deeper tissues in layers, bringing them together so that the skin is not under tension.

10. When faced with closing an abdomen which you expect to be under some pressure postoperatively, you may place deep tension sutures. These are large-gauge monofilament sutures which, when tied, are outside the circumference of your skin closure. They usually come on a large needle; be careful not to inadvertently injure yourself or the bowel. For each suture, place the first stitch in the abdominal wall that is away from you, from outside the abdominal wall to inside approximately 3 to 4 cm from the skin edge,

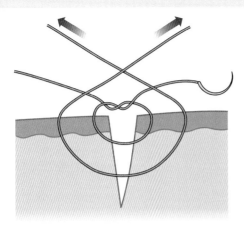

Fig. 3.49 Insert and tie a temporary stitch to take the tension while you insert and tie the definitive stitches. You need not tie it if you have your assistant cross the threads and hold them taut.

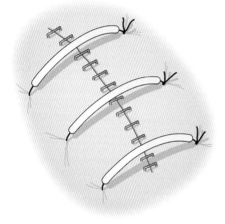

Fig. 3.50 Deep tension sutures hold the abdominal wall together without putting tension on the midline closure.

and the second stitch from inside the opposite abdominal wall to outside, mirroring the contralateral side. Narrow plastic tubing is then threaded onto one end and both ends are held with a haemostat. Complete sutures in the same fashion from the cranial end of the laparotomy wound to the caudal end, at approximately 3- to 4-cm intervals. Then proceed to close the abdomen in the usual fashion. Tie the deep tension sutures over the top of the standard close, keeping the knots on one side and positioning the plastic tubing over the wound to prevent the deep tension suture cutting into it (Fig. 3.50).

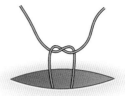

Fig. 3.51 Tying a knot in a cavity. Form the hitches on the surface to ensure the thread is sufficiently long.

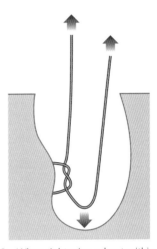

Fig. 3.52 When tightening a knot within a cavity, you must push one end in with exactly the force with which you pull the other end out. If not, you will displace the structure or pull off the ligature.

Tying knots in cavities

1. In some cases you need to tie a knot deep in a cavity. As a rule, it is most convenient to form the hitches outside the cavity (Fig. 3.51).
2. Ensure that you have a sufficient length of thread so that after you have encircled or sutured the deep structure both ends of the thread lie outside the cavity.
3. Tie a two-handed half-hitch outside the cavity without putting any tension on the threads.
4. With an extended finger, or a pushed but not grasping instrument, close the loop onto the structure.
5. Tighten the hitch by pushing down with a finger on one thread, with exactly the same force as you pull on the other thread from outside the cavity (Fig. 3.52). In some cases when you can insert both hands, you can pull the threads apart as you would on the surface.

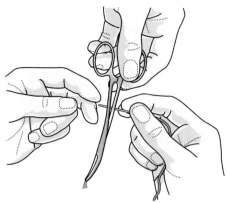

Fig. 3.53 While your assistant lifts the handles of the forceps, pass the ligature from one hand to the other behind them.

6. If you merely pull on the deep structure, you may damage it, avulse it or pull off the tie.

LIGATURES

A ligature (from the Latin *ligare* = to bind) is tied round a structure, most commonly a blood vessel or other duct, usually intended to close the lumen. Ligatures are secured by knotting the ends.

Key points

- Blood vessel ligation is one of the commonest repetitive procedures in surgery.
- Practise, practise, practise ligating vessels until you can perform it effortlessly, perfectly, every time.
- Perfection is more important than time. Indeed, two rapidly performed failed attempts take longer than a single effective ligature.

1. Synthetic polymerised, braided, absorbable threads are commonly used as ligatures and are digested with minimum inflammation by hydrolysis. Silk is soft, flexible, can be tied securely without slipping and has a limited tendency to be reabsorbed, but is used less often now. Avoid using it near the skin unless you will remove it, because it evokes a foreign body reaction, produces worrying subcutaneous nodules or even sinuses to the skin surface.

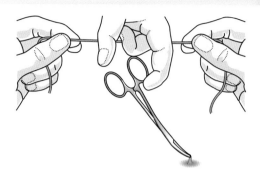

Fig. 3.54 Stretch the thread between your hands beyond the forceps and have your assistant reach over the thread to pick up the handle of the forceps.

2. Springy stainless steel and synthetic nonabsorbable materials cause minimal tissue reaction but are usually now restricted to bonding together solid structures including bone.

3. Select the finest material that will reliably hold. Position it, tie and tighten it carefully. Too tight a ligature cuts through fragile tissue; too slack and it will not occlude a thick-walled vessel or it will slip off.

4. When preparing to divide and ligate ducts and blood vessels, preferably doubly clamp and divide them first or clamp them after they are cut. In either circumstance, place the forceps with the concavity towards the cut and ensure that the tips of the forceps project a few millimetres beyond the ducts or vessels.

5. While an assistant holds up the handles of the haemostatic forceps, pass the end of the ligature under them on the side away from you, to capture it with the other hand (Fig. 3.53). Alternatively, stretch the thread between your hands on the far side of the forceps and then have your assistant reach over the thread and pick up the handles (Fig. 3.54).

6. When passing ligatures round vessels or ducts placed deeply, carry the thread stretched between the tips of your index fingers (Fig. 3.55) to reach under the tips of the forceps to avoid incorporating them in the ligature. Alternatively, use dissecting or curved artery forceps (Fig. 3.56). Warn your assistant to avoid pulling on the forceps; they will be pulled off or allow the ligature to slip over the tips of the forceps. Avoid tying in the tips of the forceps, or when they are removed, the ligature will be pulled off.

7. Tie the ligature carefully, slowly and securely.

8. Do not let your assistant undo all your safety precautions by cutting the threads too short. Have the ends of braided threads cut 2 to 3 mm long, and monofilament materials cut to 4 to 5 mm.

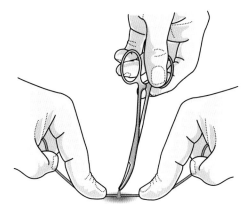

Fig. 3.55 Stretch the ligature thread between the tips of your index fingers to depress it and encircle only the vessel, without including the tips of the forceps.

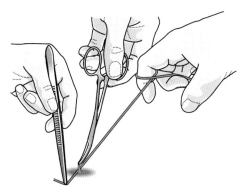

Fig. 3.56 You may pass the ligature using long-handled dissecting forceps.

STITCHES

1. Versatile thread stitches are peerless for joining together tissues that can be pierced with a needle, in spite of the development of metal clips and adhesives. Threads are carried through by the needle and secured by knotting them.

2. Suture strength is related to the diameter of any particular material and is measured by the 'knot pull strength' test—the force that can be applied to the free ends of a suture tied with a surgical knot around a quarter-inch rubber tube.

3. A portion of tissue may need to be constricted to stop or prevent bleeding or leakage of internal fluids.

4. To prevent a ligature around a divided duct or vessel from slipping, first insert a stitch across the diameter of the tube, then tie it as a suture–ligature, a so-called transfixion suture.

5. A stitch left long and untied can act as a means of exerting gentle traction. A coloured thread stitch makes a convenient marker.

6. If two materials are to be joined, insert the stitch through one, then the other, and knot the ends of the threads together.

7. A weak area or defect closed by inserting tightly drawn stitches has a high failure rate. Alternatively, it was formerly reinforced by inserting a darn (Fig. 3.57), but polypropylene mesh with or without a composite absorbable component, which is well tolerated by the tissues, has virtually replaced it. The mesh must be large enough to overlap the edges of the defect and is then sutured or clipped in place. A correctly inserted mesh creates a reliable tension-free closure of hernial and many other defects. Biological meshes are also coming into use but are more expensive.

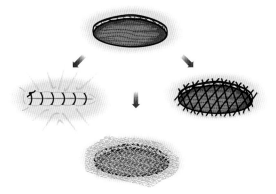

Fig. 3.57 Closing a defect. It was traditional, in order to avoid dragging the edges together under tension, as on the *left*, to bridge the defect with a darn as shown on the *right*. Because materials that are well tolerated by the tissues are now available, tension-free closure can now be achieved by inserting a polypropylene or similar plastic mesh extending beyond the margins of the defect, fixed with sutures or clips.

Key point

- The more methods of dealing with a problem that exist, the less likely it is that any of them works reliably.

Needles

1. Needles come in a variety of shapes and sizes (Fig. 3.58). Curved needles are most commonly used. As a general rule, they follow the circumference of a circle and may be a small arc or more than half the circumference.
2. Straight, handheld needles were formerly used extensively in surgery (Fig. 3.59). Surgeons are expert in handling them—flexible structures can be deformed in order to facilitate the entrance and exit of a straight needle to provide a curved passage of threads. The needles are so convenient that glove and skin punctures were accepted as a small price to pay. Recognition of the transmission of viral infections and possible prion diseases has made us change over almost exclusively to no-touch techniques.
3. There are occasions when a straight needle is invaluable. Whenever you need to pass one, always drive it by using a needle-holder (Fig. 3.60).
4. Virtually all needles are now eyeless and factory prepared. The needle is usually swaged onto the thread, although fine threads may be inserted and fixed with an adhesive into holes drilled into the shank of the needles. As a result, the hole produced by the needle is only slightly larger than the thread that will be drawn through it.
5. Sutures are supplied in sealed packets after gamma ray sterilisation.
6. A variety of points and cross-sections are available (Fig. 3.61) and the sizes range down to 3 mm for microsurgery. The needle shank is usually flattened along the section that will be grasped by the needle-holder.
7. Use a round-bodied needle to sew fragile tissue, or tissue arranged in strands that can be displaced since the strands are not cut, merely pushed aside, with minimal damage. Round-bodied needles are appropriate for sewing bowel and blood vessels because the round holes produced by the passage of the needle close by tissue elasticity around the thread, preventing leakage.
8. Skin and fibrous tissue are resistant, so use cutting needles of triangular or flat cross-section. The sharp edges of the needle cut through the tissues, so they do not contract

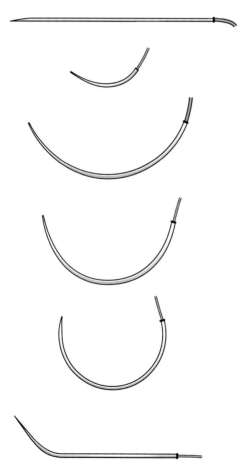

Fig. 3.58 Needles come in a variety of shapes and sizes.

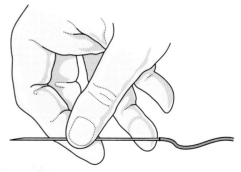

Fig. 3.59 The handheld straight needle is convenient but dangerous.

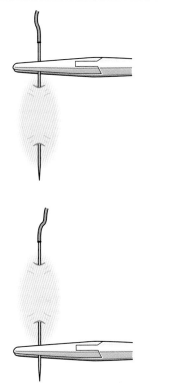

Fig. 3.60 Insert and withdraw a straight needle using a needle-holder.

onto the thread. Cutting needles of triangular section usually have the apex of the triangle on the inside of the curve. When such needles are used to insert stitches that will come under tension, in pulling two edges together, the threads tend to extend the split towards the edges with a liability to cut out. Reverse cutting needles have a flat surface on the inside of the curve and are less likely to cut out (Fig. 3.62). An alternative is a spear point, which is flat on the inside and outside of the curve.

9. Use blunt taper-pointed needles for stitching soft tissues such as the abdominal wall, excluding the skin. The needles penetrate the fascia and muscles, but surgical gloves usually resist penetration and so protect you from needle-stick injury.

10. Use blunt-ended, round-bodied needles to sew soft viscera such as liver. Sharp-edged needles create splits that are likely to extend.

11. Use a robust trocar (from French *trios* = three + *carre* = side) needle when sewing very tough tissues in which a normal needle might break.

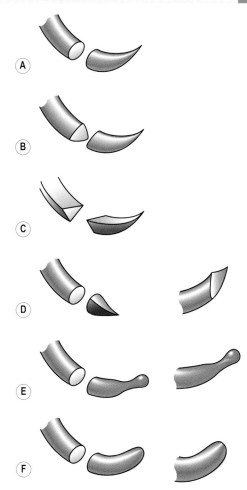

Fig. 3.61 Needle cross-sections and points. (A) Round-bodied taper-point. (B) Triangular cutting. (C) Reversed cutting. (D) Trocar pointed. (E) Blunt taper point. (F) Blunt-ended.

Key points

- Do not pick up needles with your fingers. Use needle-holders and forceps to control them. Never leave them where they could damage your patient, yourself or your colleagues.
- When not in use, place needles with other sharp instruments in a kidney dish. Never pass them from hand to hand.
- Many needle pricks occur during abdominal wall closure; the blunt taper-point needle effectively penetrates the tissues of the abdominal wall, but glove penetration is greatly reduced.

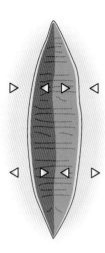

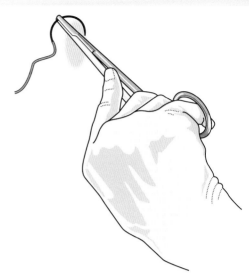

Fig. 3.62 Closing a wound that is under tension or is liable to be put under tension. Top: the holes made by a standard cutting needle with the apex of the triangle on the inside of the curve. It is liable to extend when subjected to tension. Bottom: the holes made by a reversed cutting needle present a flat face to the site of possible tension when the suture is tied. There is less likelihood of such a suture cutting out if it is placed under tension.

Fig. 3.63 Stitching with a curved needle. Start with your hand fully pronated.

Stitching with a curved needle

1. Insert, drive and withdraw curved needles exclusively with instruments. The tissues can usually be moulded to conform to the curvature.
2. Do not select too short a needle. You need to have sufficient length to allow you to push in the needle and retain a grip until the point emerges sufficiently to be gripped without damaging the point. For the same reason, do not attempt to take large bites of tissue on each side of a suture line in a single pass. Prefer to take the needle through each side separately.
3. Mount the needle in the tip of the needle-holder, approximately one-third of the way from the threaded end towards the point. If you are right-handed, with your hand in mid-pronation, the needle-holder pointing away from you, have the needle point upwards and to the left, upwards and to the right if you stitch with your left hand. Right-handed operators most easily stitch from right to left, and from away towards

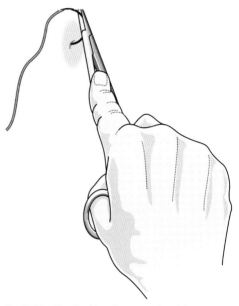

Fig. 3.64 Needle driven in a curved path by progressively supinating your hand.

you. Left-handed operators prefer to stitch from left to right, and from away towards you.
4. Start with the hand fully pronated to enter the tissues perpendicularly (Fig. 3.63, see also Fig. 3.66A). As you continue, progressively supinate the hand so that the path follows the curve of the needle (Fig. 3.64).

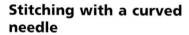

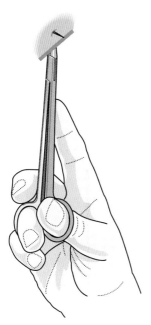

Fig. 3.65 Your wrist is fully supinated as the needle emerges.

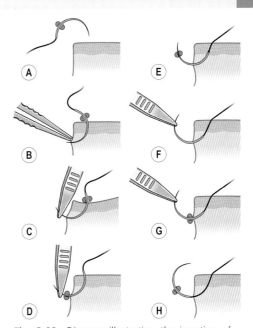

Fig. 3.66 Diagram illustrating the insertion of a stitch using a curved needle held in a needle-holder, indicated by two apposed stippled hemispheres. It shows a right-handed surgeon inserting the stitch from dominant to nondominant side. If you are left-handed the needle is inserted in the opposite direction. (A) Enter the point at right angles to the surface; your hand is fully pronated. (B) As you drive the needle through, progressively supinating your hand, apply counter pressure against the tissues as the point emerges, so helping to reveal more of the needle. (C) When sufficient needle emerges, grasp and steady it with dissecting forceps. (D) Release the needle-holder and reapply it to the emerging needle. (E) Draw through the needle along its curved path. (F) Steady the needle with the dissecting forceps. (G) Reapply the needle-holder to the emerging needle at the place you wish to grasp it for the next stitch, keeping your hand partly supinated. (H) Finally, draw the needle right through, with a fully supinated hand.

In this way the needle finally emerges perpendicularly from the tissues (Fig. 3.65).

5. The ability to pronate and supinate enables you to drive a curved needle through the tissues with minimal trauma, and with minimal force. Make full use of this human facility. The range of movement can be extended by shoulder and trunk movements.

6. If necessary, use the closed tips of dissecting forceps to apply counterpressure near, but not on, the point of emergence of the needle in order to avoid turning the needle point and blunting it (Fig. 3.66A and B). If you use too short a needle or take too great a bite, you may need to change the grasp of the needle-holder nearer the thread end of the needle to push the needle further through. When the point comes into view, grasp the shank behind it, if necessary gently pushing back the surface tissue to expose a greater length of needle, and steady it (Fig. 3.66C).

7. Relinquish the grasp of the needle-holder and use it to regrasp the emerging needle, gently pushing back the tissues to allow you to grasp it well away from the point (Fig. 3.66D).

8. Draw the needle through along its curved path (Fig. 3.66E) by further supinating your hand.

9. Again steady the needle with the dissecting forceps so you can disengage the needle-holder (Fig. 3.66F).

10. Re-grasp the needle in the correct position for making the next stitch (Fig. 3.66G), and draw it through (Fig. 3.66H). If you are inserting a continuous suture, this technique allows you to avoid the need to readjust your grasp of the needle with the needle-holder.

11. If you select the needle size correctly to match the tissue thickness and stitch depth and length, you can avoid several steps. In one

movement you may expose enough emerging needle to be able to grasp it far enough back so that you can replace the needle-holder in the correct position for the next stitch. However, if you pronate your hand before grasping the emerging needle, you will need to change your grip before inserting the next stitch. Try it.

12. If you are suturing in a deep cavity and find that the needle displaces as you release the needle-holder, you can grasp the needle coming through the tissue with forceps before you release the needle-holder. If really stuck, sometimes you may need to ask your assistant to grasp the advancing needle with another needle-holder before you release your needle-holder.

13. When stitching in difficult circumstances, you may need to stitch from nondominant to dominant hand direction, or from near to far, a so-called backhand stitch. Sometimes you can avoid this by going to the other side of the operating table. If not, take special care. You will be made aware of the difference in facility between making a familiar and unfamiliar manoeuvre.

14. Do not draw through the thread by pulling on the needle. You risk sticking the needle into an assistant or pulling the needle off the thread. Grasp the thread with a spare finger of the hand holding the needle-holder. Above all, do not draw through the thread by grasping it with the needle-holder or dissecting forceps; all the modern threads are severely weakened by being held with metal instruments.

15. Watch spare thread as you stitch. It has a fiendish propensity to catch on any projections. Have your assistant follow it and guide it; if you are using stainless steel, you must avoid producing kinks. Do not try to stitch with thread of too short length—you are tempted to take shorter stitches, tie imperfect knots, and waste time.

Types of stitch (Fig. 3.67)

1. Surgeons often adamantly claim that the type of stitch they use is the reason for their success. They are too modest (a characteristic rarely attributed to surgeons). Their success depends on the care with which they insert the stitches, appose the tissues, adjust the tension and tighten the knots. Watch a few outstanding surgeons performing—the only common factor

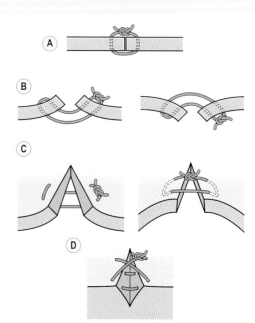

Fig. 3.67 Commonly used stitches. (A) Simple interrupted. (B) Interrupted longitudinal mattress, everting on the left, inverting on the right. (C) Interrupted horizontal mattress, everting on the left, inverting on the right. (D) Inverting 'X' stitch.

is the perfection of their technique, not the methods they use.

2. The simplest stitch to join two edges of tissue is a single thread that catches each side and draws them into contact, with both ends of the thread tied with a reef knot. This is an interrupted stitch. Pierce the tissue perpendicular to the upper and lower surfaces; otherwise it has an inverting or everting effect. If you tie it too tightly, or if it is subjected to too much tension, either the thread will break or it will cut out.

3. A mattress stitch is a double stitch. Start from one side, cross to the other side, reinsert the needle at a small distance from where it emerged and take it through to emerge on the original side a short distance from the first entry and tie the original entry and final exit thread together. If both stitches are parallel, this is a horizontal mattress stitch. Because a mattress stitch draws on a segment of tissue between the two lengths of thread joining the edges, it is much less likely to cut out. This is particularly true when you sew tissues in which the fibres run at right angles to the edges. If the entry and exit holes are perpendicular to the edges, one bite is smaller than

the other; this is a vertical or longitudinal mattress stitch. In each case, there is a bridge of suture on the upper surface which draws in the surface away from the edge so that the edge itself is everted. These are therefore referred to as everting mattress stitches. Skin sometimes tends to invert and if you allow it to do so when closing a suture line, you are apposing the dead keratinised surface cells; healing is delayed and imperfect, so the scar will be weak. When suturing blood vessels, you must appose the endothelium by slightly everting the edges, or clots will form on the internal suture line. As a rule, you can easily get the edges to turn out using simple sutures, but on occasion you may need to start the necessary eversion with one or two everting stitches.

4. In contrast, bowel should not normally be everted. The French surgeon Antoine Lembert (1802–1851) recognized that if the outer, serous coats of bowel were brought into contact, they rapidly sealed together and prevented leakage. In 1826 he described a separate row of stitches that picked up only the serous and muscular coats, placed outside the main stitches, to create an inverting effect. However, the effect can be achieved with a single row of stitches, and Lembert's stitch is less frequently used than formerly. Insert an inverting mattress stitch by passing the suture through the wall from outside in, to the mucosal surface, returning it to the surface on the same side a short distance from the entry stitch. Now cross to the opposite side and pass the suture from outside in to the mucosal surface, returning it to the exterior from the inside out, to emerge close to the entry stitch. Tie this thread to the end of thread at the original site. You have created a mattress stitch with the loop not on the surface of the bowel but on the mucosal aspect. When the stitch is tied, it tends to bring the outer, serosal surfaces together. This stitch is often named after Gregory Connell, the American surgeon who described it in 1864.

Interrupted stitches

1. These have the advantage that when used in series, failure of one does not necessarily prejudice the other stitches.
2. The potential weakness of interrupted stitches is that each one is held by a knot; even when knots are perfectly tied and tightened, they reduce the strength of the thread considerably. A roughly tied, snatched or imperfectly tightened knot may reduce the strength by over 50%. Once one knot gives way, the contiguous stitches are subjected to greater tension and may give way in turn. It is for this reason that you must form and tighten every knot perfectly, every time.
3. Moreover, tension on the stitches must be even; if it is not, the tightest stitch is exposed to excess tension and may give way, creating a domino effect. Furthermore, the overtightened stitch tends to strangle the enclosed tissue and subsequently cut out.

Continuous stitches

1. These have the advantage of being quick to insert and have knots only at the beginning and the end—but those two knots are crucial.
2. Stitching can be carried out in a continuous manner, forming a spiral within the tissues. It has the advantage that the tissues are not strangulated, although the tension is usually sufficient to be haemostatic (Fig. 3.68A).
3. You may use a variety of stitches depending on the circumstances. If you pass the needle through the loop of the previous stitch before it is tightened, you produce a locked stitch, which holds the tension while the next stitch is inserted (Fig. 3.68B)—but do not drag the thread through the loop or you will damage it. A continuous mattress stitch with the loops on the surface has an everting effect (Fig. 3.68C). In contrast a stitch leaving loops on the deep surface has an inverting effect (Fig. 3.68D).
4. In some circumstances it is an advantage to bury the stitches beneath the surface. This is especially valuable when you are sewing skin, in which case it is called a subcuticular stitch (Fig. 3.6E). This is dealt with in more detail in Chapter 6.
5. When inserting stitches that will be buried in tough tissue potentially subject to tension, the required strength may demand a very thick, stiff suture that is not only difficult to knot but would produce a large mass of foreign material. By using doubled thread, the thickness can be reduced and the suppleness increased. Needles can be supplied with both ends of a thread swaged into the needle, leaving a loop at the free end. Make

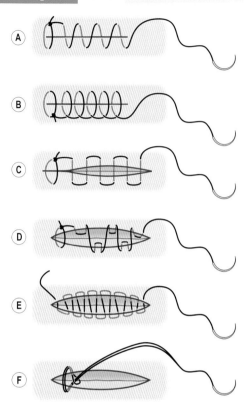

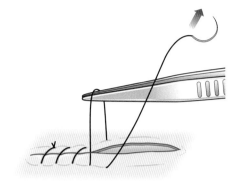

Fig. 3.69 Control the thread loop with your fingers or dissecting forceps as you tighten it, to guard against it snagging or catching on other structures and to ensure that it sits perfectly.

Fig. 3.68 Continuous stitches. (A) Over-and-over, spiral. (B) Locking or blanket stitch. (C) Continuous everting mattress stitch. (D) Continuous inverting mattress stitch. (E) Subcuticular type of stitch. (F) Starting a continuous run using a doubled looped thread.

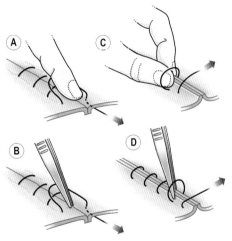

Fig. 3.70 Producing inversion and eversion using simple 'over-and-over' stitches. (A) Push in the edges and hold back the loop with your index finger as you draw the loop tight from the under surface, along the line of stitching. (B) Alternatively, achieve the same effect by the 'no touch' method, using dissecting forceps. (C) Evert the skin edges using your finger and thumb. (D) Alternatively, achieve the same effect by gently pinching the edges to maintain the eversion.

the initial stitch and pass the needle through the loop (Fig. 3.68F), anchoring the thread with the minimum bulk. Continue the stitch, and if there is sufficient length at the point of closure, cut one thread near the needle, take another stitch with the remaining thread and then tie the two threads to form a knot which is not excessively bulky.

6. When inserting continuous stitches, make sure they lie correctly; guide them by holding the loop with a finger or a closed dissecting forceps (Fig. 3.69) and carefully place the thread as you tighten it.

7. Continuous stitches cause twisting of the thread. From time to time, run your finger and thumb along the thread from where it emerges from the last stitch to the needle to allow the twists to unwind; otherwise a kink may form and snag the thread.

8. The union may be edge to edge, inverted or everted, controlled by the way in which you form and tighten the threads and place the edges (Fig. 3.70). When sewing bowel, if you hold back each tightening loop while pushing in the edges with a fingertip or dissecting forceps, the loop will retain an inverting effect, especially if you tighten the thread

only when you have inserted the stitch from without in and you are drawing the thread from within the lumen. This is because the tightening outer loop inverts the edges. When sewing skin or blood vessels, if you evert the edges between finger and thumb or dissecting forceps, the tightening stitch will retain an everting effect. Once started, the effect of edge to edge inversion or eversion tends to continue as you insert further stitches.

9. At the beginning of the run, insert the first stitch and tie it as though this is an interrupted stitch, but do not cut the thread. Continue to the end. You now have two choices to tie off this single thread. The traditional method is to hold the last loop before inserting the final stitch, using the closed loop as though it is a single thread. Having inserted the last stitch, cut off the needle and tie a knot using the final thread and the closed loop; be careful and use several throws, since knots are not as secure using threads of different thickness as when they are the same thickness (Fig. 3.71). An alternative method is to hold the loop before the last stitch, then pull a loop of the thread following the last stitch through the first loop, tighten the first loop, pass a loop of the final thread through the second loop and finally pass the needled end through that loop and tighten it. This method is used by knitters finishing off a row of knitting as a chain stitch and by fishermen when they are repairing their nets—in honour of the fishermen of Aberdeen, it is usually called an Aberdeen knot. Rarely, in order to insert stitches of an unusual material you may need to use an eyed needle. Hold on to the end of the thread before inserting the last stitch and tie this to the loop after making the stitch.

10. If you do not have sufficient thread to complete a continuous line of sutures, tie off and start again. You may leave the end of the first thread loose, insert a new stitch and tie it, then tie the loose end of the first thread to the new one.

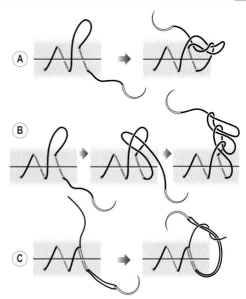

Fig. 3.71 Different methods of tying off continuous sutures. (A) Hold a loop before inserting the last stitch; use this loop like a single thread to tie to the end, after cutting off the needle—I have left it on in the drawing to identify it. (B) Hold a loop before inserting the final stitch. When you have inserted the stitch, pass a loop of the free thread through the first loop, tighten the first loop, pass a third loop through the second loop and tighten the second loop and so on three or four times. Finally, pass the needle and the free end through the last loop, tighten the loops and cut off the needle, leaving a generous free end. This is often called the Aberdeen, crochet, or daisy chain knot. (C) Very occasionally it is necessary to use an eyed needle. Hold on to the free end before inserting the last stitch, and tie this to the doubled end attached to the needle. Because the threads are of unequal thickness, tie several half-hitches and securely bed them down. Finally, cut off the needle.

CHOICE OF SUTURE MATERIAL

1. Suture material, size of thread and size of needle will depend on the tissue that you are suturing. Generally, sutures that will be removed are nonabsorbable, for instance interrupted sutures in the skin. A subcuticular skin suture may be absorbable if left in or nonabsorbable if the plan is to remove it (in which case the ends will be secured outside the skin). Internal sutures placed in tissues that will remodel (such as bowel) should be absorbable. Internal sutures placed in tissue that will not remodel (such as in a vascular anastomosis) should be nonabsorbable.

2. You should make sure you know the approximate length of time that absorbable sutures take to be absorbed, as this will impact on the integrity of the join. Bear in mind that similar sutures made by different manufacturers have different absorption times.

3. Generally the size of suture will depend on the size of the structures that you are joining. Too small a gauge and it may not hold; too large a gauge and there will be unnecessary tissue reaction.

4. The length of time that removable sutures are left in will also depend on the tissues being joined. For instance, interrupted sutures on the face, with its excellent blood supply, may be removed as early as 5 to 7 days, whereas interrupted sutures in the abdomen may need to stay in for 10 to 14 days. Interrupted sutures placed in an amputation stump, where the amputation is the consequence of ischaemia, may need to stay in for 21 days.

Chapter | 4 |

Handling ducts and cavities

The body has a variety of ducts (from the Latin *ducere* = to lead or conduct). In addition, there are many closed spaces or potential spaces. Be careful to avoid inadvertent injury to normal function:

1. Some ducts, such as the ureter, oesophagus and intestine, are capable of peristalsis. The circular smooth muscle contracts to occlude the lumen above, and relaxes below the content. An intramuscular neural plexus, named myenteric in the intestine, generates a wave of contraction preceded by relaxation, carrying the content with it. Consider the effects of any procedure on the resulting function. Other ducts, such as the common

53

bile duct, have insufficient muscle to produce peristalsis, and transmission of the content is by *vis a tergo* (from the Latin word for force from behind), often resulting from secretion into, and distension of, the elastic tube. In other circumstances transmission may result from external pressure changes; muscular expansion of the thorax expands the lungs and lowers the pressure in the trachea and bronchi, drawing air into the lungs.

2. Passage of content is often controlled by circular muscle sphincters, for example at the pylorus (from the German *pyle* = a gate and *ouros* = a watcher), at the anus and lower end of the bile duct, the sphincter of Oddi (named after Italian physiologist Ruggero Oddi, 1864–1913). There may be no anatomical, only functional evidence of a sphincteric action, for example at the gastrooesophageal junction, which also selectively prevents reflux of gastric content into the oesophagus.

3. Although tubes within the body differ in form and function, they are all transmitters of substances that are absorbed from or secreted or excreted into the lumen of glands, larger ducts such as the intestine, or to the exterior.

4. Passages and cavities are created by disease— sinuses and fistulas or spaces such as seromas, haematomas, cysts and abscesses. Potential spaces are opened up surgically. Artificial fistulas include internal fistulas such as gastroenterostomy and external stomas (from the Greek *stoma* = a mouth).

5. Wherever there is stagnation in spaces or in ducts, microorganisms collect and tend to contaminate and infect the tissues.

6. Ducts and cavities are prone to injury, stenosis, obstruction, other mechanical problems, or paralysis, and require intubation, dilatation, drainage, repair and anastomosis. Some cavities require similar management.

7. The principles of management are often common to different situations. For this reason, acquire familiarity with all the techniques, watch experts, and assiduously practise the manoeuvres to develop the necessary skills. Success often results from adapting methods from one area to another.

8. Here, examples used are procedures that are lifesaving or commonly performed to demonstrate the required technical skills; but selection, preparation and aftercare are not discussed.

INTUBATION

Percutaneous access

A number of commonly performed procedures, some of them lifesaving, incorporate percutaneous (from the Latin *per-* = through, beyond and *cutis* = skin) puncture.

1. Insert needles in a straight line; if you need to change direction it is usually better to withdraw the needle and reinsert it. If you move the needle within the tissues you risk damaging any or all of the structures between the entry point and the needle tip.

2. Hollow needles are available in varying diameters and lengths; for example, long thin 'skinny' needles are used for percutaneous liver puncture to minimise subsequent leakage. Needles are usually best connected to a syringe so that you can see what emerges or what the aspirate contains. Do not use short needles that must be fully inserted, since if they break off at the Luer connection, the thin retained shaft is difficult to identify and grasp.

3. When you intend to remove fluid, it may be convenient to interpose a three-way tap between the needle and the syringe; aspirated fluid can then be expelled through the side channel of the tap, into a receiver.

4. Some needles have an internal obturator (from the Latin *obturare* = to stop up) that is withdrawn when the needle is correctly placed, allowing contents to emerge; lumbar puncture needles have stylettes, presumably to prevent the contamination of cerebrospinal fluid by other fluids during the passage of the needle.

5. If you wish to inject fluid into a tube or space, can you confirm that the tip of the needle is correctly sited? You may aspirate identifiable fluid into a syringe attached to the needle. To minimise subsequent leakage along the needle track when performing percutaneous transhepatic biliary puncture, a long, very thin, 'skinny' needle is used. Bile can be aspirated and radio-opaque material injected to outline the biliary tract radiographically (Fig. 4.1A). You may aspirate fluid from a cyst, blood from a haematoma or pus from an abscess cavity (Fig. 4.1B). In some cases, ease of fluid injection helps confirm that the tip is in the correct place; for example, injection of sterile saline into a venous cannula. Similarly, ease of gas flow may help; insufflation (from the Latin *in* and *sufflare* = to blow) of the peritoneal cavity with

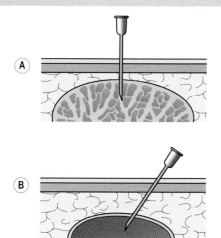

Fig. 4.1 (A) Percutaneous puncture to gain access to ducts. To guard against subsequent leakage from, for example, bile ducts within the liver, a long, thin 'skinny' needle is used. (B) Puncture of a cavity such as a cyst, haematoma or abscess cavity.

carbon dioxide to initiate pneumoperitoneum does not produce a rapid rise in pressure as would occur if the gas were infused into a closed space. In contrast, when you wish to inject into a closed space such as an obstructed tube, carefully note if the flow is freer than you expect, suggesting you have entered an extensive cavity or patent ductal structure.

6. When you have entered the tube or space, make sure you do not penetrate beyond it. One method is to mark the penetrator with a clamp or the sterile-gloved fingers or use a penetrator with a shoulder such as on a haemorrhoid injection needle, to limit its

entrance. A similar risk occurs when creating a pneumoperitoneum prior to minimal access surgery (see Ch. 13). To minimise the risk of penetrating the viscera within the potential space before they fall away from the parietal peritoneum (see Fig. 4.2 and Ch. 13), use the special Veress needle which has a sharp bevel tip but within it is a spring-loaded blunt trocar. As soon as the bevel penetrates the parietal peritoneum the trocar projects, pushing away any at-risk viscera.

7. Alternatively, an open Hasson technique may be preferable (see Ch. 13) (after Harrith Hasson of Chicago, USA); a vertical or curved transverse cut down is made just below, or sometimes above, the umbilicus. Ask your assistant to retract the skin edges with two Alliss forceps, and then, as you retract the subcutaneous fat, with two small Langenbeck retractors. Pick up the linea alba with two tissue forceps and make a 1.5-cm longitudinal incision. Apply stay sutures to each side. Then pick up the peritoneum carefully between two fine-tipped haemostats, ensuring that there is no bowel caught. Then incise this vertically for about a centimetre. You may wish to apply stay sutures to the peritoneal edges to allow you to do a finger sweep and then carefully insert the cannula, with its obturator (see also Ch. 13). In other circumstances you may not know the required depth of penetration; when entering the trachea, too deep intrusion may damage the thin posterior wall or even breach the oesophagus. Too deep insertion of the needle may cause damage during lumbar puncture or pericardiocentesis.

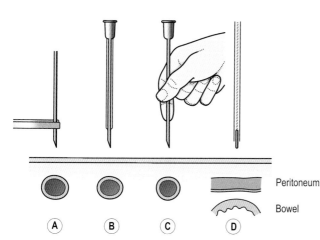

Peritoneum

Bowel

Fig. 4.2 Methods of limiting overpenetration and inadvertent damage to susceptible structures. (A) Place a nondamaging clip on the puncturing instrument. (B) Use a shouldered needle, as is used for injection of haemorrhoids. (C) Grasp the instrument at a point that limits insertion. (D) The Veress needle has a blunt, spring-loaded obturator that projects as soon as resistance is overcome, pushing away at-risk mobile structures.

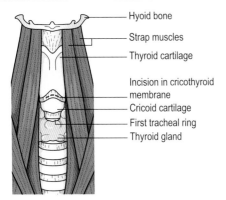

- Hyoid bone
- Strap muscles
- Thyroid cartilage
- Incision in cricothyroid membrane
- Cricoid cartilage
- First tracheal ring
- Thyroid gland

Fig. 4.3 Cricothyrotomy. The incision is shown in the broken line.

Cricothyroid puncture

Cricothyroid puncture may be lifesaving in the absence of any other means of relieving respiratory obstruction.

1. Feel for the laryngeal prominence and follow down the anterior edge of the thyroid cartilage to the gap between the thyroid and cricoid cartilages, identifying the cricothyroid membrane (Fig. 4.3).
2. Insert a needle carrying an external cannula, in the midline just above the cricoid cartilage, aiming slightly caudally, while aspirating on an attached syringe. Feel for the 'give' as you pierce the cricothyroid membrane. As soon as air enters the syringe you are in the trachea.
3. Hold the needle still, while gently advancing the cannula. If you do not have a cannulated needle, insert one or more plain needles to create an emergency short-term relief.
4. An oxygen source can be attached to the needle, though may have to be released intermittently to allow exhalation.

Cricothyrotomy

Cricothyrotomy is the preferred emergency procedure.

1. Carry it out if necessary without preliminary local anaesthesia and tracheal intubation, though if the patient is conscious you will need to use local anaesthetic.
2. Place the patient supine, head straight, in line with the body. If possible extend the neck by placing a pillow or sandbag under the upper thoracic spine.

3. Ensure that the trachea is central. Identify the thyroid cartilage. Follow the anterior border down to the gap from here to the cricoid cartilage.
4. Incise the skin transversely for 1–1.5 cm over the centre of the cricothyroid membrane and deepen it down to and through the membrane, signalled by a hiss of air.

> **Key points**
>
> - Do not extend the incision too far laterally or you may cause bleeding from the anterior jugular veins.
> - Avoid inserting the knife too deeply or you may penetrate the thin posterior wall into the pharynx.

5. It was traditional to reverse the knife, insert the handle into the laryngeal incision and turn it to open the incision, but in doing so you may not succeed in relocating and reentering the larynx. Hold the knife blade quite still and insert alongside it a haemostatic or other forceps. Now withdraw the knife blade, open the forceps to create a gap and insert the tracheostomy tube alongside it, directing it caudally. If you do not have a tracheostomy tube use whatever is available. Remove the forceps. If the tube has an inflatable cuff, gently expand it. If it has attached tapes, encircle the neck and tie them to secure the tube. Use your ingenuity to fix an improvised tube.

> **Key points**
>
> - In an emergency use your ingenuity. Many lives have been saved using penknives to insert a variety of tubes.
> - Tracheostomy is inappropriate as an emergency procedure except by an expert.

Lumbar puncture

Lumbar puncture is usually performed with the patient lying on the side, strictly horizontally, parallel to the couch, with a fully flexed spine to widen the space between the posterior vertebral arches. Have a receptacle available to collect cerebrospinal fluid if this is a diagnostic procedure.

1. Under strict sterile precautions, following an injection of local anaesthetic, insert the spinal needle with the lumen filled by stylette, between the third and fourth, or fourth and fifth lumbar vertebral spines, perpendicular to the skin surface or minimally angled in a cephalic direction. A line joining the highest points of the iliac crests on each side passes through the spines of the fourth and fifth vertebrae.
2. Feel for the 'give' as you pierce the interlaminar ligament (ligamentum flavum)—the depth for extradural (or 'epidural') puncture.
3. If you need to enter the subarachnoid space, carefully feel for the second, less obvious 'give' as you pierce the dura—the arachnoid mater is closely applied to the undersurface of the dura of the spinal canal.
4. Withdraw the stylette to watch for cerebrospinal fluid to emerge from the needle and collect a specimen for biochemistry and bacteriology.

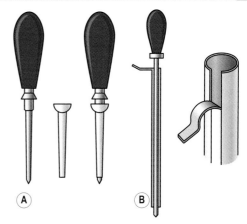

Fig. 4.4 (A) A traditional trocar, a cannula, and then the trocar fitted into the cannula. (B) A cross-section of a disposable Lawrence-type trocar and cannula, together with a close-up view of the thin panel being stripped along the length of the cannula so that it can be detached from the catheter that has been inserted through it.

Pericardiocentesis

Pericardiocentesis (from the Greek *kentesis* = puncture) should be performed with electrocardiographic monitoring.
1. Insert the needle, connected through a three-way tap to a capacious syringe, just to the left of the xiphisternum, aimed towards the tip of the left scapula. Be sensitive to the 'give' as you puncture the pericardium. Keep a close watch on the ECG monitor to ensure that you have not inadvertently pierced the cardiac muscle. Aspirate to draw fluid into the syringe.
2. If you irritate the myocardium by contact with the needle you will provoke cardiac irregularities.
3. A Seldinger technique may be used to insert a pericardiocentesis catheter.

Suprapubic cystostomy

Suprapubic cystostomy is an example of the value of distending a tube or cavity in order to enter it. A traditional method is to use a trocar (from the French *trios* = three + *carre* = side, since the sharp tip of the internal perforator was three-sided) and cannula (Fig. 4.4).
1. Carry it out with strict sterile precautions.
2. Ensure that the bladder is full, confirmed by displaying suprapubic dullness to percussion. Bladder distension peels the peritoneal

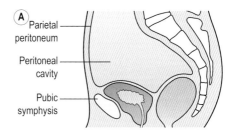

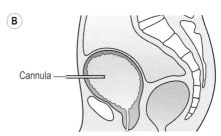

Fig. 4.5 Suprapubic cystostomy. In (A), the bladder is empty. A cannula inserted into the bladder is at risk of transgressing the peritoneal cavity. In (B), the bladder is full and the peritoneal reflexion from the anterior abdomen onto the bladder is well above the track of the cannula.

reflection from the bladder wall upwards to the abdominal wall, and so avoids the risk of puncturing the peritoneal cavity (Fig. 4.5). If there is scarring of the lower abdomen from previous surgery, there may be bowel adherent to the inner surface of the abdominal wall and the procedure should be performed under ultrasound guidance.

3. Infiltrate the skin with local anaesthetic in the midline, 3–5 cm above the symphysis pubis. Using a longer needle, inject down to and into the bladder wall. When there is a sudden 'give' and you can aspirate urine, you have entered the bladder. Do not continue unless you have confirmed this.

4. Withdraw the syringe and needle. Make a short incision with a scalpel at the site of needle entry and carefully cut vertically down to the bladder wall.

5. Gently insert the trocar and cannula along the prepared track and through the bladder wall into the lumen. Avoid sudden uncontrolled penetration that might endanger pelvic structures.

6. Withdraw the trocar, at which point urine should emerge. Immediately insert a Foley catheter through the cannula.

7. When you are confident that the tip and balloon are in the bladder, carefully remove the cannula without displacing the catheter and inflate the catheter-retaining balloon. A traditional cannula may resist being withdrawn over the bulky catheter outlet. The disposable plastic Lawrence-type cannula has a detachable strip so that it can be opened out to detach it after withdrawing it from the bladder (Fig. 4.4).

8. Attach the catheter to a drainage tube emptying into a collecting bag. The wound requires only a simple, temporary dressing. A drain-stitch suture is often placed to secure the catheter until the tract is matured.

Peritoneal diagnostic lavage

Peritoneal diagnostic lavage is useful if ultrasound or computerised tomography imaging are unavailable to determine whether or not there is intraabdominal damage. It is an alternative to diagnostic laparoscopy.

1. Pass a urinary catheter and nasogastric tube to ensure that the bladder and stomach are empty. Have a specimen tube and culture swab available in case any fluid emerges.

2. Under sterile conditions, after infiltrating local anaesthetic, make a 2-cm vertical incision at the junction of the upper third and lower two-thirds of the line joining the umbilicus and symphysis pubis, down through the linea alba to the peritoneum. Carefully pick up and lift the peritoneum between two pairs of forceps and incise it to gain access to the peritoneal cavity.

3. Insert a finger to ensure that you have safely entered the abdomen and pass in the end of a dialysis catheter, guiding it down towards the pelvis. Connect a syringe and aspirate the catheter, sending any aspirate for microscopy.

4. Connect the tube to a container of normal saline, 10 mL/kg body weight, warmed to body temperature, and slowly run it into the abdomen.

5. Gently agitate the abdomen, wait for 10 minutes, then lower the container to the floor, allowing the fluid to siphon back into the bag. Send a specimen for microscopy.

6. The test is positive if there are more than 100,000 red cells and more than 500 white blood cells per cubic millimetre, making it likely that there is intraabdominal damage. However, remember that there can be intraabdominal damage without intraperitoneal bleeding.

7. A Seldinger technique may also be used to perform the lavage, introducing the catheter over a guidewire.

Chest needle thoracentesis

Chest needle thoracentesis is a useful lifesaving procedure in the presence of a tension pneumothorax. Treatment should be immediate, and a chest X-ray should not be delayed. The clinical features of ipsilateral hyper-resonance, ipsilateral absence of breath sounds and tracheal deviation to the contralateral side are characteristic.

1. Palpate for the second intercostal space in the midclavicular line.

2. Pierce the skin with a hollow needle ensuring that you pass as close to the superior surface of the third rib, to avoid inadvertently piercing the intercostal vessels adjacent to the inferior surface of the second rib.

3. Listen and feel for the satisfying gush of air as the needle pierces the parietal pleura.

Chest drain

A chest drain allows you to remove air or liquid to achieve and maintain lung expansion (see Ch. 11).

Key point

- Do not wait to insert a chest drain in the presence of tension pneumothorax. Decompress with a needle first.

Direct access

1. Ducts, tubes, and spaces that open onto the surface, or are exposed at operation, can be intubated directly.
2. By special techniques internal ducts may be cannulated through instruments such as endoscopes, which are usually passed into hollow viscera via natural orifices. For example, the common bile duct or pancreatic duct can be cannulated through a fibreoptic upper gastrointestinal endoscope, and at ERCP (endoscopic retrograde cholangiopancreatography) the ureter can be catheterised through a cystoscope. I shall not describe these since they require special training.
3. Plastic, latex rubber, metal, and in the past gum elastic and other types of catheters have been used, having plain open ends, side holes, and straight or curved tips (Fig. 4.6). Choose one that slips in easily without being gripped by the walls or you will lose the 'feel' of the catheter. Ducts that can be directly intubated include the trachea, urethra, upper and lower gastrointestinal tracts, salivary ducts, stomas, external sinuses and fistulas, or ducts exposed at operation.

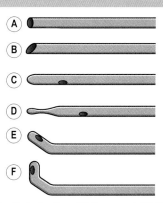

Fig. 4.6 Catheter tips. (A) Open end. (B) Flute tip. (C) Round end with side hole. (D) Olivary tip. (E) and (F) Coudé and bicoudé (derived from the French words for bent and double-bent).

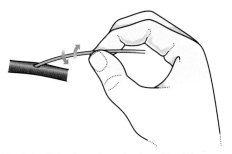

Fig. 4.7 Twist the catheter back and forth between thumb and forefinger to allow it to search out the channel.

> **Key points**
>
> - If you have difficulty in advancing a tube or catheter through a convoluted space, do not use force.
> - Slightly withdraw it and rotate it before gently advancing it again.
> - In case of difficulty, twist a flexible catheter back and forth between finger and thumb to allow it to search out the channel (Fig. 4.7).
> - When possible apply gentle traction to straighten the channel.

Tracheal intubation

Tracheal intubation can be carried out through the mouth or through the nose, although nasal intubation requires special skill. You will normally pass an endotracheal tube only on a deeply unconscious patient (ensure the patient does not have a cervical spinal injury before extending the neck).

1. Choose an endotracheal tube of the correct length and diameter and test the inflatable cuff. Lubricate the tube with water-soluble jelly. Ensure adequate preoxygenation.
2. Place the patient supine with a small cushion under the shoulders. Keep the neck straight in the line of the body, slightly flexed, with the head extended at the atlantooccipital joint and resting on a small pillow.
3. The path the tube will take is a curved one, but you must control it under direct vision; this entails temporarily straightening it. Achieve this by using a Mackintosh laryngoscope (Fig. 4.8), held in the left hand.
4. The mouth and opening of the larynx lie anteriorly but the base of the tongue and epiglottis bulge posteriorly. Lift them, and the mandible, by placing the 'beak' of the laryngoscope in the vallecula (from the Latin diminutive of *vallis* = valley) between the tongue base and the epiglottis, and gently raise them.
5. You can now look from the head of the table along one or other side of the nose and view the pharynx and laryngeal opening through the side of the mouth, alongside the tongue (Fig. 4.8).

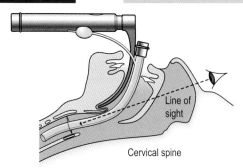

Fig. 4.8 Insertion of an endotracheal tube. The base of the tongue and epiglottis are raised with Mackintosh's laryngoscope. You would be looking past one side of the nose and through the side of the mouth to see the laryngeal opening. The curved endotracheal tube can now be inserted under vision.

6. Pass the tube of correct diameter, length and curvature, under vision, along the right side of the mouth, pushing the tongue to the left, through the laryngeal opening into the trachea. The inflatable cuff must lie beyond the vocal cords; gently expand it through the side tube just enough to completely fill the trachea.

7. Check the pressure in the cuff by feeling the small monitor balloon on the inflation tube. Collapse of this balloon warns you if the cuff leaks and deflates.

8. Now confirm that the tube is in the trachea by checking that if the chest is compressed air is ejected through the endotracheal tube; if the tube is connected to a bag which is then compressed, the chest should expand. Ensure that the tube does not lie in the oesophagus by excluding upper abdominal distension or an epigastric tympanitic note on percussion. Auscultate the lungs to ensure there is equal air entry on both sides. Secure the tube in place.

9. If you have not managed the manoeuvre within seconds, stop and preoxygenate before any further attempt.

OROPHARYNGEAL AIRWAY

If you do not feel competent to pass an orotracheal tube, or as a first resuscitative manoeuvre you may consider temporizing with an oropharyngeal (Guedel) airway and ventilating with a bag-mask. The oropharyngeal airway stops the tongue from falling posteriorly and occluding the passage of air. Size the airway by ensuring that it is the same length as the distance from the patient's own corner of their mouth to the angle of the mandible.

1. With the patient's neck straight and in line with the body, open the patient's mouth, lifting the chin forward from behind the mandible.

2. Insert the oropharyngeal airway into the mouth upside down (concave cranially) and once the tip is passed the upper teeth, rotate it 180 degrees and slide it over the back of the tongue. Alternatively, with a laryngoscope blade, tongue depressor, or if desperate your gloved thumb, depress the tongue so that it does not slide posteriorly, and slide the oropharyngeal airway the right way up (convex side cranially) over the tongue. The flange rests on the outside of the patient's mouth.

3. The bag-mask can now be positioned over the face and the patient ventilated without the tongue obstructing the airway.

NASOPHARYNGEAL AIRWAY

If your patient is semiconscious an oropharyngeal or orotracheal intubation would elicit a gag reflex and not be tolerated. To maintain oxygenation, consider a nasopharyngeal airway. Size the airway by checking that it is the same length from the tip of the patient's nose to the earlobe.

1. Check that there are no nasal polyps or other obstructions in the nasal passage.

2. Lubricate the nasopharyngeal airway and pass it into the nostril directing it posteriorly.

3. The flange will rest against the nostril.

4. The bag-mask can now be positioned over the face and ventilation can proceed.

Feeding jejunostomy

Feeding jejunostomy is an example of a catheter introduced through the abdominal wall, then into the intestine, when the abdomen is open.

1. Place a large haemostat or tissue forceps with which to lift the left wound edge of the laparotomy wound. Make a stab incision through the abdominal wall in the left upper quadrant of the abdomen well clear of the abdominal incision, umbilicus and the rib margin. Take great care to avoid injuring the intraabdominal structures.

2. Evert the wound edge and pass a haemostat through the stab wound from within out, to grasp the tip of the catheter and draw it into the abdomen.

3. Lift the greater omentum and left transverse colon. Identify a suitable segment of proximal jejunum by finding the ligament of Treitz and following the bowel distally until you have a loop long enough to reach the anterior abdominal wall without tension.

4. On the antimesenteric border, encircle the intended catheter entry site with a seromuscular purse-string suture tied with one half-hitch and kept slack. Make a small incision within the relaxed purse-string, taking care to avoid cutting the suture. Insert the tip of the catheter through the hole, pointing distally for 10 cm. Tighten and tie the purse-string but not sufficient to obstruct the catheter. You may insert a further purse-string suture, inverting the first one to create an inkwell effect.

5. Leave the purse-string suture ends long and take them back and forth around the emerging catheter (see below), tying them to hold the catheter in place.

6. Evert the abdominal wall to facilitate inserting three to four stitches, each one catching the seromuscular coat of the jejunum close to the emerging catheter and the parietal peritoneum near the stab wound in the abdominal wall. Place all the stitches, then gently tighten them to draw the jejunum into contact with the abdominal wall, forming a seal.

7. After closing the abdominal wall, place a stitch through the skin near the emerging catheter, tie it, then encircle the catheter and tie it again so that any traction on the catheter does not displace it, but is taken by the stitch. Flush the catheter with some saline to ensure that you have not occluded it with your stitches. The saline should flow freely.

8. Now close the abdomen.

Urethral catheterization

Urethral catheterization in the male is a classical example of the art of inserting tubes because it demands great sensitivity, gentleness and skill.

1. Carry out the procedure under strict sterile precautions. Check that you have available an appropriate catheter, usually Foley self-retaining (e.g., 16–18 F) with the inner sterile plastic container opened but the catheter unexposed, a local anaesthetic tube of 2% lidocaine (lignocaine) hydrochloride gel and

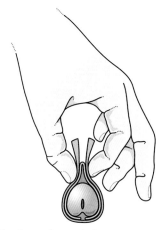

Fig. 4.9 Grasp the penis in a gauze swab sling placed just proximal to the corona. Grip the swab and a fold of loose dorsal skin between finger and thumb, leaving the other fingers free to wrap around the penis to compress the urethra during catheterization to prevent the catheter from being extruded.

sterile nozzle, forceps, towels, swabs, mild aqueous antiseptic solution, water-soluble lubricant, urine receptacle, tubing and collecting bag. Have a syringe and sterile fluid available if you are inserting a Foley-type catheter.

2. Place the patient supine, thighs separated, and pudenda exposed. With a sterile swab held in your nondominant hand grasp the loose dorsal skin of the penis just behind the corona. With another swab held in your dominant hand, clean the head and corona, pushing back the uncircumcised foreskin to expose the glans.

3. Hold up the penis and apply sterile towels– usually a single disposable sheet with a hole in the middle. Replace your grasp with a fresh swab folded lengthwise as a sling that can be held, together with a fold of loose dorsal skin, just behind the corona, between the finger and thumb of the nondominant hand (Fig. 4.9), leaving the other fingers free. Again swab the meatus and penile head with antiseptic solution.

4. Insert the anaesthetic through the nozzle and occlude the urethra to retain it for at least 3–4 minutes by compressing the undersurface of the penis through the sling-like swab, using the medial fingers of your nondominant hand.

5. Draw the penis vertically upwards, thus straightening the penile urethra (Fig. 4.10). Manipulate the opened inner sterile plastic

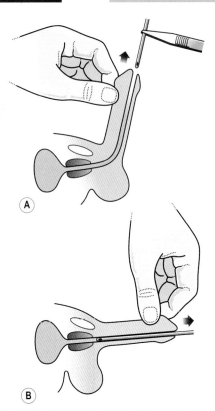

Fig. 4.10 (A) Hold the shaft of the penis dorsally, just behind the corona. First pull it vertically to straighten the penile urethra while you insert the catheter as far as the bulb. (B) Now draw the penis down towards the feet to align the penile and membranous parts of the urethra.

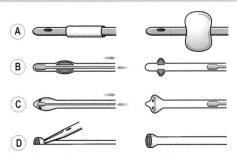

Fig. 4.11 Self-retaining catheters. (A) Foley catheter with an inflatable balloon. (B) De Pezzer and (C) Malecot catheters, both inserted after stretching over an introducer. (D) Winsbury White catheter inserted with the end folded.

8. Ensure that the catheter can be emptied into a container. Now gently advance it through the prostatic urethra into the bladder. Do this to the hilt of the catheter to ensure that the balloon is in the bladder. Success is signalled by the appearance of urine. If no urine emerges when the catheter seems to be fully inserted, try pressing on the bladder suprapubically through the sterile towel. If this fails, aspirate gently with a bladder syringe. Maintain compression of the urethra to prevent the catheter from being extruded until you have secured it by inflating the balloon.
9. Obtain a specimen of urine for microscopy and culture, then connect the catheter to a closed collecting bag.

Fixing catheters and tubes

Various tubes fulfil an important and sometimes lifesaving function. Make sure that you fix them securely and safely. Replacing a catheter that has been inserted with great difficulty and has now fallen out is challenging both for you and for the patient.

Self-retaining catheters

In the past rubber catheters were moulded with projections that could be straightened by stretching or compressing during insertion but they have been largely superseded by the invention of the Foley catheter by American urologist Frederic Foley of Minnesota (1891–1966), which has an inflatable balloon near the tip of the catheter (Fig. 4.11); the catheter can be withdrawn easily after deflating the balloon. Another useful retaining device within a small duct is the 'T'-tube catheter (Fig. 4.12).

catheter container to allow 5–7 cm of the tip to protrude. Do not touch the catheter but hold and control it through the cover. Lubricate and insert the catheter tip gently and slowly. Progressively draw back the plastic container.
6. Prevent the catheter from being extruded following each advancement by wrapping the free fingers of the left hand around the ventral surface covered by the enfolding sterile swab and compressing the urethra against the catheter. With patience, the catheter may sometimes pass through the sphincter into the bladder.
7. If the catheter is held up, draw the penis towards the feet. Without losing your grip on it, swing the penis down between the separated thighs. This has the effect of directing the tip of the catheter upwards into the prostatic urethra and bladder.

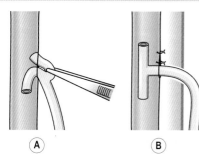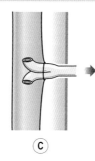

Fig. 4.12 Using a soft, flexible T-tube as a self-retaining catheter. In (A), it is being inserted through a side hole into the duct. In (B), the short limb of the 'T' lies in the lumen. It does not obstruct the lumen and allows contents to pass through it or into the long limb. (C) Traction causes the short limbs to come together in order to be pulled out. Any leak rapidly dries up.

The short limb of the 'T' lies in the duct and allows fluid to flow through it or out of the long limb. When the tube is to be removed, apply gentle traction on the long limb and the flexible cross-pieces of the short limb fold together so that it can be pulled out. The minor leakage dries up rapidly unless there is distal obstruction, and this can be excluded beforehand by radiology following injection of contrast medium through the 'stem' of the T-tube. This is a T-tube cholangiogram.

The ability to mould curves in plastic tubes creates a simple means of retaining them. Introduce a pigtailed catheter after first inserting into it a straight guidewire; withdraw the guidewire, enabling it to regain its natural shape. A double pigtailed catheter or double J stent (Fig. 4.13) resists movement in either direction, yet when pulled from either end is sufficiently flexible to be withdrawn easily.

Non-self-retaining catheters

Non-self-retaining catheters require some sort of fixation, depending on the circumstances.

1. To retain a catheter indefinitely within a narrow duct, secure it with a ligature or suture–ligature encircling the duct and catheter (Fig. 4.14); the ligature will eventually cut through the wall of the duct. It is difficult to retain a small catheter within the cut end of a wide-bore duct while preventing leakage; try entering the catheter at one side, then close the remaining duct lumen with stitches.
2. Catheters emerging through the skin can be fixed to prevent them from being dislodged in a number of ways (Fig. 4.15). Adhesive plaster or tape may suffice. A stitch inserted through the skin and the tube is a secure method but allows leakage through the stitch hole in the tube. Alternatively, place a stitch through the skin and then lace it back and forth around the tube; so-called 'English lacing', after the manner in which the ancient Britons wrapped their lower legs.

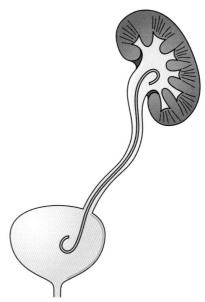

Fig. 4.13 A double pigtailed catheter lies in the ureter. One end is curled in the pelvis of the ureter, the other is curled in the bladder. It may be retrieved easily after grasping the tip within the bladder through a cystoscope.

3. An elastic catheter can be neatly fixed by a method used by Miss Phyllis George (1925- 2017); cut a small segment from the open end of the tube and stretch it to fit over the emerging catheter. Insert a skin stitch incorporating the cuff that does not pierce the emerging catheter.

DILATING DUCTS

Bougies

Bougies (derived from the French word for candle, from the town in Algeria where they were made)

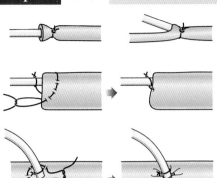

Fig. 4.14 Fixing catheters into small ducts. At the top on the left the catheter has been inserted into the end of a duct; on the right it is passed through the side, thus retaining the flow through the duct. Below are shown methods needed for fixing them into the end or side of larger ducts.

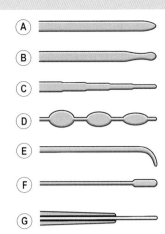

Fig. 4.16 Bougies. (A) Tapered. (B) Olivary-tipped. (C) Stepped. (D) Multiple olives. (E) Curved rigid. (F) Malleable. (G) Hollow dilator threaded over flexible guidewire.

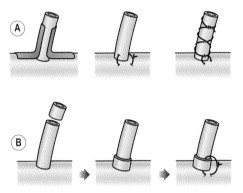

Fig. 4.15 (A) Methods of fixing catheters to the skin using adhesive plaster or stitches. (B) Method suggested by Miss Phyllis George: cut a collar from the end of the duct, slip it over the duct and insert a stitch between it and the duct to stitch it to the skin.

are usually rods or tubes of circular cross-section (Fig. 4.16) with expanded sections that dilate the channel through which they pass. They may be of rigid or malleable metal or semirigid plastic. Dilators may be straight or curved. Metal instruments introduced into the urethra or uterus to probe or dilate the passage are often termed 'sounds' (from the French *sonder* = to prove, to try).

1. Rigid instruments are damaging in clumsy hands but, when used skilfully, give a better 'feel' and the direction can be controlled. Malleable instruments are useful if the shape of the track is irregular.

2. The tip of a dilator is rounded and of smaller diameter than the shank, the transition being gradual. Once the tip has entered the stricture, advancing the instrument gradually dilates it. An olivary-tipped dilator has an oval globular end, likened to an olive; as the olive slips through the stricture its onward passage suddenly becomes easier, providing an estimate of the length of the narrowing— confirmed if necessary by withdrawing it again and noting when the grip of the stricture is suddenly relaxed. The freedom of the dilator after the olive has passed through the narrowing allows you to retain the 'feel' of the passage beyond. As you advance the dilator, it gradually expands the lumen.

3. Start with the largest dilator that is likely to pass, especially if you are using a rigid instrument, since fine rigid instruments too easily perforate the walls of the channel, which may be diseased and fragile.

4. When appropriate, apply a sterile lubricant such as liquid paraffin or a water-soluble jelly.

5. If possible straighten the channel by exerting traction so there is minimal friction with the walls and you do not lose the 'feel' of the tip. This is possible when you dilate the male urethra.

6. Try varying the direction of the tip until it engages; if this fails, try successively smaller instruments.

7. Multiple strictures require great sensitivity of touch to negotiate them. The grip of each stricture or of a tight orifice dulls your sense of 'feel' for the tip within the next stricture. For this reason, dilate each stricture as far as

possible before tackling the next one, so that the dilator lies freely until it is gripped by the new stricture.

8. When the tip of the dilator is forcefully pushed through the wall of the channel, it creates a space that may become epithelialised, remaining as a diverticulum into which a future dilator may enter as a false passage. At subsequent attempts at dilatation, the tip of the dilator easily enters into this side channel keeping it open. In the urethra, such passages usually develop just distal to a stricture, so you encounter them instead of entering the stricture.

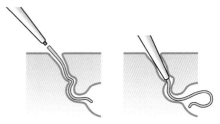

Fig. 4.17 Using a filiform leader as a pilot for the dilator.

Key points

- You are nearly always dilating a duct because it is strictured or blocked by inflammatory swelling or abnormal content.
- If you encounter resistance or bleeding, there is a reason.
- Your likeliest way of determining the cause is to hold the dilator with your fingertips and 'feel' the obstructing surface as you gently probe it.

---

9. Withdraw the dilator and advance it once more while you keep the tip pressed against the opposite wall. It is suggested that one dilator can be left in the false passage to block its mouth while a second instrument passes along the main duct. I have never succeeded with this method.

10. A filiform (from the Latin *filum* = thread, hence threadlike) flexible bougie may be induced to follow a tortuous path through the stricture. If it passes through, a dilator can be screwed to it and guided by it through the stricture; the flexibility of the filiform leader allows it to fold upon itself within a cavity beyond the stricture (Fig. 4.17), where it can be captured, drawn through with a dilator attached to follow its path.

11. *Seldinger's wire* (see Ch. 5) is a useful method of following a tortuous channel and negotiating a difficult stricture. Pass the flexible tipped guidewire through the stricture by gently rotating it back and forth as you advance it through the stricture. Radiographic monitoring of the progress of the tip of the radio-opaque guidewire is invaluable. You may be able to introduce contrast medium to outline the passage. When you have succeeded in advancing the guidewire through the stricture, thread over it a close-fitting (but not tight) dilator that has a central hole and gently advance this down to and through the stricture (Fig. 4.16G). At intervals ensure that the guidewire moves freely within the dilator; fixation of the guidewire indicates that it is trapped and kinked so the tip of the dilator is not entering the stricture and could perforate the side wall of the duct.

12. *Endoscopic guidance*, when available, allows you to visualise one end of the stricture so that you are able to negotiate a guidewire through it under vision, as in the oesophagus. You can leave the guidewire in place, remove the endoscope and pass graded dilators that have a central channel over the guidewire to dilate the stricture.

13. Occasionally it is impossible to pass even a fine guidewire through. In some circumstances, if one end of a thread is fixed proximally and the other end is introduced above the stricture, this will eventually be carried through by fluid flow and peristalsis. After retrieving the distal end, attach a thin, flexible dilator to the proximal end. Exert slight traction on the distal thread to guide and draw through the tip of the fine dilator (Fig. 4.18). I have used this method (devised by Mr Richard Franklin) using the radio-opaque marker thread of a surgical swab as a leader, with success in overcoming seemingly impassable oesophageal strictures.

14. Commonly, you can pass a series of graduated dilators, each one being slightly thicker than the previous one. As you negotiate the stricture, note the details of the passage. Do not remove it until you have the next dilator ready. Now smoothly draw out the first dilator and immediately and gently slide in the next size, and so on. The tip of each bigger dilator is slightly smaller than the shank of its predecessor. Control the direction

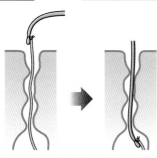

Fig. 4.18 A thread has been induced to pass the stricture and acts as a leader for the dilator.

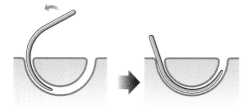

Fig. 4.19 Negotiating a curved channel with a rigid curved dilator. The handle of the dilator must be swung in an arc to direct the point along the curved path.

of insertion and passage of a rigid dilator by movement of the handle (Fig. 4.19). A rigid curved dilator cannot be rotated while it lies in a narrow channel but if it reaches a wider channel it can be rotated. Confirm that you have reached the bladder by this method when dilating urethral strictures.

15. Occasionally you may need to stretch a normal channel very gently, in order to insert instruments or substances—for example, the meatus and penile urethra—to pass a large instrument such as a prostatic resectoscope.

Key points

- Do not be too ambitious; be willing to stop before you achieve the maximum diameter, and repeat the procedure at increasing intervals, gaining a little each time.
- If you overstretch it and split the lining, usually signalled by bleeding, the stricture will recur.
- Never fail to record the size of the dilators and details of the peculiarities of the passage on each occasion, for future guidance.

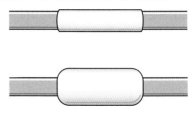

Fig. 4.20 The catheter carries a collapsed balloon, which can be placed within a stricture. When the balloon is inflated it exerts a radial dilating effect.

Balloons

When a dilator is pushed through a stricture there is a damaging shear force on the duct lining. As this heals, scar tissue is laid down, which contracts as it matures, recreating the stricture. When possible, avoid the shearing force by exerting centrifugal distension only, from within the stricture. An excellent method of achieving this is by balloon dilatation. Overdistension of the balloon may disrupt the wall; for this reason, balloons are available that reach a predetermined maximum diameter or pressure and then rupture if overinflated.

1. Negotiate a collapsed balloon across the stricture and inflate it, exerting only radial forces (Fig. 4.20). The balloons can be passed under vision, mounted on catheters threaded over guidewires, or over endoscopes. They can be accurately placed under radiological control and, for this reason, usually incorporate radio-opaque markers at each end of the balloon.
2. Balloon dilatation is sometimes used to overstretch the sphincteric muscles of—for example, the lower oesophagus—to overcome a holdup resulting from achalasia (from the Greek *a* = not + *chalasis* = relaxation), the failure to relax as a bolus of food reaches it to pass through into the stomach.

Other methods

1. Dilators that expand while they lie within a narrow channel have been used for many years. A classic method is a laminaria tent (from the Latin *tenta* = a probe) in which a cylinder of dried seaweed is inserted into a duct; it expands and dilates the channel as it absorbs water. The method has long been in use to dilate the uterine cervical canal to procure an abortion.

2. Mechanical expansile dilatation from within the lumen was devised to dilate stenosed heart valves.

3. *Stents*, named after the English dentist Charles Stent (1807–1885), are increasingly used to hold open passages that have been dilated. One type can be sited as a long, narrow tube within a stricture and then expanded by inflating a balloon within it, expanding the stent which then retains its shape, preventing restenosis.

4. Special materials have been developed in the last few years in order to produce wire mesh self-expanding stents. The mesh is compressed to produce a long thin tube that is released when it lies across the narrowing. It actively adopts a shorter and wider shape that progressively expands the narrowed segment, by exerting a radial force.

5. When the lumen of a duct is encroached on by an ingrowth of diseased tissue such as cancer, the passage can often be restored using several forms of treatment including diathermy, radiotherapy, laser therapy and chemotherapy. Photodynamic treatment of certain tumours consists of giving a sensitizing agent which is taken up by the encroaching cells, then using laser light to produce selective tumour cell necrosis.

ENDOSCOPIC ACCESS

1. Endoscopy (from the Greek *endon* = within + *skopein* = to view) and 'down the line of sight' operative procedures have been well established for many years through an extensive range of rigid and flexible endoscopes. Instruments can be inserted into natural tubes and manoeuvred by 'feel'. Advances were possible because of improvements in visualization and instrumentation. Improvements in imaging reduce the need for physical exploration.

2. A wide range of instruments can be introduced through open tubes or through special channels in more sophisticated endoscopes with good lighting and visual characteristics, into natural or abnormal channels, including catheters, dilators, balloons, diathermy wires, forceps, scissors, cytology brushes, Dormia baskets and snares (Fig. 4.21). These may be rigid or flexible and controllable.

3. Instruments with moving parts such as scissors, forceps and snares can be activated by two rods sliding on each other, or one rod sliding within a rigid tube; the moving rod can be pushed or pulled. Flexible instruments often

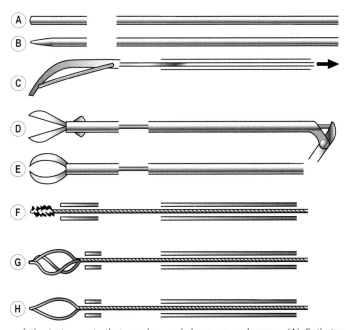

Fig. 4.21 Some of the instruments that can be used down an endoscope. (A) Catheter. (B) Dilator. (C) Diathermy wire tightened to produce a 'cheese-cutter' effect. (D) Forceps. (E) Scissors. (F) Cytology brush. (G) Dormier basket. (H) A snare.

Fig. 4.22 Methods of controlling moving tipped instruments. (A) A wire passes through a spiral wire flexible tube. This Bowden cable mechanism can be pulled but not pushed. (B) A rigid system of a rod passing through a metal tube. This allows both pulling and pushing.

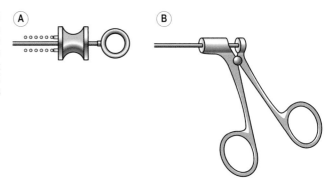

employ the principle attributed to Sir Frank Bowden (circa 1902, founder of Raleigh bicycles, for the brake cables). The inner wire can be pulled but not pushed within the outer flexible tube; if the inner wire has been pulled, release must be by some distal spring action. Handle designs vary but all rely on a gripping motion or separation of the hand or of a finger and thumb (Fig. 4.22). Because the tissues cannot be held and steadied while they are being cut with scissors, the blades may advantageously be claw-shaped (Fig. 4.21), to prevent the tissue from sliding away.

4. When introducing a rigid instrument along a convoluted channel, be extremely sensitive to the holdups. Be willing to withdraw it slightly, adjust the angle and gently advance it again. Try to keep the tip of the instrument in the centre of the lumen.

5. If a straight instrument has an angled tip it may be rotated within a flexible but twisting channel to assist the progress of its tip. A classic example is the shape of a rigid cystoscope for passage through the male urethra. Once the angled tip of the cystoscope enters the bladder cavity it can be rotated and moved—the shaft has straightened the urethra (Fig. 4.23). Although cystoscopy is now generally performed with a flexible instrument there are occasions when only a rigid instrument may be available or suitable.

6. Of necessity, rigid instruments passed under vision must be manoeuvred along the line of sight. Depth perception is limited. The point of action of instruments with an offset tip can be controlled by rotating them.

7. Flexible instruments are difficult to control within a wide channel or open tube, but their flexibility may facilitate progression along a tortuous track. However, the tip may engage

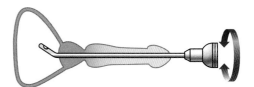

Fig. 4.23 A bent but flexible duct such as a male urethra can be straightened. The angled tip of the instrument follows the bends of the urethra because it can be rotated. Once it enters the bladder the tip can be freely rotated and advanced or withdrawn.

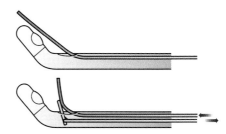

Fig. 4.24 A flexible catheter or instrument can be passed out of the side of a rigid or flexible endoscope. The angle of emergence can be controlled using an Albarran lever.

in an irregularity; if it does, withdraw it slightly, rotate it and gently advance it. Remember, there is less 'feel' with a flexible instrument than with a rigid one.

8. An instrument or catheter can be led out of a tube through a side hole to angulate it (Fig. 4.24). Some rigid and flexible endoscopes have a controllable lever to vary the angle of emergence. This was originally designed by the Parisian urologist of Cuban origin, Jacques Albarran (1860–1912). The tip of the instrument or tube can be kept in view through a side-viewing telescope.

Rigid instruments

The cystoscope was the first endoscopic instrument to reach a very high standard of development. Through it, you may inspect the bladder, take biopsies, fulgurate tumours and catheterise ureters. Fibreoptic cystoscopes can be passed relatively painlessly. Urethroscopy, ureteroscopy and percutaneous nephrostomy can be carried out. Transurethral resection of the prostate gland can be achieved using a diathermy loop, through a resectoscope.

Sigmoidoscopy

Sigmoidoscopy is now usually carried out using a flexible instrument; however, you may need to use a rigid instrument because of the circumstances. Take the opportunity to practise gentle, skilful manipulation of a tube.

1. Place the patient on the left side, buttocks overhanging the right side of the couch, knees drawn up to the chest, and feet on the far side from you as you stand on the right side of the couch (Fig. 4.25).

> **Key point**
>
> - Never insert an endoscope without first inspecting the perianal area and carrying out a careful digital examination, after explaining to the patient what you are doing.

2. Gently place the tip of the obturator within the well-lubricated sigmoidoscope (Fig. 4.26) against the patient's anus, pointing towards the umbilicus. Maintain only slight pressure until the sphincter relaxes, allowing you to insert the sigmoidoscope for about 6–8 cm when it abuts against the anterior wall of the rectum. Hold the sigmoidoscope steady while you withdraw the obturator and fit on the viewing end seal with the attached light bulb and air pump.

3. Perform all subsequent manoeuvres under vision. Insufflate only sufficient air to separate the walls and allow you to guide the endoscope safely without causing discomfort. You are now close up to the anterior rectal wall. To regain the view of the lumen you need to swing the outer end of the endoscope anteriorly to turn the internal portion into the rectum lying in the hollow of the sacrum. Concentrate initially on introducing the instrument to the intended limit, keeping the tip centred in the bowel lumen. As you withdraw it in a spiral manner you can examine every part of the interior, paying particular attention to the mucosa and any abnormalities.

4. If you wish to remove a biopsy or swab specimen, you must remove the viewing end and allow the air to escape. First of all, bring your objective into the centre of view; you can usually trap it by enclosing it and gently pressing the tip of the instrument against the bowel wall. Do not overinflate the rectum or it will suddenly deflate and the target mucosa

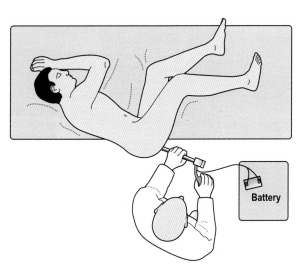

Fig. 4.25 Sigmoidoscopy seen from above. The sigmoidoscope is angled after initial insertion to view the rectum, which lies in the hollow of the sacrum.

Battery

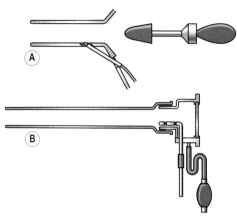

Fig. 4.26 (A) A short proctoscope, which is an open hollow tube. The obturator has been withdrawn. (B) A rigid sigmoidoscope, which is an open tube that can be closed off so the bowel can be inflated and distended. The cap has a transparent window.

will move. Insert the biopsy forceps or swab, obtain the specimen, then replace the viewing end-piece so that you can reinflate the rectum and complete the examination.

5. Deflate the rectum and warn the patient as you finally withdraw the sigmoidoscope, since it feels like an embarrassing defecation.

Proctoscopy

Proctoscopy is carried out in a similar manner but retains the obturator until you have fully introduced the instrument. Once more, remember that you must swing the handle portion forward on the patient to negotiate the almost 90° angle between the anus and rectum. Only now should you remove the obturator.

1. Carefully view the interior of the lower rectum and anal canal as you slowly withdraw the proctoscope.
2. As the rim of the proctoscope descends into the anal canal, the sphincter attempts to extrude it; apply slight counterpressure to prevent this while you examine the lower anal canal.

Haemorrhoids

Treatment of haemorrhoids depends on the grade of haemorrhoids and whether they are symptomatic or not. There are four grades: Grade 1 is when the haemorrhoids are seen within the anal canal without any extra anal protrusion, grade 2 haemorrhoids prolapse outside the anal canal during

defaecation or straining but return back spontaneously, grade 3 haemorrhoids protrude out on defaecation but have to be manually reduced and grade 4 are those which cannot be reduced and remain prolapsed outside the anal canal.

Grade 1 haemorrhoids are treated with laxatives and dietary modification which consists of high fibre and plenty of fluids.

Grade 2 haemorrhoids are treated with either injection sclerotherapy or band ligation.

1. During your first introduction and withdrawal of the proctoscope take careful note of the situation of the haemorrhoids as they prolapse over the lip of the withdrawing endoscope. Traditionally they were recorded as though the patient lay supine in the lithotomy position at 4, 7 and 11 o'clock related to a clock face. Since the patient now usually lies on the left side, they are usually at 1, 4 and 8 o'clock.
2. As you withdraw the proctoscope until the piles prolapse into the lumen, they obscure your view of their bases. You must now remove the proctoscope, replace the obturator, fully reintroduce it and again remove the obturator to inject at the base of each haemorrhoid.
3. Slowly withdraw the proctoscope until a rim of anus appears, and the sphincter begins to extrude the proctoscope. Resist this but angle the proctoscope to reveal a complete ring of about 0.5 cm of the anal canal. If the haemorrhoids prolapse you are too low; withdraw the proctoscope, reinsert it and start again.
4. Band ligation is the preferred choice. Banding can be performed either by using a special suction apparatus or a forceps ligator. In the former, the haemorrhoid is sucked into the banding apparatus and a rubber band is released at the base of the haemorrhoid. The forceps ligature method employs a ligator which has a rubber band applicator and forceps to grasp the haemorrhoid.
5. Injection with sclerosant must be made into the perivascular tissues around the upper pole of each pile.
6. Taking each site in turn, insert the shouldered needle attached to the filled haemorrhoid syringe. Aspirate. If blood enters the syringe you are within the vessel. Fully withdraw the needle and reinsert it in a slightly different site until you cannot aspirate any blood.
7. Inject approximately 5–10 mL of 5% phenol in almond or arachis (peanut) oil into the submucosa at the base of the pile. Watch as you inject. You should produce a slight swelling; if the swelling blanches, you are too

superficial, if there is no swelling you are too deep. If it is very painful, you are too superficial.

8. Grade 3 and 4 haemorrhoids: Some grade 3 haemorrhoids may be treated with rubber band ligation but most of them and grade 4 are treated with surgical haemorrhoidectomy which involves dissection of the haemorrhoid through an incision at the anal orifice and dissection of the pedicle, ligation and excision. When the wound is closed, the method is called closed haemorrhoidectomy and when left open, open haemorrhoidectomy.

9. Newer methods of treating haemorrhoids are infrared coagulation (Grades 1 and 2), stapled haemorrhoidectomy (Grades 3 and 4) and doppler-guided transanal haemorrhoidal dearterialisation.

Key points

- Haemorrhoid injection cannot be performed with a single insertion of the proctoscope.
- Injection must be perivascular, into the base of each pile, and never into the vessel.

Other rigid instruments

Laryngoscopes, auriscopes (from the Latin *auris* = ear), colposcopes (from the Greek *kolpos* = sinus or pocket, but applied to the vagina), hysteroscopes (from the Greek *hysteros* = womb) and many other endoscopes are used. In some cases, the instrument is called a speculum (from the Latin term for a mirror, from *spectare* = to look) since a mirror was inserted. Nasal and vaginal specula are in common use.

Key points

- Safe passage of instruments for the various forms of single access to tubes and spaces, requires specialised training, especially in order to interpret the findings and perform procedures that sometimes demand skills at the limits of technical accomplishment.
- Some procedures, such as laryngoscopy, proctoscopy and sigmoidoscopy, should be well within the capability of the surgical trainee. Take every opportunity to learn how to use these endoscopes safely and effectively.

Flexible endoscopes

Fibreoptic endoscopy became possible following the development of coherent glass fibre bundles by Harold Hopkins (1918–1994) in Reading, UK (Fig. 4.27). Basil Hirschowitz of Birmingham, Alabama improved the fibres and introduced gastrointestinal endoscopy.

A variety of controllable, flexible endoscopes can be passed into the upper and lower gastrointestinal tract (Fig. 4.28), the trachea and bronchi, urinary and gynaecological tracts, and other tubes, blood vessels, joints and tissue spaces. The instruments are remarkably versatile and allow, for example, inspection, biopsy, snaring, dilatation and diathermization, and facilitate the capture, ultrasonic shock and laser beam fragmentation of stones, among other specialised procedures.

Your patient is usually in the left lateral position. For an upper gastrointestinal endoscopy, your patient is nil by mouth and will have local anaesthetic sprayed to the back of the oropharynx. A mouth guard is then inserted. Sometimes intravenous sedation is also given, in which case pulse oximetry is mandatory.

Hold the control end of the endoscope in your nondominant hand. Lubricate and pass the flexible end through the mouth guard with your dominant hand keeping the lumen in view. Once the endoscope has passed through the pharynx it may help to ask the patient to swallow gently.

When passing a flexible endoscope, insufflate gently and aim for the centre of the lumen. If you cannot see the lumen you should not advance.

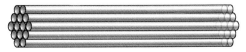

Fig. 4.27 A coherent bundle of glass fibres. They transmit light in a constant relationship within the fibres throughout the bundle.

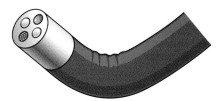

Fig. 4.28 The end of a flexible controllable fibreoptic endoscope. There are two light-carrying ports and one optical port. Top right is a channel for biopsy forceps, cytology brush, catheters and other instruments. Suction, insufflation and lens spraying facilities are also incorporated.

There are many simulation-based flexible endo-scopes and if you have access to these you should practice handling them again and again before embarking on their use in patients.

For a lower gastrointestinal endoscopy, your patient will have had bowel preparation in the form of strong laxatives to empty the colon.

DISPLAY

Some ducts, such as the bowel, lie free while others, such as intrahepatic bile ducts and bronchi, are buried in connective tissue. Take every opportunity to recognise ducts by gaining an intimate knowledge of the anatomy, appearance and feel. For example, the ureter has a character-istic vermiculating peristalsis. Ducts opening onto a surface, such as the urethra and salivary ducts, can be catheterised to delineate their paths. Fistulous tracks can be followed by inserting a probe or injecting dye.

Radio-opaque media can be injected through catheters, administered orally or parenterally and may be secreted or excreted into ducts to be displayed on X-rays, such as cholecystograms and urograms. Other imaging methods may also be used to aid identification and location.

1. When seeking a duct lying in homogeneous tissue, always cut in the expected line of the duct rather than at right angles to it, to avoid the risk of transecting it.
2. If you wish to display a long segment of duct take care not to damage any tributaries or divisions and respect its blood and nervous supply.
3. Remember that a collapsed and empty duct may be imperceptible but can be made more prominent by gently distending it with fluid, catheterizing or cannulating it.
4. Protect a fragile duct from injury as you display it by separating overlying tissues with care. Gently insert the rounded tips of nontoothed dissecting forceps superficial to the duct, allow them to open, and cut between the separated blades (Fig. 4.29). Blunt-nosed haemostatic forceps are valuable dissecting instruments when freeing ducts; insinuate the closed blades next to the duct and gently open them parallel to the duct (Fig. 4.30). If the duct has tributaries or if it branches, it is sometimes preferable to open the forceps at right angles to the duct (Fig. 4.31).

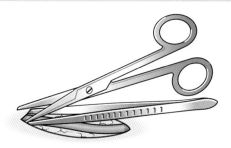

Fig. 4.29 Display a duct by placing dissecting forceps superficial to it, allow the forceps blades to separate, and cut between them.

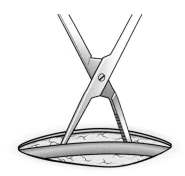

Fig. 4.30 Displaying a duct by opening haemostatic forceps parallel to it.

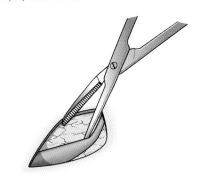

Fig. 4.31 Displaying a duct by opening haemostatic forceps at right angles to it.

5. It may be possible to inject methylene blue dye into a duct, such as a thyroglossal fistula, so that if it is inadvertently entered or tran-sected, dye leaks out to warn you; however, in my hands, it has usually leaked and caused general staining. Another method is to pass in a probe or catheter; for example, the ureter can be catheterised through a cystoscope if you need to preserve it from injury when subsequently dissecting structures nearby in difficult circumstances.

OCCLUSION

Divided duct

1. The duct may be divided deliberately or accidentally.
2. Diathermization under compression creates a weld in a small duct but check that it has been effective. Ultrasonic welding is an alternative method of closure (see Ch. 2).
3. If it is important that the channel does not reform, as when carrying out vasectomy or female sterilization by occluding the fallopian tubes, divide them after doubly ligating or clipping them and separate the ends. Folding the end of the duct back on itself and then ligating the two thicknesses of it together may secure the ligature more effectively (because the loop is bulkier) and also serves to move its transected ends further away from each other to prevent recanalization. This is particularly helpful in vasectomy (Fig. 4.32).
4. Ligation is usually safe and effective but do not tie it too tightly or it may cut right through. Do not apply the ligature too near the end or it may slip off or be gradually rolled off if the duct undergoes peristalsis (Fig. 4.33). As a safeguard against this, insert a transfixion suture–ligature (Fig. 4.34). If spillage of contents is a risk, apply double ligatures before transecting the duct between them (Fig. 4.35).
5. Close a supple large-bore duct using a simple ligature reinforced by invaginating the end within a purse-string suture (Fig. 4.36).
6. Flatten a supple but thicker-walled duct and close it with a linear suture (Fig. 4.37). This can be reinforced by invaginating it within a second layer of sutures (Fig. 4.38).
7. A single metal or absorbable clip is sufficient to occlude a small duct. Close the flattened end of a larger duct with a linear stapler (Fig. 4.39).

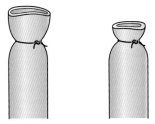

Fig. 4.33 Do not apply ligatures too near the end of a duct. The one on the right may slip off or be rolled off by peristalsis.

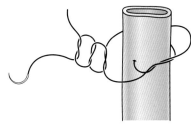

Fig. 4.34 Transfixion suture–ligature. The needled thread has been passed through the duct before being tied.

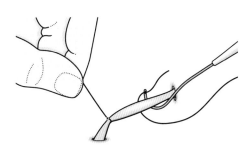

Fig. 4.35 If there is a risk of spillage, do not transect the duct until you have applied two ligatures at a distance from each other, then cut between them.

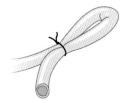

Fig. 4.32 Folding the end of the vas back on itself in vasectomy secures the ligature more effectively and moves the transected ends farther apart.

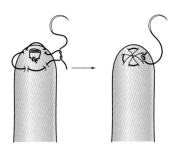

Fig. 4.36 On the left a ligature has been tied to close the end of a large duct. On the right the closed end has been invaginated with a purse-string suture.

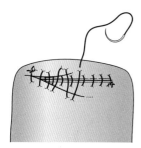

Fig. 4.37 Closing a wide-bore tube with a row of sutures after flattening the end.

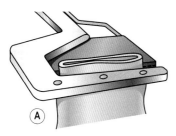

Fig. 4.38 A linear suture-closure (or staple closure) of a duct can be reinforced by invaginating the first suture line with a second layer of sutures.

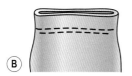

(A)

(B)

Fig. 4.39 Closing a deformable tube with a double row of staples. (A) Apply the stapler across the duct and actuate it. (B) When the stapler is removed, the double line of staples can be seen.

Key point

- When there is a choice, prefer sutures to clips; they are more versatile and less likely to catch in other tissues, instruments, or materials and be dragged off.

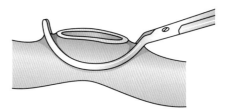

Fig. 4.40 The curved Satinsky-type clamp allows flow along the lower part of the duct as the open upper part is isolated to control leakage.

In continuity

If you wish to occlude a small supple duct without dividing it, apply a ligature, or a metal clip. Larger supple tubes cannot be occluded in this manner and must be flattened and closed with a line of stitches or a line of staples.

Control of leakage

1. Achieve temporary control of an actual or potential leak from a duct by simple compression, constriction with a thread or tape ligature, or by applying one of the large variety of noncrushing clamps to occlude the flow of content upstream of the site of the leak. The curved Satinsky-type clamp does not obstruct flow along the duct but isolates a potential source of leakage while it is being repaired, joined or closed (Fig. 4.40).
2. Alternatively, occlude the lumen using a balloon obturator such as a Foley catheter, which can be deflated and withdrawn at the last minute before final closure. If necessary, fluid can be introduced into, or drained from the duct through the main channel of the catheter.
3. The principle of a cuffed tube is employed when an endotracheal tube is passed to inflate the lungs during anaesthesia or to provide respiratory assistance (Fig. 4.41). Inflate the cuff, lying in the trachea, to prevent leakage around the tube during respiratory inflation.

DISOBLITERATION

A duct can be blocked as a result of many factors or a combination:

Intraluminal: the contents, for example inspissated (from the Latin *spissare* = to thicken) contents,

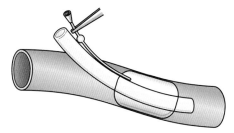

Fig. 4.41 The tube has an external cuff that can be inflated through a side tube. This channels all fluids through the tube lumen. The technique facilitates inflation of the lungs through a cuffed endotracheal tube (see Fig. 4.8).

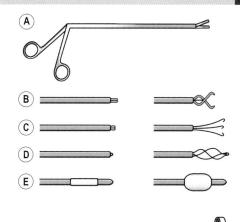

Fig. 4.42 Instruments for removing obstructions. (A) Rigid 'alligator' forceps. (B) and (C) Flexible grasping forceps, shown closed and open. (D) A Dormier basket, shown closed and open. (E) A balloon catheter, shown deflated and inflated. (F) An internal ring stripper.

worms, flukes in the bowel, stones in the ureter, bile duct or salivary duct, polyps and various foods or bezoars (Persian–ingested concretions), block the lumen.

Intramural: (from the Latin *murus* = wall) such as a stricture, tumour, or failure to transmit the contents by peristalsis. The presence of a tumour in the wall of the intestine may obstruct the passage by blocking the lumen or, by its rigidity, stop the run of peristaltic waves, often generating the classical 'change of bowel habit'.

Extramural: external factors such as adhesions, bands, hernial orifices and external tumours.

> **Key points**
>
> - How you manage the blockage depends upon its cause–is it likely to recur?
> - If the cause is progressive—for example, malignant obstruction—you need to isolate any corrective procedure from encroachment by the disease.

1. If obstruction results from a stricture it may be dilated. A tumour can be shrunk by external radiotherapy, local irradiation–brachytherapy (from the Greek *brachys* = short, short range) or chemotherapy.
2. Stones can often be pulverised (from the Latin *pulvis* = powder) by shock-wave lithotripsy (from the Greek *lithos* = stone + *ripsis* = rubbing), ultrasound or laser therapy. Accessible stones can be crushed, and with other obstructions, can often be removed using forceps or other instruments passed through an endoscope (Fig. 4.42). In some cases, disobliteration can be carried out endoscopically either by excision, as in diathermy loop

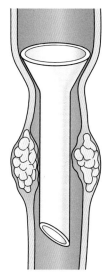

Fig. 4.43 A plastic hollow stent has been impacted in a tube to hold it open. The flared upper end is designed to prevent the stent from passing through the stricture.

transurethral resection of the prostate, or by vaporization with a laser beam, as with oesophageal carcinoma.

3. The lumen can often be restored by inserting a splinting tube or stent (Fig. 4.43). This may be placed after first dilating the narrow segment and leaving in a bougie, then passing over this a plastic tube advanced through the

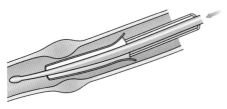

Fig. 4.44 The safest way to introduce a stent is to dilate the stricture and leave a bougie within the lumen. Slide the stent over the bougie, using a 'pusher', to advance it into position, then remove the pusher and bougie.

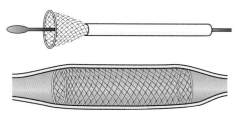

Fig. 4.45 Expanding stent. The springy wire stent is compressed, making it long and thin. When it is correctly placed across the stricture it is released and expands its diameter while shortening its length, expanding the narrow segment.

narrow segment with a 'pusher' tube (Fig. 4.44). Insertion of such tubes often demands immediate and extensive preliminary dilatation. This can be avoided in many sites by inserting a tube stent made of springy metal that can be introduced across the narrowing in a compressed state and allowed to expand spontaneously (Fig. 4.45).

Key points

- Inserting a stent into a tube or duct that normally passes on the contents by peristalsis creates an aperistaltic segment.
- Transmission is seriously prejudiced and viscous or solid contents may obstruct within the stent.

---

4. It may be necessary to deal with an obstruction by open operation. On occasion noninvasive methods have failed or are inappropriate. For example, normal or diseased bowel may be obstructed by a swallowed foreign body, impacted food, a gallstone that has ulcerated into the bowel, or a ball of intestinal worms. Do not immediately open the duct. Soft material may be disimpacted, broken up and

manoeuvred through a narrow segment and allowed to pass through normally. If this is impossible, consider massaging it proximally and opening the duct where the wall is less likely to have suffered damage. Remove the cause of the block and carefully repair the opening. This is now rarely required for impacted stones in the ureter, bile ducts or salivary ducts. Especially when removing salivary duct stones guard against them slipping back into the gland by encircling the duct with a thread or a gently closed tissue forceps, before opening the duct (Fig. 4.46).

5. Obstruction of the bowel commonly results from pressure or kinking by adhesions—originally fibrinous, often becoming fibrous strands—usually but not always resulting from a previous inflammation or an operation. A second cause is herniation in which the intestine protrudes through a restricted hole within which the entrapped bowel becomes blocked. Infrequently, the bowel is blocked by spontaneous twisting, and also by intussusception in which the bowel draws itself within the lumen and passes it along.

6. A narrow segment of a supple duct can be widened by a plastic (from the Greek *plassein* = to form) procedure. It was originally devised to overcome strictures resulting from long-standing ulceration at the pylorus and named *pyloroplasty*. It has been adapted as a stricturoplasty for dealing with the small bowel strictures resulting from *Crohn's inflammatory bowel disease*. Make a longitudinal incision through the full length of the stricture, open it out and close the defect as a transverse suture line (Fig. 4.47).

7. It may be preferable to excise a narrow segment and bring the ends together directly to bridge the defect (Fig. 4.48A). The circumferential suture line that results may narrow the lumen; if so, minimise this by cutting the duct diagonally at each end of the stricture, producing a longer oblique line of closure (Fig. 4.48B).

8. *Immovable or recurrent obstruction* can be dealt with in many ways. You may accept the blockage; an example is blockage of a ureter below a poorly functioning kidney with good function of the other kidney. One method of relief is bypass, creating an internal stoma (from the Greek word for mouth) with the duct below the obstruction or with another channel, for example draining a blocked bile duct or ureter into the bowel (choledochoduodenostomy

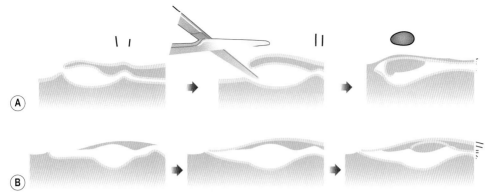

Fig. 4.46 Removing an obstructing stone from a superficial duct. A stitch prevents the stone from escaping proximally. In (A), the stone is near the orifice, which can be opened up with scissors to release the stone. In (B), the stone lies some distance from the orifice. Cut down onto the stone through the overlying epithelium, leaving the duct orifice intact. Pull the thread through after removing the stone.

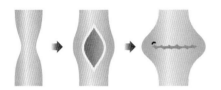

Fig. 4.47 Overcome a longitudinal stricture with an incision along its whole length. Open it out, draw the two ends of the incision together and close the defect as a transverse incision, creating a shorter but wider tube.

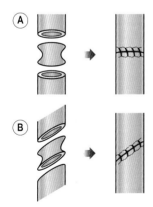

Fig. 4.48 (A) Excise the stricture and join the cut ends. (B) End-to-end anastomosis with a circumferential suture line may leave a constriction. This can be avoided by cutting the ends obliquely and joining them.

and ureteroileostomy respectively). A duct that is merely a transmitter, not secreting any substance into the lumen, may be divided above and below the obstruction, with the proximal and distal cut ends united; an irremovable obstructed segment is left in situ. For example, in the case of the bowel, which secretes substances such as mucus, an irremovable segment cannot usually be left undrained. The creation of an *external stoma* may be valuable because it not only clears the secretion but also allows the output to be measured.

Key points

- Differentiate between a duct that is merely a conduit and one that secretes or fills with content; for example, the bowel secretes enzymes and mucus.
- If the duct secretes into the lumen, you must not leave a closed segment or loop, which will become distended with its own secretions.

9. Methods of bypass are shown in Fig. 4.49. It may be possible without transecting the duct (Fig. 4.49A1). Draw up a distal loop proximally and unite it above the obstruction, to carry on the obstructed contents (Fig. 4.49A2). Contents may stagnate in the segment between the obstruction and the stoma. An external stoma can also be created without transecting the duct (Fig. 4.49A3); again, content may stagnate in the segment between the obstruction and the external stoma. The duct may be transected below the obstruction (Fig. 4.49B1), allowing you to draw up the distal cut end above it (Fig. 4.49B2), and close off the stump below the obstruction. Do not close off the stump if it is likely to

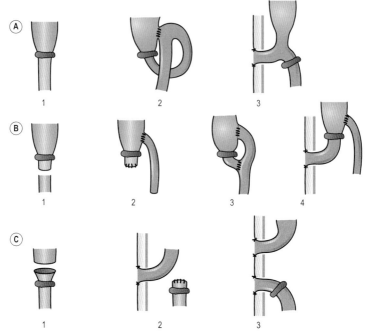

Fig. 4.49 Possibilities for dealing with an irremovable obstruction. (A) (1) Do not transect the obstructed segment above or below the blockage. (2) Draw up a distal loop from beyond the obstruction and form an anastomosis proximal to the obstruction. (3) Bring the segment above the obstruction to the surface to form an external stoma. (B) (1) Transect the distal duct below the obstruction. (2) Draw the lower cut end proximally to unite it above the obstruction. Close off the distal stump beyond the block. (3) If there is a risk of the remnant below becoming distended by local secretions and it is closed, join it into the draining loop or (4) bring it to the surface as a draining fistula. (C) (1) Transect the bowel above the obstruction. (2) Bring out the upper cut end to the surface as a terminal stoma and close the stump above the block. (3) If the closed stump is likely to become distended, bring the stump to the surface as a draining fistula.

become distended (or it will blow out); prefer to join the cut end into the draining loop (Fig. 4.49B3) or bring it to the surface (Fig. 4.49B4); this is often termed a draining fistula (from the Latin word for pipe) to distinguish it from a stoma that drains the whole duct content. The duct may be transected above an irremovable obstruction (Fig. 4.49C1) and brought to the surface as a stoma (Fig. 4.49C2). If a secreting remnant above the obstruction is closed off, it may become filled and rupture. One solution is to create a loop stoma (Fig. 4.49A3) but to prevent any flow down the loop, separate stomas can be created (Fig. 4.49C3), so the proximal duct is drained but also the duct between the distal cut end and the obstruction. If you cannot drain the segment internally or bring it to the surface as a stoma, consider inserting a tube to bridge the distance between the loop and the surface (Fig. 4.50). If the tube points upwards it tends

to drain downwards and can be collected into a bag. If it points downwards, the contents may need to be sucked out. If the tube remains in position for a considerable period, a fistulous track may form so that the contents reach the surface even when the tube is withdrawn.

10. **Strangulation** (from the Greek *strangos* = twisted) implies cutting off the blood supply by twisting or by constriction, as may occur in herniation of the bowel through a rigid orifice. Content may flow in, but if outflow is restricted, the bowel distends and is liable to become irreducible. Inflow at arterial pressure in the presence of venous compression and restricted outflow causes vascular congestion, stagnation, capillary distension, rupture and extravasation. At this stage the bowel is still viable but appears black, like a bruise, the serosa is shiny, and the arterial pulse is still palpable, but of course the

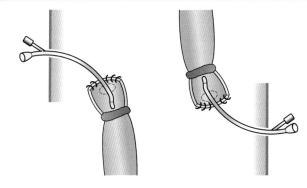

Fig. 4.50 If you need to leave a fixed, closed compartment that may fill up and cannot be drained internally, insert a self-retaining catheter. Bring the catheter to the exterior. A drain inserted upwards can be connected to a bag for collection, but one inserted downwards may require suction drainage.

subserosal haematoma will take many days to be reabsorbed. If the bowel is not released the arterial inflow ceases and anoxic blood stagnates. The mucosa, which is the most metabolically active part, begins to die and bacteria, flourishing in the lumen, pass through it as gangrene spreads through the wall. The serosal sheen is lost as the colour changes to grey and green. Colic continues in the bowel above but there is a continuous underlying pain and tenderness.

> **Key points**
>
> - Recognise incipient strangulation.
> - Urgently release and if necessary resect strangulated bowel.

REPAIR

Ducts may be damaged accidentally or deliberately as when performing a surgical manoeuvre to gain access or as part of a radical resection of spreading disease.

> **Key point**
>
> - To achieve success, carry out the repair perfectly, without tension, on a healthy duct with an adequate blood supply and protect it during the healing phase.

Gastrointestinal tract

1. If the bowel has been injured, assiduously search for every possible blunt or penetrating wound. Check the mesentery for potential threats to the blood supply.
2. The area of the folded mucosa is far greater than the area of the submucosa and seromuscularis, particularly in the small intestine. When the bowel wall is acutely breached, therefore, the mucosa tends to evert. This brings into apposition the mucosal surfaces, forming a channel for leakage of contents (Fig. 4.51). If it is difficult to replace the mucosa, use an inverting mattress stitch, often referred to in this context as a *Connell stitch*, after the 19th-century American surgeon who popularised it.
3. In contrast, a breach resulting from chronic ulceration or inflammation is associated with fibrosis that fixes the mucosa, so that it does not protrude. As a rule, you can safely bring the margins together with a simple all-coats suture as in closing a *perforated peptic ulcer*, although many surgeons include an overlying tag of omentum in the closing stitch.
4. In some cases, a large, chronic, rigid, adherent ulcer cannot be closed. A leaked anastomosis will often break down again if you attempt to close it. In both cases, it is safer to insert a catheter into the hole and drain it to the surface. A track will form and when you remove the catheter, the hole will close, provided there is no distal obstruction! Occasionally you can deal with the problem by diverting the bowel content to prevent it from reaching the defect, either by creating a proximal stoma or by forming an anastomosis proximal to the defect. Alternatively, that part of the bowel may need to be resected.

Other ducts and cavities

1. Because many ducts are of small calibre, repair of defects or injuries may result in a stricture;

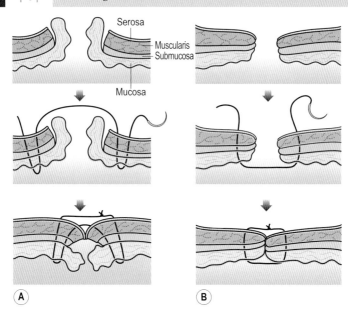

Fig. 4.51 Repair of traumatic rupture of bowel. (A) Section through an acute traumatic puncture of the bowel wall often results in pouting of the mucosa; this can be corrected using an inverting (Connell) mattress suture. (B) A chronic cause has resulted in fibrosis with fixation of the layers; it can be closed using a simple stitch, producing an edge-to-edge union.

this becomes more likely if you fail to appose the lining epithelium with every stitch. Carefully excise all necrotic tissue or the repair will break down. In many cases, the best option is reanastomosis or anastomosis to a large duct such as a bowel. It is best to use interrupted rather than continuous suturing in these cases. Sometimes, as in the ureter, spatulation can increase the circumference of the ends being anastomosed; a small longitudinal slit is made in the end of one end to be anastomosed and a similar slit made on the opposite side of the other end to be anastomosed. Thus, when opened up the two ends will look like two spoons (spatulae) with the concave parts of the spoons facing each other and the spoon handles (the two ducts) lying in opposite directions.

2. Recognise iatrogenic (from the Greek *iatros* = physician) injuries and repair them immediately, especially bile ducts and ureter. The pancreatic duct is not usually repaired but drained into the bowel.

3. Repair of the ovarian tubes, vas deferens, salivary and lachrymal ducts demand microsurgical methods (see Ch. 5), in order to preserve or regain tubal patency.

4. Repair of a cavity wall, such as the urinary bladder, is less critical because there is more available tissue. Urologists usually employ stitches that exclude the mucosa–extramucosal stitches. The bladder can contract very powerfully, so it is usual to insert a suprapubic or transurethral catheter to ensure that pressure does not build up.

RESECTION

Bowel

Bowel needs to be resected without leaking of contents, so crushing clamps are placed across the ends of the segment to be excised, which seals them. You must doubly ligate and divide blood vessels supplying the segment in the mesentery, sometimes recreating the mesentery of bowel, which is described as retromesenteric; in fact, the mesentery has fused with the posterior parietal peritoneum. You may need to repair the mesentery following resection.

Other ducts

When mobilizing small ducts, take great care not to damage the blood supply, which is often tenuous (from the Latin *tenuis* = thin). For this reason, do not try to free it excessively. In some cases, the adventitia—the loose tissue surrounding the duct—carries small vessels and the duct is deprived if this tissue is stripped off. Even blood vessels have their own blood supply. Autonomic nerves, which carry motor impulses to peristaltic muscle and also have an important trophic impulses effect, are also stripped off. Make certain the repair will not narrow the duct and cause obstruction.

ANASTOMOSIS

Galen (AD 131–201) used this term (from the Greek *ana* = through + *stoma* = a mouth, hence a coming together through a mouth). Ducts of the same or different types can be joined together.

Principles

1. Ducts of all types must retain or gain an adequate arterial blood supply and venous drainage, in order to heal.
2. Ensure that the anastomosis is performed between disease-free ducts. Inflammation, infection, neoplasms or foreign bodies all threaten healing.
3. Do not join ducts without excluding distal obstruction.
4. Some ducts, notably the bowel, have autonomous directional peristalsis. If you forget this, drainage of the contents may be impaired.
5. Ensure that there is no tension, no twisting or excessive constriction when ducts are joined.
6. Avoid back pressure and stagnation; bacteria rapidly flourish in stagnant contents.

Bowel

1. Ensure the bowel ends match. If they do not, be willing to angle the end of the narrower end, to enlarge it. Cut back on the edge opposite the entrance of the blood supply—the antimesenteric edge (Fig. 4.52). Alternatively, create a Cheatle slit (after English surgeon Sir George Cheatle, 1865–1951); make a slit in the antimesenteric border of the smaller calibre end to increase its available free edge.
2. You may apply noncrushing bowel clamps to steady the ends and prevent leakage of

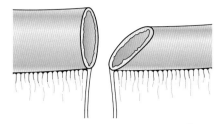

Fig. 4.52 If the ends are disparate in calibre, cut back the narrower end on the side opposite the mesentery or the entry of the blood supply.

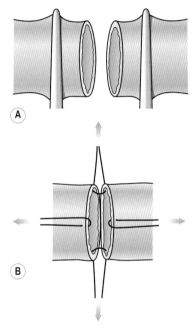

Fig. 4.53 Preparing to form an anastomosis. (A) Noncrushing bowel clamps steady the ends and prevent leakage of content. Some clamps can be locked together. (B) The ends are held together with traction sutures. If the bowel cannot be rotated, insert these not at the ends but slightly onto the back wall, so that when they are distracted they tauten the apposed back walls, leaving the anterior walls slack so that the back wall stitches can be easily inserted. (I was taught this method by Mr John Cochrane.) You may distract the anterior walls with stitches or tissue forceps to improve access to the posterior walls.

content. Alternatively, insert sutures at each end uniting the ends but clipping instead of tying them ('stay' or 'traction' sutures, Fig. 4.53). If you need to suture the back wall first when the bowel cannot be rotated, insert the traction sutures just posterior to the junction of the back and front walls, so that the anterior walls remain slack when the sutures are distracted, allowing easy access to the back wall. Some surgeons distract the middle of the anterior walls with traction sutures or tissue forceps to provide the best possible access while they insert stitches in the back wall.

3. Types of stitch are determined by your beliefs, training and current fashion since no satisfactory controlled trials have been carried out comparing popular methods. The strongest and therefore most important layer to include is the submucous, collagenous coat—the coat from which catgut is made. The traditional stitch takes in all coats (Fig. 4.54), attributed to William Halsted (1852–1922), the great American surgeon. Another method is an extramucosal or serosubmucosal technique; all layers are included with the exception of the mucosa. A seromuscular stitch apposing and sealing the serous layers was described in 1826 by the Parisian surgeon Antoine Lembert (1802–1851), to prevent leakage; it does not incorporate the submucosa and is usually considered suitable only as a second-layer stitch.

4. Use a synthetic absorbable 3/0 suture mounted on a curved, round-bodied eyeless needle. Smooth monofilament material, having no interstices where organisms can reside, is safer in the presence of contamination but is a little stiff to tie. A braided multifilament suture is supple and forms reliable knots.

5. The method of stitching depends on personal choice and on the need to control the apposition of the edges. Use continuous, interrupted simple or mattress stitches passed vertically through all coats, 3–4 mm from the edge and 3–4 mm apart. Full-thickness interrupted and spiral continuous stitches are more haemostatic than mattress stitches. In either case, carefully pick up and ligate bleeding vessels before starting the anastomotic suture.

6. The anastomotic line may lie in the sagittal or coronal planes. If the line of sutures lies in the sagittal plane it is usually easier to work from far to near; if it lies in the coronal plane it is usually easier to start at the end from your nondominant to your dominant side.

7. It is also usually easier to drive the needle progressively from far to near when it lies in the transverse plane, and from dominant to nondominant side when it lies in the sagittal plane. In each case, your hand starts fully pronated and drives the curved needle through by progressively supinating.

8. Your intention must be to appose the edges perfectly, just bringing into contact the same layers of each edge. The stitches cause inflammation, producing oedema. If you have pulled the stitches too tight, they cut off the blood supply and result in delayed healing, ulceration of the mucosa, or worse, cutting out with potential anastomotic leakage.

9. The methods I shall describe are applicable throughout the bowel but be prepared to practise the methods of your trainers.

10. On completion, check that the lumen is patent; carefully confirm that you can invaginate the walls from each side through the anastomotic ring. It should feel like a small doughnut.

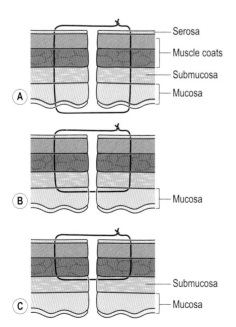

Fig. 4.54 (A) The all-coats stitch. (B) An extramucosal or serosubmucosal stitch. (C) The seromuscular or Lembert stitch. The knots are offset from the joined bowel edges.

Key points

- Check the colour of the bowel, the integrity of the blood supply, the lack of tension, the luminal continuity and the circumferential perfection of the union.
- If there is a mesentery to be closed, exclude haematoma that may subsequently prejudice healing.

11. Repair any defect in the mesentery with fine, interrupted sutures carefully inserted to avoid pricking any of the vessels or including them in the sutures and thus obliterating them. Failing to close a mesenteric defect may result in internal herniation of the bowel and subsequent bowel obstruction.

Alternative methods

Used depending on the circumstances and on individual choice.

Mobile bowel, edge to edge, single layer, interrupted stitches

1. Insert sutures joining the anterior walls. Carefully avoid picking up the back wall. Tie the knots on the outside of the bowel.
2. When you have completed the anterior wall, turn the bowel over to bring what was the back wall to the front and insert a series of sutures to close this, completing the anastomosis (Fig. 4.55).
3. If you used stay sutures, cut out or tie them.
4. Carefully check the mesenteric and antimesenteric edges of the bowel—the junctions of the anterior and posterior suture lines are the most likely to have defects. Insert extra sutures if necessary.

Edge to edge, single layer, continuous stitches

1. Starting on the back wall, insert a stitch at one end from outside in on one side, inside out on the other side and tie it. Clip the short end, insert the needle back through into the lumen and introduce a continuous, unlocked, spiral stitch joining the back walls as far as the other end.
2. If the line of anastomosis lies in the sagittal plane, start at the near end, complete the stitching of the back wall, continue around the far corner and close the anterior walls from far to near, to reach the starting point. If you continue the spiral stitch onto the anterior wall you will discover you have to stitch with an unnatural action, starting with your hand held supine and pronating it to drive the stitch through. For a right-handed surgeon, to avoid this, at the far end, having passed the needle through to the left side, reverse the needle and pass it from within out, creating a loop on the mucosa—a single 'Connell' stitch. You can now continue to sew naturally, driving the needle from right to left along the anterior wall, to reach the starting point. Remove and discard the needle and tie the free end to the clamped short end. Reverse this if you are left-handed.
3. If the line of anastomosis lies in the transverse (coronal) plane, start at the right end (Fig. 4.56). Insert the first stitch from without in, then from within out, tie the stitch and clamp the short end. Reinsert the needle from without in on the near side. Carry on with the over and over spiral stitches, uniting the back walls from right to left. Again, at the left end, having taken the last stitch from far to near, reverse the needle to create a single Connell (mattress stitch with a loop on the mucosal aspect) stitch, coming out on the

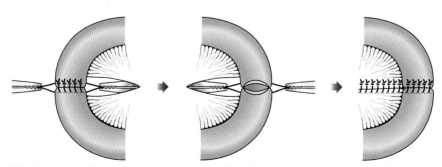

Fig. 4.55 If the bowel is mobile, suture the front wall, taking care to avoid the back wall. Now turn over the bowel to bring the previous back wall to the front and close it. If the bowel has a mesentery, carefully close the defect.

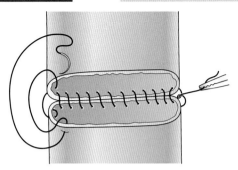

Fig. 4.56 Bowel anastomosis by continuous suture. The anastomotic line lies transversely. Start at the right side, insert an all-coats stitch and tie it. Enter the needle from without in on the near side. Unite the back walls with a spiral over-and-over stitch. At the left end insert a single Connell stitch on the near side and then continue from left to right on the anterior wall, to reach the first stitch and tie off. If you rotate the drawing 90° to the right (clockwise) it demonstrates the method when the anastomotic line lies in the sagittal plane.

near side. You can now continue on the anterior suture line from left to right, inserting stitches from far to near. When you reach the right end, cut off the needle and tie the free end to the clamped short end.

4. Check that the anastomosis is patent.

Fixed bowel, single layer, interrupted stitches

1. This method is particularly applicable in the large bowel to anastomose it with the rectum, which lies against the sacrum and cannot be rotated. In addition, access is limited, so you must fashion the anastomosis not at the surface but in the depths.

> **Key points**
>
> - Do not unite the bowel ends under tension or they will surely distract.
> - Take particular care when inserting and tying sutures in situations that are inaccessible following completion of the procedure. This applies particularly to the posterior layer sutures in colorectal anastomoses.

2. Unite the posterior layers using carefully placed all-coats stitches, with the knots tied within the lumen. If the bowel is fixed, and subsequent access will be greatly restricted, place

and tie these stitches with the bowel ends apart, clipping but not tying them until they are all inserted. Now, keeping the sutures taut and in the correct order, slide the mobile end down to lie accurately apposed to the fixed edge of bowel and tie them (Fig. 4.57). This is the 'parachute' technique. Leave the outer ligature ends long for the present but cut the ligature ends of the remainder, leaving the knots on the interior of the bowel.

3. Many colorectal surgeons use inverting, longitudinal (vertical) mattress sutures for the back wall (see Ch. 3). These pass out through all coats at a distance from the edge, enter the other bowel end at a similar distance from the edge, then take a small bite of each of the edges before being tied within the lumen.

4. Insert interrupted inverting anterior stitches to complete the anastomosis. These may be simple or inverting longitudinal mattress stitches. Because I was taught that bowel must be sutured using all-coats stitches as a basis, I should favour these. Many colorectal surgeons employ extramucosal or even seromuscular stitches with success.

5. There are no absolute tests of perfection of the colorectal anastomosis but since it transmits solid faeces, many surgeons try to exclude defects or leaks that might disrupt the union or allow leakage with consequent infection. A reliable assistant may insert a finger through the anus to feel the integrity of the anastomosis and insert a narrow-bore rigid sigmoidoscope and inspect it. Finally, the pelvis may be filled with sterile saline and the rectal stump is gently inflated with air through the sigmoidoscope. If no bubbles appear, this suggests the anastomosis is satisfactory.

Two-layer anastomosis

In the past, the stomach and bowel were routinely and very satisfactorily sutured using two layers. The inner, all-coats stitch inverts the bowel wall. This is reinforced with an absorbable or nonabsorbable outer seromuscular Lembert stitch. Although most surgeons have converted to single-layer techniques, many senior surgeons, adept in the two-layer technique, continue to use it and obtain good results with it.

Stapled anastomosis

Mechanical stapling devices are now more often used for joining bowel. You should familiarise

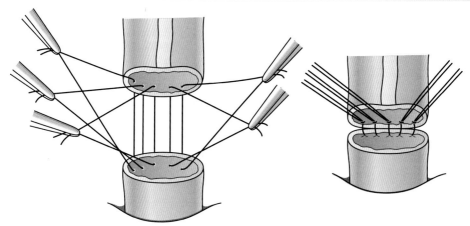

Fig. 4.57 If the bowel cannot be rotated, insert the back wall stitches, tying the knots within the lumen. In case of difficulty, leave the ends apart while you insert all the back wall stitches, slide the mobile end along the stitches and only then tie the knots. This is the 'parachute' technique.

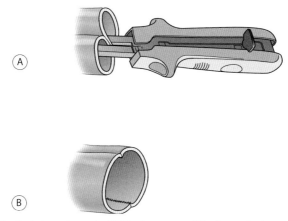

(A)

(B)

Fig. 4.58 Side-to-side stapled anastomosis. (A) The two arms of the linear stapler are inserted into the two respective lumina, away from the mesenteries, and the stapler locked and deployed. (B) The stapler fires two rows of staples and cuts between the two joining them with a wider lumen. It then remains to close this opening transversely by firing the linear stapler across the opening, maintaining a lumen within.

yourself with the mechanism before using it. Staplers can be used to transect and at the same time close the two cut ends each with a row of staples. Thus, the stapler can be used to resect a segment of bowel by stapling either side of the portion being resected.

1. For a side-to-side anastomosis, position the two ends of the bowel side by side with the open ends facing the same way and the mesenteries away from the stapler, ensuring there is no twist. Apply an absorbable stay suture. Insert the two arms of the stapler into the respective lumina and then lock the stapler together. If you have used the stapler to resect the intervening bowel, you will first have to make a small incision on each side close to the staple line to admit the respective arms of the stapler. Discharge the stapler using the sliding mechanism. This will staple the two ends together with two parallel rows of staples and at the same time cut the bowel between the two rows, which will serve as the new lumen (Fig. 4.58).

2. You now need to close the transverse defect that allowed insertion of the stapler. Steadying the free ends with two Alliss forceps, apply the stapler across the outside of the two free ends of the bowel. Ensure that you can see

the full circumference of both ends of bowel at one side of the stapler before locking it into place. Also ensure that you are not stapling across a large vessel in the mesentery. Discharging the stapler will again release two parallel rows of staples, one that closes the end of the anastomosed bowel and one that attaches the two free ends together. At the same time, the bowel will be cut between the two staple lines, thus transecting the redundant bowel ends. Discard the free ends of bowel.

3. Palpate the lumen in the side-to-side anastomosis to ensure that it is patent.
4. Many surgeons will apply a row of hand-sewn interrupted sutures to invert and bury the row of staples, in particular at the corners.
5. Staplers come in varying sizes (e.g., 25 mm, 38 mm, 48 mm) and lengths (60 mm, 80 mm, 100 mm).

Variations

1. Anastomoses can be made not only end-to-end but also end-to-side and side-to-side (Fig. 4.59). In each circumstance ensure that the holes match each other.
2. The circular stapler can be used to create an end-to-end anastomosis, for instance in an anterior resection. It inverts the bowel and applies a double row of metal staples. A 'doughnut' of redundant tissue is removed after the ends are joined. Do not assume that

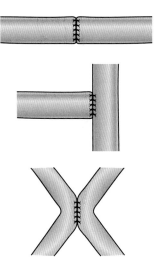

Fig. 4.59 In addition to end-to-end anastomoses, the bowel can be joined end to side and side to side.

mechanical devices can always be used more rapidly or more effectively than hand sewing. They demand careful placement.

> ### Key points
>
> - Successful surgeons who employ techniques that work well for them often attribute their success to the method, but other successful surgeons using different techniques also pay tribute to their method.
> - What is the explanation?
> - These surgeons are too modest. Their success depends more on their skilful application of different but sound methods than on the techniques themselves.
> - A good anastomosis is dependent on attention to detail, tension-free anastomosis, healthy tissue and good vascularity.

Other ducts

1. Ureters undergo peristalsis to transmit the content. This may be impaired if the myenteric nerves or vascular supply are damaged. It is often worth cutting the ends obliquely or spatulated to obviate producing an annular, constricting anastomosis.
2. Bile ducts have insufficient muscle in their walls to constrict, so they transmit contents passively by *vis a tergo* (force from behind). If they are injured, they often require to be united to another conduit, such as the jejunum. Bile is extremely penetrating and leaks if the anastomosis is imperfect.
3. Anastomosis of the fallopian tubes and vas deferens in order to restore continuity following disease or previous division is usually carried out using magnification.
4. Anastomosis of small ducts is almost always performed using a single row of interrupted, all-coats sutures, with the knots placed outside the lumen. The fear is that a continuous encircling suture may have a constricting effect.

> ### Key point
>
> - Every stitch must unite the epithelial linings of the anastomosis. Fail, and a leak or stricture will follow.

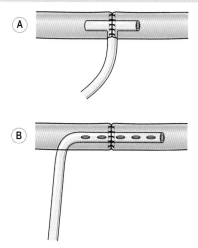

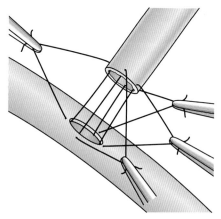

Fig. 4.61 Epithelium-to-epithelium anastomosis of small ducts is achieved by inserting the stitches while the ducts lie apart, then sliding one duct down onto the other.

Fig. 4.60 (A) Insert a T-tube at the site of the anastomosis to splint the union. This channels the contents through the anastomosis or drains it externally. (B) The same effect is achieved by inserting a straight tube with side holes.

5. Use a fine needle and suture to produce a perfect leak-free union. A straightforward end-to-end union produces a potential annular constriction ring. The postoperative oedema may block the lumen and rising pressure can then rupture the anastomosis with subsequent leakage. To avoid this, the anastomosis can be made over a 'T-tube' or straight tube (Fig. 4.60). If necessary, check the anastomosis and the 'run off', using radio-opaque contrast medium before you withdraw a splinting tube. The leakage from the side hole will rapidly heal provided there is no distal obstruction. A double pigtailed catheter can conveniently be inserted into a repaired ureter with the upper loop in the pelvis of the ureter and the lower one in the bladder (Fig. 4.13); it can be captured and extracted using a cystoscope.

6. If access is difficult as in the depths, place the stitches while the ducts lie apart before sliding them together—the 'parachute' technique (Fig. 4.61).

7. Be willing to slit the end of a small duct so that you can join it into a similar duct that has also been slit. The slit duct can also be joined to the end or side of a wide duct (Fig. 4.62). If necessary, use stay sutures to hold the ducts in apposition while you insert the stitches.

8. You may close the end of a large open-ended duct until it will fit the end of a small duct. Alternatively, close the end completely, joining

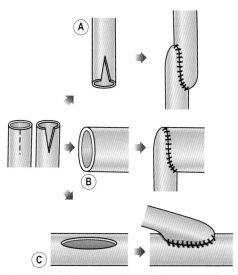

Fig. 4.62 Slit the end of a small duct to produce a wide opening. (A) Join it to another small duct, similarly split. (B) Join it to the end of a wide duct. (C) Join it into the side of a wide duct.

the small duct into a freshly made side opening (Fig. 4.63). Very small ducts are best cannulated with a plastic catheter which is tied in, before using the catheter as an introducer. If you leave the needled suture intact following ligation, pass the needle into the accepting hole and out nearby, so you can tie

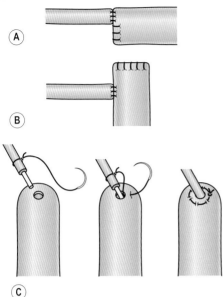

Fig. 4.63 Joining small ducts into larger ones. (A) End-to-end. (B) End-to-side. (C) Using a plastic cannula to aid union of a small duct with a large one.

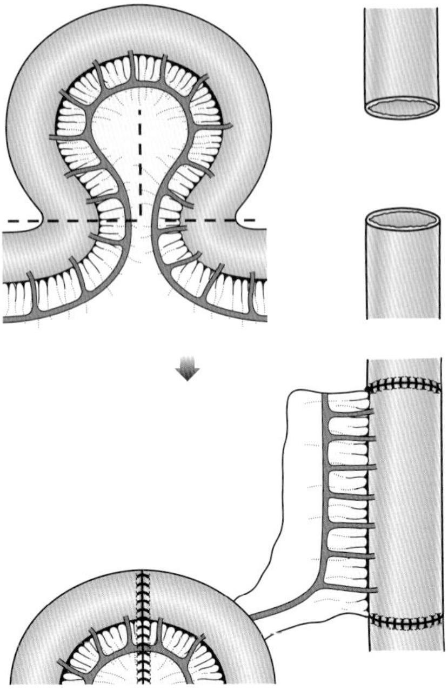

the end to the other end of the ligature to fix the duct in place. To prevent leakage, insert a purse-string suture around the anastomosis, gently push in the duct and tie the purse-string suture, producing an 'inkwell' effect.

BOWEL TRANSFER

Bowel, which has a rich blood supply, can be transferred to a different site but must retain or regain a blood supply to survive. A segment of bowel can be transferred elsewhere, while preserving its blood supply, by opening out the arching blood vessels that run in its mesentery to supply it from one end. The other end can be extended (Fig. 4.64). This was first described by the brilliant Swiss surgeon César Roux (1851–1934) in 1908. Small bowel can be refashioned to form an ileal conduit following cystectomy and colon can be transposed into the thorax to replace the oesophagus after oesophagectomy. If it is necessary to transfer the segment at a distance, the blood vessels can be divided and reimplanted into vessels near the recipient site (Fig. 4.65). This demands highly skilled microvascular surgery (see Ch. 5).

Fig. 4.64 Transferring bowel while retaining its blood supply. At the top on the left, the dotted lines show the lines of section, retaining the arterial circuit; on the right is a gap in the bowel to be bridged. At the bottom, the loop has been straightened out and joined in to bridge the gap on the right. The cut ends of the supplying bowel have been united to restore continuity on the left, with closure of the mesenteric defect.

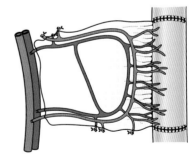

Fig. 4.65 Bowel removed from one site has its blood vessels joined into those at the new site. As a rule, two veins are anastomosed for each artery.

SPHINCTERS

Localised segments of specially controlled circular muscle meter and regulate the rate and direction of flow. These are sphincters (from the Greek *sphingein* = to bind tightly). They may or may not be anatomically obvious.

Inadvertent damage to the muscle or nerve supply may be irrevocable. Dilatation or overstretching often puts the sphincter out of action. It can be achieved in a similar manner to correcting a stricture, by passing graded bougies or balloon dilatation. The method may be used for achalasia (from the Greek *a* = not + *chalaein* = to relax) of the gastrooesophageal cardia and to temporarily overcome anal sphincter spasm from anal fissure. If the sphincter is overstretched, the muscle is disrupted and may never recover. If the muscle is torn, the resulting fibrosis may produce stenosis.

Myotomy

1. Divide a clearly defined circular muscle forming a sphincter, using a longitudinal incision while leaving the lining intact (Fig. 4.66). Perform this when the sphincter is overdeveloped or fails to relax so that the contents cannot pass.
2. *Infantile hypertrophic pyloric stenosis* can be treated by pyloromyotomy, described by Karl Ramstedt of Munster in 1912. Gently lift out the pylorus with fingers or tissue forceps. Hold it steady while carefully incising the thickened muscle, leaving the mucosa intact and bulging into the gap. Gently elevate the remaining fibres using a hook or fine nontoothed forceps and cut them. Pick up each side of the cut edge using gauze swabs to improve your grip and gently separate the edges or use round-nosed forceps to lever the edges apart.

Sometimes you can collect a little air into the segment to bulge the mucosa and exclude or identify any leak. If there is a break in the mucosa, carefully suture it, perhaps drawing over it a tag of tissue such as omentum.

3. Myotomy of the lower oesophageal sphincter overcomes the condition of achalasia of the cardia of the stomach. Like pyloromyotomy, it is intended that the underlying mucosa remain intact. The operation was described by Ernst Heller of Leipzig in 1913.

Sphincterotomy

1. Divide the whole thickness, including the duct lining, when the sphincter controls the termination of a spouted duct (Fig. 4.67). The ampulla of Abraham Vater (1684–1751 of Wittenberg in Germany) usually accepts both the common bile and pancreatic ducts. It can be divided to allow small gallstones to pass. This type of sphincterotomy is now usually performed through a fibreoptic endoscope, using a diathermy wire.
2. *Fistula in ano* is usually between the rectum or anus and the skin of the perineum and may require sphincterotomy to treat it (see below).
3. *Anal fissure* can sometimes be successfully treated by the application of local anaesthetic combined with stool-softening agents, application of glyceryl trinitrate (GTN) or nifedipine or injection of type A botulinum toxin (Botox) 20 units

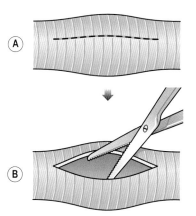

Fig. 4.66 Myotomy. Divide the sphincter (A) along the dotted line. Split the edges apart (B) to ensure that the circular muscle is totally divided. Leave the mucosal lining intact.

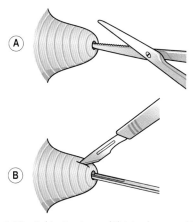

Fig. 4.67 Sphincterotomy. (A) Introduce one blade of the scissors into the mouth of the duct to cut through the encircling sphincter. (B) Introduce a grooved probe into the duct and cut down onto it with a scalpel.

diluted to 50 units/mL. If these fail it can usually be successfully treated by dividing the lower internal sphincter. The fissure nearly always lies in the midline posteriorly but carry out the sphincterotomy on the lateral wall. Insert a proctoscope with an open slot that reveals the lateral anal wall. Make a small circumferential incision at the anal margin. Through this insert closed blunt-ended scissors beneath the mucosa and gently open them to separate the mucosa and lower internal sphincter. Withdraw the scissors, close them and again insert them, this time deep into the lower internal sphincter, and open them to separate it from the external sphincter. Remove the scissors and introduce a straight haemostat, one blade superficial to, one blade deep to the internal sphincter, clamp it, open it and withdraw it. With the scissors now cut vertically through the crushed sphincter to the upper level of the fissure.

4. *Episiotomy* (from the Greek *epision*, meaning pubic region, and *tome*, meaning a cutting). There is no closure sphincter at the lower end of the vagina but during parturition (from the Latin *parare* = to bring forth), the skin and circular muscle of the lower vagina may be torn, with a risk of uncontrollable extension. To avoid this the obstetrician (from the Latin *ob* = before + *stare* = to stand) may deliberately cut the tissues to divert any tear clear of the anus, carefully repairing it after the baby is delivered.

Sphincteroplasty

If you perform sphincterotomy, the raw edges may rejoin. However, if you join the inner and outer epithelia with sutures, the opening will remain patulous (Fig. 4.68). When a sphincter surrounds a duct in continuity, such as the pylorus, incise longitudinally through it, widely separate the walls and suture the defect as a transverse suture line. At the pylorus, this manoeuvre is referred to as a *pyloroplasty*. It is a method of overcoming stenosis that results from chronic peptic ulcer in the proximal duodenum with consequent scar contracture.

Sphincter repair

A sphincter may need to be cut deliberately. Repairs of old sphincteric defects or tears are usually less successful; it is occasionally effective to excise the edges of the old, scarred sphincter and carry out a fresh repair (Fig. 4.69).

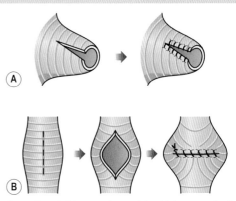

Fig. 4.68 Sphincteroplasty. (A) Divide a terminal sphincter and stitch the inner and outer linings together. (B) Divide the sphincter longitudinally, widely separate the edges and sew up the defect as a transverse suture line.

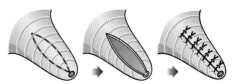

Fig. 4.69 Sphincter repair. Excise the edges to expose the fresh, raw ends of the sphincter before suturing them together.

Sphincter reversal

Some sphincters act unidirectionally, rather like valves. Indeed, as a rule, though not always, the direction of peristaltic action in the bowel is unidirectional so that it acts like a one-way valve. In order to slow down the passage in the hope of allowing more time for absorption following massive bowel resection, it is possible to take out a segment, still attached by its blood and nerve supply, reverse it, and restore it into continuity (Fig. 4.70).

ACQUIRED CHANNELS AND CAVITIES

These are varied in origin including developmental, traumatic, infective, resulting from the presence of foreign material, and neoplastic.

Sinus

A sinus is a blind-ending channel lined with epithelium (from Latin for something hollowed

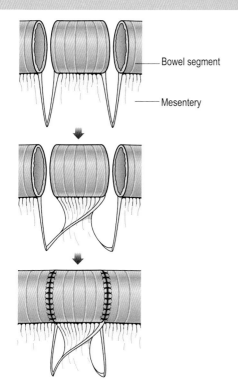

Fig. 4.70 Sphincter reversal. Take out of continuity the sphincteric segment, still attached to its blood supply, reverse it and restore it into continuity.

Bowel segment

Mesentery

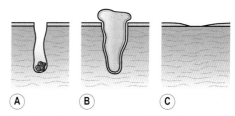

Fig. 4.71 Sinus. (A) A sinus with foreign material, diseased tissue, or hair within a pilonidal sinus. (B) The irritant cause of chronicity has been removed, the opening has been widened and the cavity packed so that it fills the base. (C) The base has filled with granulation tissue, which contracts while epithelium grows in to heal over.

out; a bay). It is often a tract from the skin into other tissues.

1. The lining of the channel may be granulation tissue, but it may become epithelialised. In some cases, removing the cause may suffice; the whole track needs to be excised in others.

2. The most common sinus you will see is a *wound sinus*. A superficial stitch often acts as a foreign body, especially if it has a long, stiff cut end lying beneath the skin which eventually protrudes. In some cases, it may be caused by a piece of necrotic tissue or missed foreign material. Initially try to insert sinus forceps or fine 'mosquito' artery forceps, gently open the blades and attempt to capture the stitch or other cause and remove it. If this fails, be willing to explore the sinus under local anaesthesia, enlarging the opening until you can see the cause and remove it.

3. A classical condition is *pilonidal sinus* (from the Latin *pilum* = hair + *nidus* = nest). Hair driven beneath the skin over the coccyx forms a source of chronic irritation and often infection. It has an external opening. In the past, it was often widely excised as though it was a malignancy. It is now usually treated successfully by opening up the channel to the surface, scrupulously removing all the hairs and the lining of the sinus and keeping the mouth widely open while the cavity fills up from the depths (Fig. 4.71) to obliterate itself.

Fistula

1. The term fistula (Latin for pipe) is used in medicine to signify a pipe forming an abnormal communication between two epithelial surfaces. In some cases, removing the cause may succeed but if the track becomes completely epithelialised it will never close spontaneously. When the lobe of an ear is pierced and an earring inserted, epithelium grows through and lines the track, so that it will remain open for life. If there is infection (foreign material), neoplasia and a high rate of flow through the track it is unlikely to heal, especially if the discharge is irritant. This applies if a fistula develops from, for example, the biliary system or the bowel. The fistula will never heal if there is distal obstruction and the fistulous track is acting as a safety channel.

2. In some circumstances, such as when a fistulous tract relieves an impassable or unresectable obstruction, the fistula is beneficial. If a serious leakage occurs into a large compartment such as the peritoneal cavity, containment as a result of the development of a fistulous track spares the patient possible generalised peritonitis.

3. A *fistula in ano* results from inflammation usually in or near the lower bowel, although

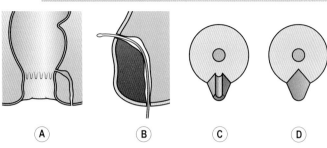

Fig. 4.72 Fistula. (A) Diagram of an anal fistulous track communicating between the anal canal and the perianal skin. (B) A malleable probe has been passed through the track and the intervening tissue has been divided (shaded portion), exposing the track in the bottom of the cleft you have created (C) when seen from the perineal aspect. (D) As a result of the packing and other measures to prevent the edges from bridging over, the cleft is shallow, smaller, and will shortly heal.

it may develop from a more proximal intestine. Infection may result in an abscess which sometimes 'points' towards the perianal skin so that a track develops between the bowel and skin. A probe can usually be passed from the external orifice, through the track into the bowel. If the track is now laid open (Fig. 4.72) and subsequently kept open until new tissue has filled the defect it may heal. This cannot always be achieved if the internal opening is high because it entails dividing too much of the anal sphincter muscles that maintain anal continence.

The standard method is to pass a probe through the track, usually from the perianal skin into the anus, then cut down onto the probe so that the whole length of the track is exposed. Such treatment transects intervening sphincteric muscle. The operation demands skill and experience to avoid excessive damage to the sphincteric muscle layers, rendering the anus incompetent. In some cases, extensive muscle division can be averted by first constricting the tissue to be divided within a ligature (a seton), which causes fibrosis so that when the muscle is transected the fibres are held by the scar tissue and do not retract.

4. Notwithstanding the definition of a fistula above, an arteriovenous fistula is an abnormal communication between two endothelial lined surfaces. This may be intentional as in an arteriovenous fistula fashioned for the purpose of haemodialysis in end-stage kidney disease, or unintentional such as following trauma. The latter would require a vascular surgeon to repair the injury and separate the two abnormally joined vessels.

Stoma

1. The term stoma (from the Greek word for mouth) applies to a natural or artificial mouth between an internal duct and another duct, another part of the same channel, or to the exterior. For example, the mouth is a natural stoma; a surgical union of the stomach and intestine is a gastroenterostomy (derived from the ancient Greek and Latin *enteron* meaning intestine and *intus* meaning within), and the exteriorization of the colon to the skin is a colostomy.

2. Provided the lining of the two surfaces fuse, the stoma is stable. If fusion does not occur, or if the epithelium is destroyed, fibrosis develops and as this matures it contracts so that the stoma constricts. For this reason, if you wish to form a permanent stoma as when joining the intestine at an anastomosis, joining ducts, or uniting a duct into the bowel, ensure that the epithelium and mucosa are sutured into perfect contact. When forming a colostomy (Fig. 4.73), mucosa and skin must be carefully united. In the past surgeons often brought bowel to the surface without uniting the mucosa to skin. As a result, a frequently performed operation was the 'refashioning of colostomy'.

3. A bowel stoma may be a small bowel stoma or colonic. A colonic stoma is made flush with the skin. At laparotomy, first, using a small scalpel or cutting diathermy cut the desired hole in the skin. Continue cutting through the fat until you reach fascia. Make a cruciate incision in the fascia and then use the points of a pair of Mayo scissors to separate the underlying muscle. If you have an assistant, two Langenbeck retractors can be used to

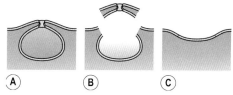

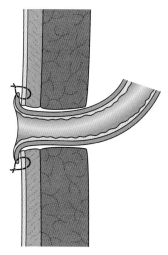

Fig. 4.73 External stoma. Diagram through a stoma in which the end of the bowel has been brought to the surface through a hole made in the abdominal wall. The end of the bowel wall has been everted so that the mucosa can be stitched directly to the skin.

Fig. 4.74 Deroofing a cyst. (A) A retention cyst: the secretions cannot escape because the mouth of the glandular cyst is stenosed. (B) The overlying epithelium and the roof of the cyst have been removed. (C) The lining of the cyst and the epithelium have fused at the edges and the surface gradually becomes uniform.

widen the orifice. Placing your nondominant hand on the peritoneal surface of the anterior abdominal wall where the stomal orifice lies, lift it away from the underlying bowel and using cutting diathermy make a cruciate incision in the peritoneum. With a Babcock, gently pull the bowel end that is going to form the stoma through from inside to outside.

4. Ensure that the bowel is not twisted or under too much tension. Allow for the fact that the patient may develop an ileus with some bowel distension postoperatively, which may place your stoma under further tension. Suture the bowel to the skin around the circumference with interrupted absorbable sutures. Ensure that the stoma is pink and shiny.

5. If you are applying a stoma bag, you will need to cut the opening to size. It often helps the bag to stick if the flange of the bag is slightly warm. Alternatively, Friar's balsam (tincture of benzoin) can be applied to the skin before sticking it on.

6. A small bowel stoma is formed with a spout to prevent the enzyme-rich small bowel effluent from causing skin excoriation; once the end of the small bowel is exteriorised, use a Babcock to gently grab the mucosa and some of the muscle wall approximately 3 cm from the free end. Stabilising the Babcock with your dominant hand, gently ease the free edge of the bowel back over itself, everting that part of the bowel held by the Babcock. When suturing this to the skin, take a bite through the free edge, a

seromuscular stitch, the now adjacent outer bowel wall and a third bite in the skin to which it is being attached. Continue these interrupted stitches around the full circumference, ensuring that there is good apposition of the free edge of the bowel to the skin.

7. A urostomy, or ileal conduit, is made in much the same way as a small bowel stoma, with a spout that prevents urine from excoriating the skin.

Cysts

1. Some cysts (from the Greek *kystis* = bladder, bag or pouch) are developmental, such as a *branchial cyst* (from the Greek *branchion* = gill). If an epithelium such as skin is detached and buried, it grows until it meets other cells of the same tissue, resulting in an *implantation cyst*. Some diseases, including neoplasms, result in cyst formation.

2. One method of dealing with a cyst is to excise it without opening it, avoiding spilling the contents. This applies to *ovarian*, *branchial* and *epididymal* (from the Greek words *epi* = upon and *didymos* = twin; it was an old term for both testes and ovaries) cysts. A retention cyst such as a sebaceous cyst can usually be excised under local anaesthesia; prefer to use a fairly large volume of dilute anaesthetic injected not into but around the cyst. This separates the capsule from the surrounding tissue, greatly facilitating the subsequent sharp dissection and reducing bleeding. If you fail to excise all the secretory lining of a cystic gland, it is liable to reform.

3. The most common cyst with which you will have to deal is a *sebaceous cyst* (from the Latin *sebum* = fat, suet; see Ch. 6).

4. A retention cyst near a surface can often be deroofed by removing the overlying tissue. The epithelium of the surface rapidly fuses with the lining of the cyst (Fig. 4.74). Salivary cysts within the mouth are amenable to this treatment.

5. A cavity such as a cyst can be occasionally treated by introducing a tube attached to a suction device which draws the walls together so that it collapses and shrivels.

Abscesses

See Chapter 12.

REFERENCE

1. Hasson HM. A modified instrument and method for laparoscopy. *Am J Obstet Gynecol.* 1971;110:886–887.

Chapter | **5**

Handling blood vessels

1. The anatomical arrangement of the main blood vessels provides general protection from injury and overstretching. Those in the trunk lie posteriorly close to the bony skeleton and are cushioned anteriorly by the viscera. In the limbs they lie on the flexor surfaces of joints. They are thus protected when the body is in a cowering or foetal position.

2. Transmission of blood is by *vis a tergo* (from the Latin *vis* = force, compulsion + *tergum* = the back; hence, compulsion from behind), propelled by the heart beating. Blood vessels are neither rigid nor undergo peristalsis. Luminal flow is largely as a result of autonomic nervous system control. Furthermore, blood flow is faster in the centre of the lumen than the periphery, where interaction of luminal contents can occur with the endothelial wall. The smooth flow of blood may be disturbed by turbulence, especially if there is irregularity of the intimal lining, such as by atheroma or an intimal dissection flap.

3. The internal surface of blood vessels is lined with endothelial cells forming a continuous surface. If these intimal cells are damaged, destroyed or separated by overdistension to expose the subintimal collagen, platelets adhere and trigger clotting factors. In the presence of local inflammation, the intimal cells release a number of cytokines and chemokines, and additionally express cell adhesion proteins (such as ICAM-1 and VCAM-1); monocytes and T-cells are attracted and become instrumental in an ensuing inflammatory process. Therefore, you should remember to handle

all vessels as little as possible because surgical trauma will render the vessel thrombogenic.

4. Arteries (from the Greek *arteria* = windpipe—after death, the arteries are empty and were thought to transmit air) have a substantial medial layer of smooth muscle cells. In susceptible areas such as at sites with disturbed blood flow and in particular in patients who smoke, have high plasma LDL, diabetes or hypertension, atheromatous plaques may form (from the Greek *athara* = porridge + -*oma* = tumour or swelling). Here, cytokines cause monocytes to differentiate to macrophages which may produce pro-inflammatory cytokines such as IL-6, IL-12 and TNF α. The macrophages become lipid-laden, so-called foamy macrophages. Intimal thickening may be seen, and proliferation of smooth muscle cells. The atheromatous plaques serve to narrow the lumen (Fig. 5.1). Calcification may also occur, rendering the vessel less elastic and potentially difficult to control with a vascular clamp. Veins are affected only when they are substituted as arterial grafts, bypasses and at arteriovenous fistulas. If the intimal cells are swept off the plaques, platelets adhere and expose the vessel to thrombus formation and possible stenosis or obstruction. If blood undermines the exposed intimal edge, a flap may be progressively raised that results in blood flow in a true and false lumen; a dissection. The texture of the vessel becomes irregular, friable and difficult to suture securely. In addition, in aneurysm formation (*ana* = up + *eurys* = wide) there is loss of smooth muscle cells, depletion of elastin and alteration in collagen distribution in the arterial wall; the wall becomes weaker and may rupture.

5. Vein walls have a thin smooth muscle media, since the pressure within them is normally low. Many are valved so that they transmit blood in only one direction. Because the blood flow is usually slower than in arteries, there is an increased tendency for clotting to occur if the endothelium is damaged, if there is stagnation or if there is a clotting diathesis (from the Greek *diatithenai* = to dispose; a predisposition). Obstruction to venous return causes distension. During pregnancy, intrapelvic pressure from the enlarged uterus compresses pelvic veins, dilating lower limb veins, widening the valve rings, so the valves become incompetent, creating varicose veins; the congestion may also distend the haemorrhoidal veins. Hepatic portal venous obstruction distends the portal-systemic anastomoses especially at the gastro-oesophageal junction.

6. During and following surgical operations on the blood vessels, clots are likely to form because of trauma, minute breaks in intimal continuity, stagnation, the presence of sutures and clotting diathesis.

7. Local anticoagulation reduces the likelihood, especially in arterial surgery, using 500 mL normal saline containing 5000 international units (IU) heparin to flush (10 IU/mL).

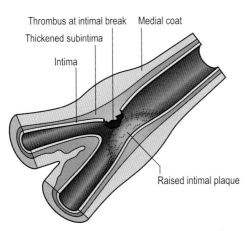

Thrombus at intimal break   Medial coat
Thickened subintima
Intima
Raised intimal plaque

Fig. 5.1 Atheroma at site of arterial division producing turbulence. Macrophages containing low-density lipoproteins accumulate in the subintima. The medial smooth muscle layer thickens and may dilate. At breaks in the intimal plaques, platelets and thrombus adhere to the subintimal layer.

PERCUTANEOUS PUNCTURE

Veins

Key points

- Your skill in gaining access to veins is frequently called upon, often in emergency circumstances with collapsed deeply placed veins. Practise, practise, practise.
- Ensure that you know the local anatomy to avoid damage to adjacent arteries and nerves.
- Repeated failure erodes your confidence and that of your patient. Seek help.

1. Veins are most easily cannulated when they are distended. They constrict in hypovolaemia, exposure to cold, and as a result of local trauma. Veins distend if they are warm, if they are placed dependently, or if mildly congested; this can often be achieved by simple finger pressure restricting venous return. For superficial veins in the limbs, having identified a vein to cannulate, place a tourniquet (preferably disposable) that obstructs venous return but not arterial inflow to distend the vein. If you tap on the vein, allow it to become dependent and ask the patient to exercise the distal muscles (such as clenching the fist repeatedly for the upper limb), the vein may distend more. Veins will also distend better in a warm environment and under general anaesthesia.

2. Do not overcongest veins, especially in elderly people; they rupture spontaneously or when punctured.

3. Ensure that the lighting is adequate; tangential lighting may be helpful by producing shadowing of the dilated vein. Be prepared to shave overlying hair to improve the view. A deeply sited vein can often be identified if you place one finger over the likely site. Gently tap proximally or peripherally, or for some sites ask the patient to cough. Your 'watching' finger detects the thrill. Some veins can be identified because descriptions exist of their anatomical position, with recommendations of site, direction and depth of needle insertion; for instance, the internal jugular, subclavian and femoral veins.

4. Veins that are not visible or palpable should be cannulated under direct vision with portable ultrasound. Near infra-red machines are now available that shine an infrared light on the skin identifying the veins underneath. Haemoglobin absorbs infrared light, so less light is reflected where there are veins which can then be detected by the machine and demonstrated by shining a light back on to the skin surface.

5. If you must insert a large needle, or carry out a subsequent manoeuvre, and especially if the patient is apprehensive, do not hesitate to inject a small volume of local anaesthetic intracutaneously through a fine needle; a 29-gauge needle attached to an insulin syringe has been suggested. Form at first a superficial bleb at a spot you can identify when the fluid has been absorbed. Allow a few minutes for it to take effect, then insert the needle through the site of the bleb. Before

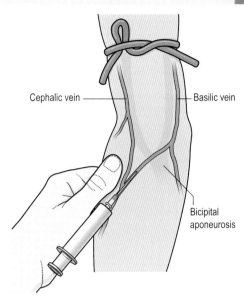

Fig. 5.2 The medial basilic vein, separated from the brachial artery by the bicipital aponeurosis, is a popular site for venepuncture. The proximal quick release tourniquet congests the veins; your left thumb to one side of the vein steadies it without compressing it. The right hand is omitted. Hold the syringe and needle almost flat with the skin, needle bevel uppermost.

inserting a large needle or one carrying an external cannula, first make a small incision with a pointed scalpel. The needle then slides easily through the superficial tissues and the 'feel' is not lost, as it is when the needle is tightly gripped by skin (Fig. 5.2). Apply a finger or thumb just beside the vein and draw it distally, slightly stretching the vessel to keep it in line. Alternatively, you may find it easier to pierce the skin a few millimetres distal to your intended venipuncture site so that as you advance the needle or cannula you are already through the skin and not impeded by its tethering. This also allows you to feel for the 'give' as the needle perforates the vessel wall.

6. Elderly patients often may present two difficulties. As some veins are distended and then punctured, they rupture and bleed into the tissues, obstructing the view. Avoid overdistending them. Others are thick-walled, slippery, and difficult to fix while puncturing them. Look for a junction which tethers the vein (Fig. 5.3) or apply traction distal to your venipuncture site to steady the vein.

7. If you press too close to the vein or apply too strong traction, you will collapse it and

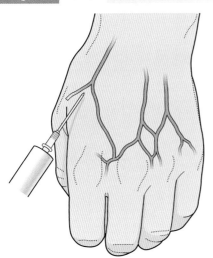

Fig. 5.3 The needle is about to enter a superficial vein at the junction of tributaries, where the draining vessel is relatively fixed. The right hand holding the syringe is omitted.

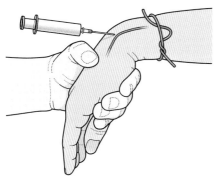

Fig. 5.4 If the vein lies near a joint you can flex it. This slightly stretches and fixes the vein, offering you a clear view along it.

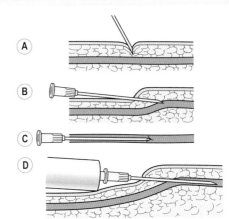

Fig. 5.5 (A) Pierce the skin almost vertically. (B) Align the needle almost parallel to the vein and prepare to 'squash' it into the vein. Notice the bevel is uppermost. (C) View from above shows the needle in the line of the vein, exactly over it. (D) The needle enters the vein, accurately lined up with it.

> ### Key point
>
> - Do not withdraw the needle until you have removed the tourniquet or there will be more bleeding and it will be more painful for the patient.

9. Apply gentle pressure through a sterile swab over the puncture site while you extract the needle and maintain the pressure for 3 minutes, timed by the clock.
10. Ensure that you dispose of sharps safely and preferably at the point of care. Do not resheath a needle unless it is the type that comes with a fold-over cover that is attached at the base of the needle. If you resheath a used needle you run the infection risk of inoculating yourself with the patient's blood.
11. When you require repeated venous access, such as for administering long-term antibiotics or chemotherapy, you will need to insert a central line or tunnelled line. These are inserted by venous access teams in many UK services. Haemodialysis patients with chronic renal failure will have an arteriovenous fistula created, anastomosing the radial or brachial artery to the cephalic vein. The increased pressure in the vein distends it so that it can be repeatedly cannulated.

your finger obstructs the line of needle insertion. When the site of insertion lies near a joint, exert gentle traction by bending the joint (Fig. 5.4).
8. Insert the needle, with the bevel uppermost, almost vertically through the skin, since the longer its track within the skin, the more uncomfortable the prick. Now direct it so that it lies close to, and parallel to, the vein. Angle the tip so that it 'squashes' gently into the vein to enter the lumen (Fig. 5.5). Check this by gently aspirating blood into the syringe, then advance the needle within the vein but avoid introducing the whole needle; if it breaks at the Luer connection the shaft cannot be grasped and withdrawn.

Arteries

1. Arteries are often mobile and if they are thick walled in elderly or hypertensive people they

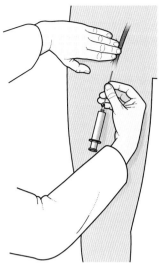

Fig. 5.6   Percutaneous puncture of an artery. Locate and fix it with your nondominant hand.

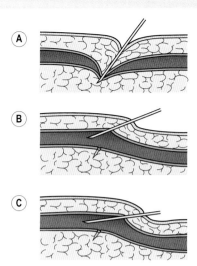

Fig. 5.7   Percutaneous arterial puncture. Rather than make repeated damaging attempts (A), transfix the artery, gradually withdrawing the needle (B) until blood spurts into the syringe, then (C) advance the needle within the lumen of the artery.

may slip from under a needle or be difficult to puncture.

2. Raise a bleb of local anaesthetic in the skin at the site of puncture and infiltrate the tissues around the artery.
3. Fix the artery if possible by pressing it against a firm base (Fig. 5.6).
4. Insert the needle with the bevel uppermost until it lies on the artery, then enter the artery at an angle, when small spurts of blood enter the syringe. The pressure required to puncture a thick-walled artery may collapse it, so make short jerky movements.
5. In case of difficulty it may be less damaging to transfix the artery cleanly and then slowly withdraw the needle until blood spurts into the syringe, rather than repeatedly stabbing into the thick wall (Fig. 5.7).
6. When you withdraw the needle have a sterile pad available to press on the puncture site; maintain this for at least 5 minutes timed by the clock, depending on the patient's clotting status.

PERCUTANEOUS CANNULATION

Cannula (from the Latin word for reed) suggests a stiff tube. Most modern vascular cannulas are commercially produced plastic sheaths fitted closely on needles; the distal part of the cannula being chamfered smoothly onto the shank of the needle (Fig. 5.8). A disadvantage of this cannula is that it cannot be longer than the needle. However, it has the advantage over a needle in that the plastic cannula is unlikely to damage or perforate the vessel wall from within. Moreover, if it is of sufficient calibre, it provides an adequate channel for the passage of a variety of catheters, guidewires and other instruments.

> **Key point**
>
> • Never reintroduce a partially or completely withdrawn needle into the cannula. The needle may penetrate the plastic cannula wall, detach it, and create a foreign body embolus.

Veins

1. To introduce the cannula, proceed as for percutaneous puncture. First raise a bleb of local anaesthetic, then wait 5 minutes. When you enter the vein, gently advance it against the increasing resistance as the tip of the cannula smoothly expands the hole to enter the lumen. Be careful to maintain the tip of

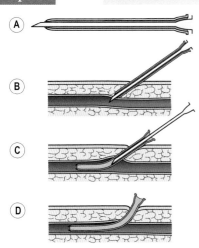

Fig. 5.8 (A) The closely fitting cannula is smoothly chamfered distally onto the needle. (B) The needle enters the vessel; then hold it steady. (C) Advance the cannula over the needle. (D) Withdraw the needle, leaving the cannula in place.

the needle central within the vein, to avoid damaging or perforating the wall. If you are cannulating a major vein such as the internal jugular or common femoral, then you should use an ultrasound to guide you.

2. When you are confident that the cannula has entered the vein, hold the needle still while gently advancing the cannula. Now withdraw the needle. For a superficial vein, with your nondominant hand, compress the vein just beyond the cannula as you withdraw the needle to prevent a brisk backflow of blood. Either place a lock, a three-way luer tap or connect up the cannula, maintaining control to stop it falling out. Secure the cannula with appropriate adhesive tape or dressing.

3. If you are in doubt about the correct siting of the cannula, connect a syringe and confirm that blood can be aspirated.

Arteries

Key point

- Do not start until you have confidently identified the artery.

1. Proceed initially as for percutaneous venous cannulation. When you enter the artery, gently advance the cannula against the increasing resistance as its tip smoothly expands the hole to enter the lumen.

2. Be careful to maintain the tip of the needle central within the artery, to avoid damaging or perforating the wall.

3. Watch carefully for incipient leakage producing a haematoma, while you are trying to insert the needle and cannula. Withdraw the cannula and compress the site for 5 minutes by the clock. Move to a fresh site.

4. When you are confident that the cannula has entered the artery, gently advance it while holding the needle still. Now withdraw the needle after preparing to connect or control the cannula.

5. Confirm that blood spurts into the syringe.

6. Secure the cannula and flush it with 5 mL of heparinised saline.

PERCUTANEOUS CATHETERIZATION

Hippocrates used the term catheter (derived from the Greek *kata* = down + *hienai* = to send) for an instrument for emptying the bladder. Like cannulas, they were also stiff tubes until the French surgeon Auguste Nélaton invented the rubber catheter in 1860. Intravenous catheters are made of plastic tubing. They may be inserted into veins or arteries. They can be passed through needles or cannulas, provided their external diameter is less than the internal diameter of the needle or cannula (Fig. 5.9). When the needle is withdrawn it cannot be removed from the catheter if this has an external Luer connection unless the needle is of a special type that can be split longitudinally and opened.

Whereas cannulae that fit on the outside of needles are usually limited in length, catheters that can be introduced through a large-bore needle or cannula can be of unlimited length, so they can be introduced at a convenient site and passed for long distances to the required site.

Seldinger technique

1. The Swedish radiologist Sven-Ivar Seldinger (1921–1998) devised in 1953 a technique for percutaneous introduction of a catheter. Originally developed for arteries, he extended the technique to be valuable in almost every system for entering blood vessels, ducts, hollow viscera, and natural or pathological spaces.

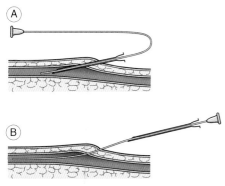

Fig. 5.9 Inserting a blunt catheter percutaneously using a sharp needle as a pilot. (A) A catheter passed through the lumen of the needle. (B) The needle withdrawn.

2. Initially inject local anaesthetic at the introduction site and make a small incision through which you will pass the needle, guidewire, and the catheter.
3. Introduce a hollow needle percutaneously into the vessel. If the internal calibre of the needle is insufficient, select one that carries an external, close-fitting, plastic cannula and withdraw the needle, leaving the cannula within the vessel (Fig. 5.10).
4. Through the needle or cannula pass a flexible, floppy-ended, round-tipped, guidewire into the lumen. Withdraw the needle or cannula, leaving the guidewire.
5. Pass over the guidewire a close-fitting but easy sliding catheter with a chamfered tip that will pass through the wall of the vessel. Ensure that you have control of the tip of the wire outside the patient before you advance the cannula over it in earnest.
6. If you need to pass a wide-bore catheter, either make a small cut in the skin adjacent to the guidewire or first pass a series of graded plastic dilators so the largest one can carry the selected catheter (Fig. 5.11). Alternatively, insert a small catheter and exchange over the wire.
7. Advance the guidewire and catheter, usually under imaging control, to the target site. If you are injecting contrast to perform an angiogram, ensure that all personnel are wearing lead aprons, and that the patient is on an X-ray translucent operating table. You will have checked the patient's renal function, and if impaired will select a low ionic contrast agent. Be sure to adhere to local radiation regulations.

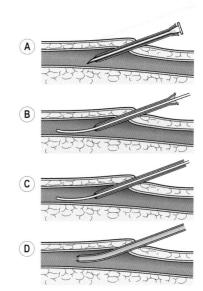

Fig. 5.10 Seldinger's guidewire technique. (A) Cannulate the vessel. (B) Withdraw the needle and replace it with the guidewire. (C) Withdraw the cannula and replace it with the plastic catheter. (D) Remove the guidewire.

8. A simple development of the technique has greatly increased the versatility and guidance of the catheter. If a catheter has a bend incorporated into the tip, the degree of bending can be reduced by inserting a straight guidewire. As the guidewire enters the curved portion, this is straightened (Fig. 5.12). The straightened catheter can be advanced, rotated and then allowed to regain curvature in order to enter, for example a side channel. A range of preformed catheter shapes and shaped guidewires are available for passage through stenoses, occlusions, often at awkward angles; for example the superior mesenteric, renal and intracerebral arteries.
9. Catheters can be inserted for long distances and guided to specific points. Locate the tip by aspirating and identifying the contents of the lumen. If the catheter tip is radio-opaque it may be visible on plain X-rays, or an imaging medium may be injected through it and identified on X-rays.
10. The technique has opened up a large number of possible minimally invasive investigations and therapeutic procedures within the circulatory and other systems. An expert interventional radiologist can collect specimens,

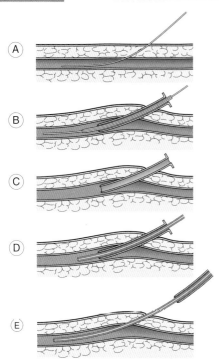

Fig. 5.11 (A) The Seldinger wire has been passed into the vessel. (B) Pass the dilator, carrying the insertion cannula into the vessel and over the guidewire. (C) Withdraw the guidewire and dilator, leaving the cannula in place. (D) Pass the catheter through the cannula into the vessel. (E) Withdraw the cannula.

deliver substances, obtain pressure measurements and make a radiological or imaging diagnosis often with the aid of injected contrast medium. In addition, vessels can be selectively embolised, ablated and controlled (see below).

Key points

- Never lose control of the guidewire. If you do it may be swept into the vessel and become irrecoverable.
- The guidewire maintains your access channel. Do not remove it until the procedure is complete.
- Recognise the value of acquiring skill in manipulating the Seldinger wire and catheters. It is a classical illustration of a versatile technique applicable in a wide range of uses. Skills are transferable.

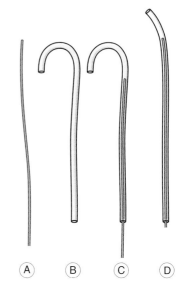

Fig. 5.12 (A) The straight guidewire alongside (B) the preformed curve-tipped catheter. (C) A catheter with a guidewire inserted through the straight portion of the catheter. (D) The straight guidewire is pushed into the preformed curved portion of the catheter, partially straightening it.

ENDOVASCULAR PROCEDURES

1. Many vascular procedures are approached by endoluminal methods.
2. The balloon-tipped catheter devised by Thomas Fogarty in the early 1960s can be introduced proximally into a blood vessel and passed distally through and beyond a soft clot or embolus. The balloon is inflated and then when the catheter is gently withdrawn it brings the clot with it. If necessary it can be introduced over a guidewire. For adherent clot, especially in prosthetic vessels, Fogarty has introduced corkscrew-like clot-removing wires.
3. Selective angiography can be performed by negotiating the catheter tip to the specific site and injecting contrast medium for imaging. In the presence of bleeding as from, for example, subarachnoid haemorrhage or Dieulafoy lesion (after French surgeon Dieulafoy, 1839–1911), the bleeding vessel may be identified by angiography and platinum coils injected to occlude it.
4. Angioplasty balloons carried by catheters can be sited across stenoses and inflated to dilate the vessel. The catheters will distend to a

predetermined diameter and rupture if over-inflated. Sizes extend from 1 to 2 mm diameter for distal lower limb vessels to occlusive balloons for the aorta. Coronary arteries can be dilated for the treatment of cardiac ischaemia.

5. After successful balloon angioplasty, endovascular stents may be inserted to maintain the channel. These may be self-expanding or balloon expanded. Reactive intimal hyperplasia may cause restenosis in half of patients. Drug eluting stents and drug eluting balloons are used with the aim of reducing this.

6. Endovascular aneurysm repair is performed using stent grafts made of polyester or polytetrafluoroethylene (PTFE) attached to a metal stent comprising either stainless steel or nickel titanium (nitinol). The grafts are introduced via the femoral arteries and deployed within the aneurysm. The metal stent provides radial and longitudinal support. The aneurysm is excluded from the circulation by the graft material.

7. Bleeding from gastro-oesophageal varices in portal venous hypertension resulting from hepatic cirrhosis can usually be controlled by transjugular intrahepatic portasystemic stent shunt (TIPSS). Under imaging control, a catheter is passed over a guidewire through the right internal jugular vein and superior and inferior venae cavae to the right hepatic vein, through which a needle and then a guidewire connect it through the liver substance to the portal vein. A self-expanding metal stent is then placed across, creating a portal/systemic shunt. The procedure is usually performed under local anaesthesia.

8. Varicose veins are treated by endovenous ablation. The Seldinger technique is used to cannulate the long saphenous vein and either laser or radiofrequency thermal energy used to coagulate the vein before removing the wire (see below).

SUTURES

1. Monofilament polyethylene or polyester-coated braided material are nonabsorbable, as is PTFE, which is used when suturing grafts made of that material. Sutures are mounted on curved, round-bodied, taper-pointed, eyeless needles. For the aorta size 2/0 or 3/0 is used, with diminishing sizes as small as 8/0 for small arteries and veins as a rule of thumb 2/0 in the abdominal aorta, 3/0 in the iliacs, 4/0 in the femorals, 5/0 in the popliteal, 6/0 at the mid-crurals and 7/0 at the distal crurals. Sutures can be supplied with an attached needle at each end—'double-needled' (often referred to as 'double-ended')—to enable you to complete an anastomosis with a single suture.

2. If the smooth surface of extruded, synthetic suture material is damaged, it is seriously weakened. Monofilament material is at greatest risk because a single break in the surface puts the whole thread at risk. Never grasp sutures with metal instruments except in segments that will be discarded, or drag them over hard, rough surfaces, or jerkily snatch them; you will reduce the strength by up to 50%. Extruded monofilament plastic threads have 'memory' and imperfectly locked knots tend to slip.

3. Insert sutures, whenever possible, from within the vessel lumen out. Especially when suturing diseased arteries there is a danger that a needle passed from without in (Fig. 5.13) will separate the intima from the media. Blood can then insinuate itself beneath the endothelium, diverting the flow away from the lumen and causing progressive endothelial stripping; a 'dissection'. The danger is greatest when the intima is lifted on the peripheral side of a break in continuity in the direction of blood flow and therefore most likely to lift the endothelium. For this reason, when suturing a transverse defect in an artery, start from the outside in on the upstream side, and from the inside out on the downstream side.

4. Bear in mind when suturing diseased arteries that atheromatous plaques make the wall fragile. You may need to vary the regularity of the stitches to maintain both the integrity and haemostasis of the suture line.

5. Carefully follow the curve of the needle by rotating your needle-holder; if you do not

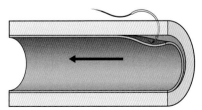

Fig. 5.13 Creation of a dissection. The arrow indicates the direction of blood flow.

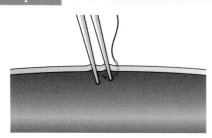

Fig. 5.14 Use slightly open dissecting forceps for counter pressure as you drive the needle through the vessel wall, not as graspers.

you may tear out the needle or thread, or enlarge the hole, so creating a point of leakage, so-called stitch hole bleeding.

6. Use nontoothed dissecting forceps held in your nondominant hand to assist you when inserting sutures. A DeBakey forcep is an ideal choice (after Michael DeBakey, 1908–2008, a pioneering cardiovascular surgeon who himself suffered an aortic dissection). Avoid gripping the vessel, and especially avoid grasping the endothelium. Use the forceps for counter pressure when inserting the needle; it is often convenient to allow the blades to separate slightly while you drive the needle through the vessel wall to emerge between them (Fig. 5.14).

7. Every stitch must pick up the endothelium and all layers. Every knot must be formed correctly and tightened correctly. The distance from the edges and between stitches depends on the size of the vessels.

8. Stitches may be:
   - Continuous: unlocked stitches are the standard method of suturing. Since they form a spiral around the circumference of an artery, each distending pulsation of the vessel tightens the spiral. Recovery of blood pressure following operation with arterial distension similarly tightens the spiral stitches, reducing the likelihood of leakage (Fig. 5.15A).
   - Interrupted: single stitches are appropriate for small vessels and in paediatric surgery because they do not restrict increase in vessel circumference as growth proceeds (Fig. 5.15B). However, because stitch separation is increased when the vessel distends, there is an increased risk of bleeding if the stitches are not correctly placed, correctly tightened and tied.

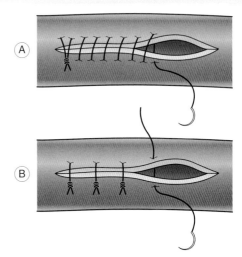

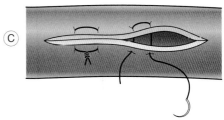

Fig. 5.15 (A) A single continuous spiral stitch. (B) Simple interrupted stitches, necessary when suturing very small calibre vessels. (C) An everting mattress stitch bringing together the endothelium from each side; it may be used to initiate eversion and can then often be continued using simple stitches.

   - Provided you can obtain perfect apposition of the intima, you should not evert the whole arterial wall with mattress stitches (Fig. 5.15C), which narrow the lumen (Fig. 5.16). Very occasionally it is valuable to start with a single mattress stitch to initiate eversion, or when suturing diseased arteries if a single stitch may cut out, or to start an anastomosis from the inside of the back wall of a fixed artery that cannot be rotated.

9. It is usually easier to insert sutures on a curved needle mounted in a needle-holder from far to near or from your dominant side to nondominant side. You insert the needle with your hand fully pronated, progressively supinating it to drive the needle through to emerge near you, or to your nondominant side. Follow the curve of the needle by a series of small 'pushes' through the tissue. If you merely drive it through,

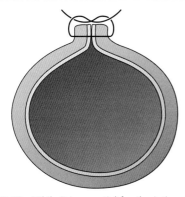

Fig. 5.16 While it is essential for the intima to be picked up with every stitch so the edges on both sides meet, the whole vessel wall should not be everted, or the lumen will be reduced.

you will produce a large stitch hole, resulting in bleeding. Until you are skilled, be willing to move to the other side of the operating table in order to suture in a comfortable, practised manner.

10. The skill of inserting stitches and drawing them to the correct tension to seal the vessel cannot be transmitted indirectly—you must assiduously watch your masters and learn the correct tension—do not let them loosen. Pass the emerging thread to your assistant to hold without changing the tension. Repeated slackening and retightening of the thread exerts a sawing effect on the vessel wall, with a tendency to cut out. It also damages the thread surface, weakening it. If you do find the suture to have become slack, you can gently pull the suture through, loop by loop with a fine nerve hook, before tying your knot (do not use a skin hook, as this may cut the thread).

Key points

- You cannot acquire the necessary skill to suture blood vessels from this or any other book.
- You must assiduously watch, and practise under the eye of your masters.

11. Knots are invariably placed on the external surface. They are potential causes of failure if they are improperly tied, either because they are imperfectly formed or tightened, or there is an insufficient number of half-hitches, or

because the material has been damaged by rough handling. The more knots, the more potential sites of failure. Tie as many as seven or eight correctly formed and fully tightened half-hitches, each successive one forming a reef knot with the previous one. Leave the ends long.

EXPOSURE AND CONTROL (SEE ALSO CH. 10)

1. Revise the anatomy beforehand but remember that blood vessels do not always follow the usual path. Disease processes may distort and weaken vessels and surrounding tissue. Blood vessels and nerves frequently run together within a sheath. In exposing individual blood vessels avoid damaging other structures.
2. On many occasions veins are exposed for partially cosmetic reasons. Never fail to mark the intended site of incision beforehand. Place the incision to produce the best possible postoperative appearance compatible with safe exposure, preferably parallel to the skin tension lines.
3. When exposing veins to act as arterial bypass vessels, handle them as little as possible. It appears that leaving the cuff of adventitia intact with the vein and manipulating the vein by grasping this rather than the vein itself reduces the tendency to spasm.
4. Gently open round-nosed haemostatic forceps on each side to expose first one side and then the other, to reveal any deeply placed branches or tributaries (Fig. 5.17).
5. Pass around the vessel proximal and distal tapes, untied ligatures or Silastic tubing (Fig. 5.18). They may, depending on the size of the vessel, be merely drawn upon to angle and occlude the vessel, or made to encircle it so that it can be constricted. Alternatively, control the vessel by applying nondamaging clamps or, for very small vessels, 'bulldog' clips (Fig. 5.19). In this way you can occlude and isolate a segment.

INCISION

1. Avoid damaging the intima when incising veins and arteries. This may occur if you make a rough incision that penetrates to or through the back wall.

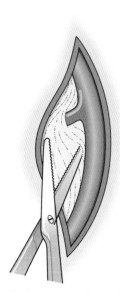

Fig. 5.17 Gently open round-nosed forceps at right angles to the artery to displace it and ensure that there is no deep branch at risk of damage.

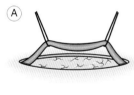

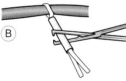

Fig. 5.18 (A) Encircle the vessel proximal and distal to the site of the procedure so that you can exert traction to tighten the tubing and occlude the lumen. (B) A tape encircles the vessel. The ends are passed through rubber tubing. If the tape ends are pulled tighter and forceps clamped across the tube, the vessel is occluded.

2. Diseased arteries may have loose plaques which can be dislodged; ensure that you make the incision as far as possible in a healthy segment. The scalpel blade may also dislodge the intimal coat, separating it from the media, potentially starting a dissection. A size 11 or 15 blade is preferable. Gently palpate for a soft portion of artery before making an arteriotomy (*arteria* = windpipe or artery + *tomi* = cut) or you may have

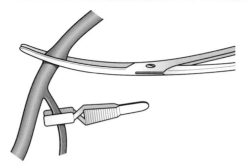

Fig. 5.19 Control of blood vessels. The larger vessel is controlled by an arterial clamp, the smaller by a spring 'bulldog' clip.

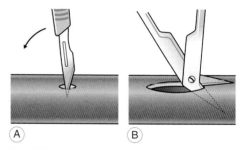

Fig. 5.20 (A) Start the incision with a pointed scalpel. (B) Extend the incision with Potts scissors.

difficulty suturing the hardened edges together afterwards.

3. Having entered the vessel, enlarge the incision using Potts scissors, ensuring the deep blade does not damage the posterior wall (Fig. 5.20). Cut cleanly without removing and reintroducing the internal scissors blade, to avoid producing a ragged incision.

4. Because veins are thin walled they usually accommodate to longitudinal or transverse incision. Large and medium-sized arteries may be opened transversely or longitudinally but smaller arteries are usually best opened longitudinally. When the vessels are closed, clot usually forms along the suture line. The lumen is less impinged upon by a longitudinal suture line than it is by a circumferential suture line at one point (Fig. 5.21). However, be aware that a longitudinal suture line is more likely to reduce lumen diameter.

VEINS—DIRECT PROCEDURES

1. Access to veins is a valuable means of obtaining venous blood for diagnostic purposes. They make valuable substitutes for arteries that are

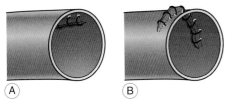

Fig. 5.21 Any clot forming on the longitudinal suture line in (A) is unlikely to cause serious obstruction, but clot forming on the circumferential suture line in (B) causes marked narrowing.

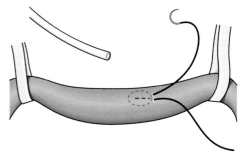

Fig. 5.23 A purse-string suture has been inserted into the vein and the straight dotted line within this indicates the site of a stab incision to accept the catheter.

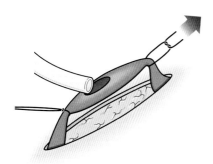

Fig. 5.22 The vein has been tied off behind the catheter. Apply traction with the ligature thread. The other ligature is left untied until you have introduced the catheter beyond it. Then tie the ligature around the vein and contained catheter to retain it.

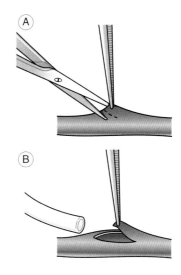

Fig. 5.24 (A) The vein is opened obliquely to produce a 'V' flap. (B) The flap is raised so that the catheter can be inserted under it.

stenosed or blocked. The most common venous disease you will encounter is varicose veins, which are lengthened, dilated and with incompetent valves.

2. Before inserting a catheter that will fill the lumen and remain, place and ligate a distal ligature and leave the long thread by which to steady and manoeuvre it. Place an untied ligature proximally. You may occlude the intervening segment by gently lifting, distracting and angulating the threads. Make a longitudinal or transverse incision in a large vein. Insert the tip of the catheter (Fig. 5.22) and relax the proximal ligature to allow the catheter to pass through. Tie the second ligature around the vein and catheter to retain it.

3. To introduce a small catheter into a large vein without occluding the lumen, first insert a small purse-string suture, with a formed but not tightened half-hitch, around the site of insertion. Control the vein using proximal and distal tapes, loops or nondamaging clamps. Carefully make a small stab into the vein and insert the catheter (Fig. 5.23). Fully advance it by partially releasing the appropriate occlusion device. Tighten and tie the purse-string and cautiously relax the occlusion, ensuring that there is no leakage.

4. Incise small veins by lifting a small portion of the wall and cutting obliquely with scissors to raise a 'V' flap. Hold this up while slipping the fine catheter underneath it and into the lumen (Fig. 5.24).

5. To insert a needle into an exposed very fine vein, utilise the ligatures on each side of the point of insertion to hold the vessel steady. It is sometimes an advantage to hold the needle in a gently closed needle-holder or haemostatic forceps for better control (Fig. 5.25).

Key points

- Do not allow air to enter large central veins for fear of causing air embolus to the heart and circulatory arrest.
- When tying off tributaries of main veins take great care not to narrow the main vein by applying the ligature too closely. Conversely, do not leave a cul-de-sac, which encourages turbulence, stagnation and consequent thrombosis (Fig. 5.26).

Varicose veins

These can be treated in a number of ways. First line treatment is conservative (elevation, support hosiery and lifestyle changes) but if this fails intervention may be considered.

Endovenous ablation

Endovenous ablation is first-line intervention following conservative management of varicose veins. This may use either laser or radiofrequency ablation

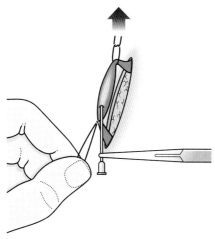

Fig. 5.25 Cannulating a very fine vessel with a needle held in a needle-holder or a haemostatic forceps.

to apply thermal energy resulting in irreversible occlusion and fibrosis of the vein. Laser ablation requires special laser protection and a dedicated environment. The procedure is done as a day case and may be done under local anaesthetic.

1. Use the Seldinger technique, under ultrasound guidance, to pass the laser or radiofrequency probe into the long saphenous vein in the thigh. Care must be taken not to cause damage to the femoral vein, so it is best to position the probe tip 1.5–2.0 cm away from the saphenofemoral junction. This is identified by looking for the three vessels the femoral vein, femoral artery and long saphenous vein in the transverse section of the groin (they appear like the head of Mickey Mouse, where the femoral vein is his head and in the right leg, the saphenous vein is his right ear and the femoral artery is his left ear); turn the ultrasound probe through 90 degrees and move the catheter caudally for 1.5–2.0 cm.
2. Tumescent anaesthesia is achieved using a spinal needle; inject diluted local anaesthetic (0.1% lignocaine in normal saline) around the vein using the ultrasound as a guide. This not only provides anaesthesia but, with good tumescence, also serves to protect the overlying tissue (the skin in particular) from thermal burns and compresses the vein onto the probe.
3. Tilt the patient into Trendelenburg position (see below) before applying thermal energy.
4. Two cycles of energy are used at the top, followed by single cycles until the exit of the probe. Remember to pull the cannula out before the last cycle and ensure that the heating part of the probe does not burn the skin at exit. Cover the entry site with an adhesive skin strip.
5. Avulsions can be done immediately after (see below).

Intravascular sclerosants

Intravascular sclerosants can be injected into minor veins after marking them. Approximately

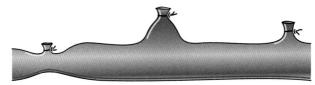

Fig. 5.26 Tying off side branches of a large vein that will remain as a conduit or be transferred to replace or bypass an arterial block. On the left, the ligature is tied too close to the main channel, constricting it. In the middle, the side branch is tied off too distally, leaving a cul-de-sac. On the right, the main channel lumen remains constant.

1–2 mL sodium tetradecyl sulphate 1% (range 0.5–2.0%) can be injected, preferably while the leg is elevated, then bandaged. Foamed sclerosant injected under ultrasound control is used for larger veins. Avoid injecting near the saphenofemoral or saphenopopliteal junctions because of the risk of embolization.

Local avulsions

Local avulsions are suitable for small varicosities as an alternative to injection therapy. It can be performed at the time of treating the truncal veins.

1. If few avulsions are required, you may use local anaesthesia. Raise a small bleb using a fine needle. Allow sufficient time for it to act, then inject more, insinuating the needle between the vein and the overlying skin to aid the separation.
2. Make a small incision over the vein, parallel to the skin tension lines. Gently open the incision, taking care not to tear the vein; then pick up the vein with a vein hook in one hand and clamp a small haemostat around it just below the hook to grasp it, ensuring that you have not grasped the skin. The vein can then be pulled out either by gentle pulling in the direction of the vein or by rotating the haemostat so that the vein wraps around the end of the haemostat much like a string of spaghetti on a fork. The vein will break off when no more can be avulsed through that incision. Apply pressure with a dry swab for two to three minutes to stop the back bleeding. Close the skin with sterile adherent paper strips.
3. As an alternative to avulsion, you may tie the vein after freeing it. This may be the case for a perforator. Dissect the vein as above and separate it from the tissues until you have encircled it. Pass a fine absorbable ligature around it using a curved haemostat and tie it off.

> **Key point**
>
> - Before operating on varicose veins, ensure that you have performed the appropriate tests, that you are thoroughly familiar with the anatomy, and that the veins are carefully marked. If you use a permanent marker to mark the veins ensure that you do not make your cuts over the ink, or you will tattoo the patient. It may be preferable to mark tram lines (on either side of the vein), to mark circles along the vein or if you do mark on the vein, to make your incisions just lateral to the vein.

Saphenofemoral ligation

Saphenofemoral ligation described in 1890 by the great German surgeon from Leipzig, Friedrich Trendelenburg (1844–1924), disconnects the long saphenous system from the common femoral vein. To facilitate the procedure by emptying the leg veins, he placed the patient head down, feet up; this is now called the 'Trendelenburg position'. Open saphenofemoral ligation is now third-line intervention and not commonly done. The principle is to remove the vein over a stripper which gathers the vein behind the head or olive (Fig. 5.27).

Arterial replacement with vein

Vein is frequently used as a conduit for diseased peripheral and coronary arteries. Because a healthy vein has one-way valves it may be reversed or if used in situ, the valves are destroyed.

1. A length of vein is harvested, the tributaries are tied off, avoiding narrowing. The vein is reversed so the valves do not obstruct the flow, and it can now be used as a bypass graft. Alternatively, if the vein is left in situ (with

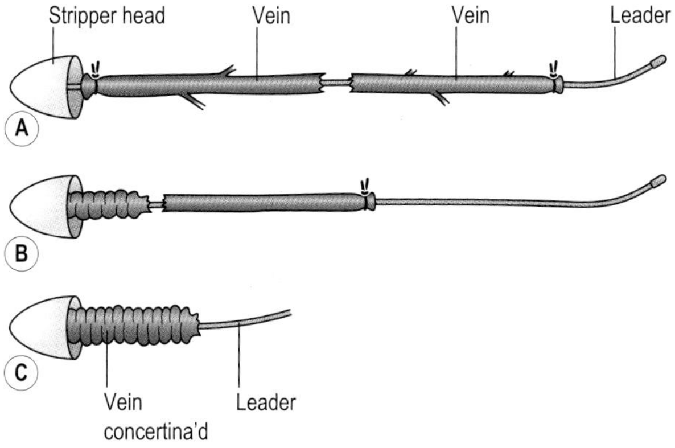

Stripper head   Vein   Vein   Leader

(A)

(B)

(C)

Vein   Leader
concertina'd

Fig. 5.27 Principles of vein stripping. (A) After transecting the vein on the left, pass the leader through the vein. On the right the vein has again been transected so that the leader can emerge and be brought out of the wound. (B) After ensuring that the stripper head lies safely in the subcutaneous tissues, exert traction on the leader in a controlled manner, drawing it to the right. (C) The segment of vein emerges, concertina'd on the stripper.

all the tributaries divided) a valvulotome can be used to disrupt the valves allowing blood flow.

2. It is important to handle the vein gently, avoid overdistending it and preserve the adventitia around it to minimise the likelihood of it developing spasm.[1]

Key points

- Damage caused by unrecognised overdistension is a cardinal cause of failure.
- Separation of endothelial cells exposes the subepithelium to platelet adhesion.
- It is one of the factors that make the difference between the success of one surgeon and the failure of another, even though they appear to have carried out the same manoeuvre.
- Keep it in mind when you are tempted to treat the tissues roughly.

3. Alternatively, in the leg a segment of saphenous vein can be used in situ after passing a special instrument (a valvulotome) to destroy the valves and united to the artery above and below the occlusion to bypass it. In this case the tributaries must be isolated and tied to prevent an inadvertent arterio-venous fistula.

ARTERIES—DIRECT PROCEDURES

During arterial procedures it may be necessary to inject or apply local topical heparin; in this case make up 500 mL isotonic saline containing 5000 international units (IU) to instil locally.

Incision and closure

1. First isolate the artery and obtain control using encircling tapes, untied ligatures, Silastic tubing, or placed but not tightened clamps.
2. Longitudinal incision and closure is usually suitable for medium-sized arteries but would seriously narrow smaller vessels, since eversion of the edges to obtain intimal contact increases the narrowing. Large vessels can be incised longitudinally and transversely without seriously narrowing them.

Direct cannulation

The exposed, intact artery can be cannulated or catheterised directly, either proximally or distally. First ensure that you have proximal and distal control. A wide-bore artery may be opened transversely but use a longitudinal incision for a narrow vessel. Insert the tip of the catheter and relax the controlling tape, tube or clamp while fully advancing the catheter.

Embolectomy

This is typically performed by direct insertion of a balloon catheter, invented by the American surgeon Thomas Fogarty (while he was still a medical student), to remove an embolus or clot, for example lodged in a peripheral artery.

1. Fully heparinise the patient with systemic heparin, 70 units/kg.
2. Control the vessel proximally and distally. Pass the catheter first proximally and then distally and withdraw it after gently inflating the balloon to fill the lumen and act as an extractor. As the catheterization is extended distally, use finer catheters.
3. Inject heparin in saline into the cleared vessels, prior to suturing the arteriotomy and releasing the clamps or tapes.

Vein patch

This offers a valuable means of avoiding serious narrowing of the lumen when closing a longitudinal incision in an artery. The patch must smoothly and slightly enlarge the diameter of the vessel. If it is too small it will not have achieved its aim. If it is too big it will so enlarge the lumen as to cause turbulence and possibly result in local thrombus formation and intimal hyperplasia. If you use saphenous vein select a proximal segment which better withstands the higher arterial pressure. Biopatches made from treated bovine pericardium are also available. Synthetic patches made of standard graft materials are also used.

1. Excise a suitable segment of peripheral vein just longer than the defect and split it longitudinally to form a flat sheet. Trim one end to form a rounded ellipse that will fit into one end of the incision. Take a double-needled suture of suitable size and insert both needles side by side through the elliptical cut end of the graft from outside into the lumen (Fig. 5.28). Bring them from inside to the outside, just beyond and on

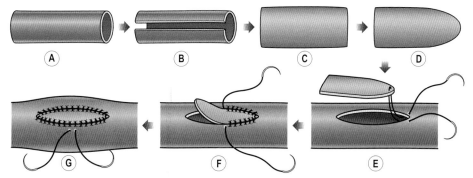

Fig. 5.28 Inserting a vein patch. (A) Excise a segment of peripheral vein. (B) Split it longitudinally. (C) Open it out. (D) Trim one end into a rounded ellipse. (E) Insert stitches in the patch and into the end of the arterial incision. (F) Continue round, keeping ahead on the back wall. Trim the end to fit into the remaining defect. (G) Carry the back wall suture around the end and continue to join the anterior suture and tie them off.

each side of one end of the incision, so that the suture is halved. When the suture is tied, it initiates an everting effect.

2. Continue from here, taking one suture along the back wall and one on the front wall as continuous over-and-over sutures. Each stitch passes in through the patch, out through the arterial wall. On the back wall, you may need to suture from near to far; as a beginner, be willing to change sides in order to sew from far to near. The flexibility of the vein patch makes it relatively easy to ensure that there is sufficient eversion to achieve intimal contact. As you reach the halfway point, leave the sutures on either side, while ensuring that the tension on them is not slackened, and direct your attention to the open end.

3. Trim the end of the vein patch into a rounded ellipse to fit into the remaining defect. Carry on inserting sutures on the back wall until you have rounded the end and continue on to meet the anterior wall sutures. As the stitching is completed, both sutures emerge on the arterial surface and if adjacent sutures are tied together, they form an everting mattress suture. Do not insert sutures in such a manner that at the end you cannot be sure that the stitches have picked up the endothelium. If necessary, have the tension maintained up to a point about 1 cm before you reach the stitch from the other end. Insert the last three or four stitches slackly, under direct view. Temporarily remove the clamps proximally and distally to allow blood flow to clear any debris and small blood clots. Flush copiously with heparinised saline. Reapply the clamps. Now you can tighten the sutures seriatim to the correct tension and confidently tie the thread to that inserted from the other end.

4. An alternative method is to start on the anterior wall near one end, with a simple running stitch and proceed around the corner onto the back wall. Continue along the back wall, trim the patch and carry the suture around the second corner, back onto the anterior wall. Insert stitches along this wall until you reach the starting stitch and tie off.

5. An alternative to using the patient's own vein for the patch is to use a commercially available biopatch. These are usually made of glutaraldehyde-treated bovine pericardium.

> **Key point**
>
> • Avoid finishing and tying the sutures at the end of an ellipse.

ARTERIAL ANASTOMOSIS

End-to-end anastomosis

A circular suture line results in some narrowing. This can be overcome by cutting the ends obliquely (vide infra). Any clot that forms on a transverse suture line impinges on the lumen through its whole circumference (Fig. 5.21).

1. When joining two arteries of equal diameter end-to-end, you can usually rotate the vessels, so enabling you to suture the circumference totally from the outside by taking one-third

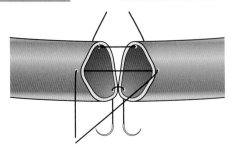

Fig. 5.29 Triangulation method of vascular anastomosis; the Carrel manoeuvre.

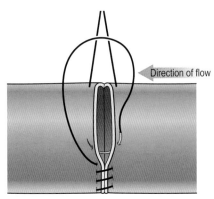

Fig. 5.30 When suturing an end-to-end anastomosis with a continuous running or interrupted stitch, insert the needle from without in on the upstream side, from within out on the downstream side.

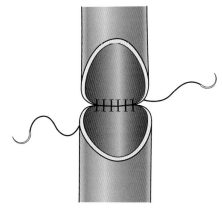

Fig. 5.31 End-to-end suture of fixed vessels starting on the back wall, identifying and picking up the full thickness including the intima in every stitch, and working towards the front.

at a time. Insert stay stitches between the two ends at one-third of the circumference intervals (Fig. 5.29). This manoeuvre was devised by the French founder of vascular surgery, Alexis Carrel (1873–1944), who won the Nobel prize in 1912. By picking up two of the three sutures and slightly distracting them, the intervening edges are brought together and straightened to facilitate stitching.

2. Begin by rotating the vessels in order to insert the first of a series of sutures, starting at the most inaccessible posterior part. Work on both sides to come around towards the anterior surface, using the traction stitches to rotate the vessels.

3. Use unlocked stitches, which form a spiral around the circumference; the suture is smooth and unlocked and can accommodate arterial pulsatile distension. The suture tightens as the artery distends, reducing the tendency for leakage at the anastomosis.

4. For small vessels and in children, use interrupted stitches. The continuous spiral in children restricts arterial growth in diameter.

5. Place and tie each stitch as though you will not be able to approach it subsequently. Take care to achieve intimal contact for every stitch. Insert the stitches from outside to inside on the upstream side and from inside out on the downstream side (Fig. 5.30). If the intima is separated on the upstream side, it will separate only to the anastomosis. If it is lifted on the downstream edge, the dissection may spread distally.

6. The interval between stitches depends on the size of the vessels but for medium-sized arteries place them 2–3 mm apart and inserted 2–3 mm from the edges.

7. Aim to finish on the superficial face and insert the last few stitches before tying them, while ensuring that the intima is caught on each side. Only then carefully tighten them seriatim,

using a nerve hook if necessary. When you are sure that every suture is perfectly placed, carefully tie them.

8. If it is not possible to mobilise and rotate the arterial ends, first insert the posterior stitches under direct vision (Fig. 5.31).

9. If necessary, leave the vessels apart; use a continuous, unlocked, double-needled suture; tighten the stitches seriatim starting with the posterior central stitch working outwards alternately on each side towards the most recently inserted ones, then continue round to the front. Ensure that everyone has a perfect grasp of the intima. This is the 'parachute' technique (Fig. 5.32). You can then continue on to the sides until the suture lines meet at the front.

10. In some situations, it is valuable to cut each end obliquely (Fig. 5.33), carrying the suture

line partially along the vessels, so that the incursion of the suture line into the lumen is less localised.

End-to-side anastomosis

When joining arteries, take care to avoid narrowing the lumen and also aim to reduce turbulence to a minimum. One way to achieve this is to insert a Taylor patch or Wolfe boot made with vein. Alternatively, you can make the anastomosis oblique angles—not at right angles—and make the anastomosis about twice the length of the arterial diameter.

1. Cut a longitudinal opening in the recipient artery approximately twice the length of its diameter. Slit the end of the tributary artery to open it and shape it to fit the opening in the main artery (Fig. 5.34).
2. Insert both needles of a double-needled suture from the outside in on the tributary 'heel' to inside out on the heel of the recipient. Proceed from here on both sides towards the toe. Prefer to insert stitches on the posterior wall first so

that you can view the internal suture and ensure that it picks up the intima every time, before commencing the anterior stitching. Stop when you have reached the halfway point towards the toe on the posterior and anterior walls.

3. Trim the toe of the tributary vessel to fit the remaining defect.
4. Now insert a double-needled stitch with both needles passing from outside to inside, just posterior to the end of the toe and from inside to outside in the corresponding end of the longitudinal hole in the recipient. Insert, with great care, the sutures around the extremity of the toe under vision. Suture the posterior wall up to the sutures running from the heel and tie the posterior suture, then complete the anastomosis along the front wall.

Key point

- The critical points are at the heel and toe. Aim to have 5–7 stitches at the curve of the heel and the toe in order to open them up.

MICROVASCULAR SURGERY

Take every opportunity to gain experience with magnification techniques. Over the years the instruments, materials and success rate for vascular surgical operations have all improved. The instruments have become more delicate, the suture materials and needles have become finer and smoother, and the techniques have been refined. As a result, vascular surgeons can confidently operate on smaller and smaller vessels. The trend will undoubtedly continue.

You do not need to undertake microsurgery to benefit from acquiring the techniques. They demonstrate a level of gentle tissue handling and

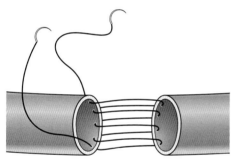

Fig. 5.32 Continuous suture anastomosis using the 'parachute' technique of placing the back wall sutures while the ends lie at a distance, then tightening the threads to bring the ends together.

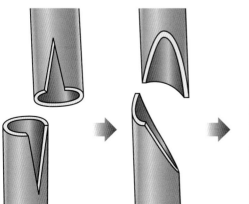

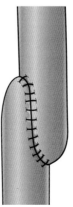

Fig. 5.33 Two small vessels are united after slitting the ends and opening them out to create a wide anastomosis.

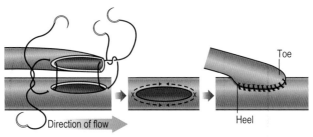

Fig. 5.34 A small vessel has been slit before joining it into the side of another vessel. The first stitch, a double-needled thread, unites the graft to the proximal opening in the recipient vessel. Unite the graft toe to the distal end of the opening with a second double-needled thread. The back edges are first united. Stitch from each end so the back wall stitches from each end meet in the middle. Stitch the anterior wall in a similar manner.

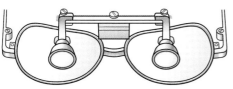

Fig. 5.35 A loupe fitting onto a spectacle frame provides you with magnified central vision and wide normal peripheral vision.

perfect apposition that can be transferred to the generality of surgery.

When you have the opportunity, examine a standard vascular anastomosis using magnification. What looked very neat is likely to appear coarsely fashioned.

Basic technique

1. The simplest form of magnification is a loupe (a French word with two disparate meanings—a knob or a magnifying glass). It may be fitted to a spectacle frame (Fig. 5.35). Try the effect of performing a procedure naked eye and compare it with a similar one carried out while wearing the loupe. You will be impressed by the greater accuracy you achieve with magnification. If you are starting out and do not normally wear spectacles for vision you could try some simple magnified reading glasses at x2.5 or x3.5 magnification to see the difference in vision.

2. Higher magnification is achieved using an operating microscope (Fig. 5.36). Ordinary

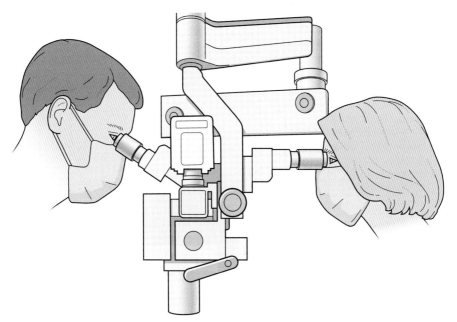

Fig. 5.36 Binocular operating microscope provides shadowless illumination. Operator and assistant can view simultaneously.

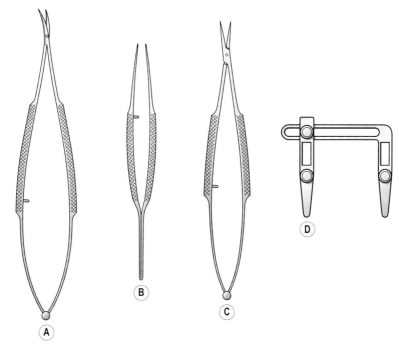

Fig. 5.37 Microsurgical instruments. (A) Scissors. (B) Dissecting forceps. (C) Needle-holder. (D) Vascular clamp.

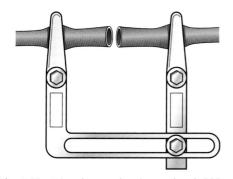

Fig. 5.38 Bring the vessel ends together, held by the double clamp.

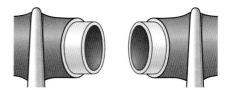

Fig. 5.39 Trim back the adventitia.

instruments appear crude using this, so special instruments have been devised (Fig. 5.37).

3. Blood vessels of 1 mm diameter or less can be anastomosed with nearly 100% success. They are conveniently held in apposition using gentle microvascular clamps (Fig. 5.38). Dissect off a cuff of adventitia since any tags falling into the lumen attract platelets and provoke thrombosis (Fig. 5.39). Intimal damage inevitably generates clotting. Never grasp it with forceps; instead, manipulate the vessels by grasping the media. You cannot produce eversion, so join the vessels end-to-end. Insert a suture through the anterior wall,

ensuring that it does not pick up the posterior wall. Pick up the other anterior wall and tie the suture just to appose but not constrict or distort the continuity (Fig. 5.40). Use interrupted sutures. Space stitches every 0.3 mm in arteries and 0.6 mm in veins, with three or four on each side. After completing the anterior wall, flip over the clamp to expose what had been the posterior wall and repeat the procedure. Irrigate the vessel throughout with heparin in normal saline or Ringer's solution (Sidney Ringer, 1835–1910, was an English physiologist), 1000 units in 100 mL. When the anastomosis is complete you may irrigate it with 0.5% bupivacaine. Remove the distal clamp, then the proximal clamp. Gently lift the vessel, slightly obstructing it and watch for a 'flicker' as blood flows across the constriction, confirming the patency. Apply local, gentle pressure for a

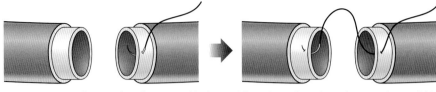

Fig. 5.40 Penetrate the vessel wall on one side from without in and on the other pass from within out, ready to tie the suture apposing the two edges.

few minutes if there is a leak. Occasionally you will need to insert an extra stitch after reclamping the vessel and washing out any blood adhering to the edges.

Key point

- If there is no flow, remove a couple of stitches, carefully wash out any clot and resuture it. If there is still no flow, carefully excise the ends and start again.

4. If you wish to create an end-to-side anastomosis, make an arteriotomy in the side of the recipient vessel one-third longer than the end of the vessel that will enter it.
5. Nerves can be accurately united using similar microsurgical techniques; fallopian tubes and vas deferens can be reconstructed in a similar manner.

REFERENCE

1. de Souza DSR, Pinheiro BB. Advantages of harvesting the saphenous vein for coronary artery bypass surgery using the 'no touch' technique. In: Abraham D, Handler C, Dashwood M, Coghlan G, editors. *Vascular complications in human disease.* London: Springer-Verlag; 2008:150–157.

FURTHER READING

Ramji DP, Davies TS. Cytokines in atherosclerosis; Key players in all stages of disease and promising therapeutic targets. *Cytokine and Growth Factor Rev.* 2015;26:673–685.

Chapter | 6 |

Handling skin

Skin is often referred to as our largest organ. It is our interface with the outer world. Among its many functions are protection from trauma and pathogens, temperature control and sensory appreciation, with the sense of touch being particularly specialised on the palmar surface of the fingers. It varies in thickness in different parts.

STRUCTURE

1. The epidermis (from the Greek *epi* = upon + *dermatos* = skin), up to 1 mm thick, consists of a basal layer producing keratinocyte daughter cells which progressively lose their DNA and become keratinised (from the Greek *keratos* = horn), and squamous (from the Latin *squama* = a scale). Average cell life is estimated at 27 days before the surface cells are shed; turnover is rapid, being estimated at 4 million cells per minute in some conditions such as inflammation and psoriasis. There are no blood vessels within the epidermis.

2. The dermis contains blood vessels, nerve receptors, sweat and sebaceous glands and hairs. The papillary layer lies beneath the ridged epidermal basal layer and where these are prominent, as on the finger palms, they form friction ridges corresponding to 'fingerprints'. The deeper layer is reticular (from the Latin *rete* = net) formed from interlacing connective tissue.

3. In most parts of the body skin blood supply is from the underlying muscle, vessels crossing the subcutaneous fat and forming loops at the

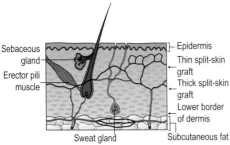

Fig. 6.1 Structure of skin showing epidermis and dermis. Note the levels, indicated on the right, at which to cut a thin or thick split-skin graft. The arterial supply is from the deep vessels directly or through deep structures such as muscles. They form angiosomes (see text) with linking small-calibre 'choke' vessels.

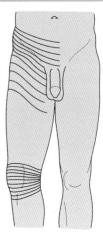

Fig. 6.2 Tension lines tend to run parallel to the creases seen at joints.

junction with the reticular dermis, supplying the capillary network. Composite blocks of tissue are supplied by the same source artery, each block being called, by analogy with dermatomes, an 'angiosome'. The angiosome arteries are linked by small-calibre 'choke' arteries that can open up to equalise the skin supply (Fig. 6.1). Likewise, the matching veins are unvalved, allowing blood to flow in either direction. Mobile skin is supplied by a few large arteries, and tethered skin by small dense vessels. The vessels are controlled by the autonomic system and shunts may bypass the dermis, notably in the ears, nose and fingertips.

4. Skin is unforgiving if it is overstretched, crushed, deprived of blood supply, or irradiated. Elasticity gradually disappears in old age and disease. The underlying orientation of the dermal fibrous tissues produces lines of skin tension identified by the Viennese anatomist Karl Langer (1819–1887). They usually run circumferentially around joint lines (Fig. 6.2). On the face they run at right angles to subcutaneous muscles and can be identified by asking the patient to grimace. Particularly on the face try to detect the relaxed skin tension lines that follow the furrows of the relaxed skin; they often follow the line between prominent underlying bones. If you gently pinch the skin between thumb and forefinger and the loose wrinkles of the skin lie perpendicular to the line drawn between your pinching thumb and finger, the wrinkle lines are a good approximation of Langer's lines for that area of skin. Incisions made and closed along these lines heal with less distortion and scarring than those made across the lines of tension.

5. Skin vitality is often difficult to judge by inspection. Viability in skin flaps can be assessed by administering sodium fluorescein intravenously and the perfusion rate measured with a surface fluorometer. Until we know all the factors involved, and how they interact, it is not always possible to predict the outcome following an injury, operation or disease process. Plastic surgeons have accumulated a great deal of practical experience of value to the generality of surgeons who need to cross the skin barrier to deal with their own special system of expertise. Take every opportunity to watch and learn from them.

HEALING

Open wounds

1. Healing is achieved through a complex series of overlapping developments: haemostasis, inflammation, proliferation and remodelling.

2. Initially, haemostasis is achieved by platelet adherence to the exposed extracellular matrix, forming a platelet-fibrin plug. Platelet chemotactic factors attract macrophages and neutrophils which are central to the inflammatory process. Inflammation is generated by many factors including ATP and nucleic acids released from damaged cells, cytokines released from platelet granules, and immune cells recruited by the fibrin matrix, bradykinin (from the Greek *bradus* = slow + *kinin* = to move), creating vasodilatation and loss of endothelial cell contact, with increasing permeability of vessels.

Neutrophils are established within a couple of hours of tissue trauma and phagocytose debris, as do monocytes, some of which convert to macrophages. These also secrete growth factors attracting endothelial cells, fibroblasts and epithelial keratinocytes. The fibroblasts become activated as myofibroblasts. Macrophages, reach maximum levels at three to five days and in addition to phagocytosis stimulate granulation tissue and angiogenesis. Cellular proliferation starts with the laying down of a provisional extracellular matrix (from the Greek *mater* = mother; womb, ground-mass or skeleton in or on which anything is developed). The complex matrix is composed of numerous molecules including fibronectin (from the Latin *nectere* = to bind) and hyaluronidase. This complex extracellular membrane is not a mere inert skeleton but involves integrins adhesion molecules controlling the attachment of cells to it and to each other—and ligands which bind to receptors and alter function. The provisional extracellular membrane facilitates cell migration and is gradually replaced with collagen.

3. During primary skin repair, keratinocytes are seen to proliferate. They release vascular endothelial growth factor, which stimulates endothelial cells to migrate and form capillary blood vessel loops, resulting in granulation tissue.

4. Epithelialization results as the daughter cells of basal cells flatten and migrate across the granulation tissue, guided by cell adhesion glycoproteins with fibroblasts laying down a basement membrane.

5. Remodelling occurs once the myofibroblasts begin wound contraction and can take weeks or months. Healthy granulation tissue forms a good base on which keratinocytes can migrate and on which skin grafts can be placed. Among the fibroblasts which accompany the new capillaries so formed are the myofibroblasts containing smooth muscle actin and cytoplasmic microtubules which draw the wound edges centripetally. This is wound contraction. It can be prevented by applying a skin graft.

Key points

- Wound contraction provides a natural method of closing wounds.
- Wound contracture, from the maturing and shortening of collagen formed as a scar, often results in loss of function.

6. The remodelling process takes weeks to years. Type III collagen is gradually replaced with stronger type I collagen, reaching 20% of its tensile strength at about 3 weeks and 80% at twelve months. A well-healed scar has only 80% of the strength of the original skin.

7. Intensive investigation is underway of foetal wound healing in which regeneration of epidermis and dermis occurs without scarring. Many differences from adult healing have been identified to include the influence of many cytokines (from the Greek *kytos* = vessel, cell + *kinein* = to move), small protein molecules acting as intercellular mediators. An important one is transforming growth factor-β released by platelets, which promotes the laying down of an extracellular matrix and influences fibroblast proliferation.

8. The influence of extracellular matrix is being extensively studied. Preparations such as sheets and powder applied to wounds are claimed to influence the regeneration and reconstruction of tissues instead of scar repair.

WOUND MANAGEMENT

1. A wound (from the German *Wunde*) is an open injury. From the history of the injury, sedulous clinical examination, and if necessary from appropriate imaging, assess the damage before starting the repair. Determine whether there is coincident damage to nerves, vessels, bones, tendons and soft tissues; in penetrating injuries, look for exit wounds. Do not blindly explore the wound if you intend to open it up at operation, for fear of causing further injury.

2. Remember that many injuries have legal, compensation and insurance implications, so immediately make careful notes, drawings and photographs if possible. Medical photography requires the patient's express permission.

3. Under sterile conditions carefully, and if necessary, widely, clean and prepare the area.

4. Explore the wound with fingers and probes, extending it when appropriate.

5. Completely stop bleeding.

6. Dirty wounds and those of doubtful viability should be debrided. Assiduously clean the wound. Irrigate it with plenty of sterile saline. In the presence of contamination, use only mild, aqueous-based antiseptics; strong and

alcohol-based ones damage the tissues. Take time to remove all the dead and foreign material. If you leave ingrained dirt, healing is severely prejudiced.

7. Search for and remove all foreign material and dead tissue. Do not leave dead muscle. Recognise it as being soggy and homogenised; it does not bleed when cut and does not contract when gently pinched with forceps or electrically stimulated with the diathermy.

8. Search for and identify deeper damage to vessels, nerves, bones and joints. Do not hesitate to enlarge the incision in these circumstances. If you do need to extend the wound in a cosmetically important area, consider following the tension lines. Make lazy-S incisions across the flexor surface of joints (parallel to the skin crease of the joint across the joint and extended perpendicular at each end with the perpendicular components joined to the transverse component with a gentle curve). Carry out appropriate repair of deep tissues before deciding whether or not to close the skin.

9. Finally recheck haemostasis, repeat the irrigation of the tissues and once more check for foreign material and dead or ischaemic tissue.

10. Do not close the wound if swelling has produced tension. You may be able to reduce swelling within a limb by first elevating it for 24 hours.

11. Unless the wound is clean, tidy, looks healthy and has recently been acquired, do not close it. Leave it open and determine to carry out delayed primary closure when it appears healthy. It is difficult to assess tissue perfusion and viability by appearance; the oxygen tension beneath a closed wound falls rapidly but is at atmospheric levels if the wound is left open.[1] If there is skin loss, loosely maintain the tissues in their correct position and defer attempts at reconstruction. If you are experienced you may cover a clean wound with a split-skin graft (see later).

12. If it is safe to close the wound but it is irregular and sited in a cosmetically important place such as the face, take the greatest care to align the skin correctly to avoid producing a distorted scar.

13. A wound of dubious viability or suspicious of ongoing infection may need a second look at 24 hours.

> ## Key points
>
> - Do not attempt immediate primary closure of doubtful wounds.
> - In the presence of delayed presentation, trauma, contamination, foreign material or ischaemia and tissue loss, be prepared to monitor the wound for 24–48 hours to allow you to exclude infection or impending necrosis, allow oedema to settle, and then carry out delayed primary closure.
> - Do not attempt to close the wound under tension.

Wound closure

1. The aim of closure is to appose the tissues in layers without tension or compression. The progressively complex steps of reconstruction are:
   a. Primary closure–suture
   b. Secondary closure/delayed primary closure (secondary intention)
   c. Local flap
   d. Distant flap
   e. Free flap

2. Provided you cause minimal trauma, and achieve perfect haemostasis, the risks of haematoma, inflammation and infection are reduced.

3. The result is rapid linking across the wound by fibroblasts and rapid healing with minimal scarring.

4. Secondary closure is spontaneous skin closure by a combination of wound contraction and reepithelialization. In the case of extensive skin loss, scar tissue is laid down and contracts as it matures, drawing in skin from the area, often resulting in loss of function. Continuous remodelling takes place while a defect exists and after healing has occurred.

5. Closure with a graft or flap is sometimes referred to as tertiary closure.

6. The healing of some open wounds may be aided by vacuum-assisted closure with a negative pressure dressing. The wound is covered with an absorbent foam layer. A drainage tube is inserted into, or laid on, the foam and the part is then covered with impermeable film. Suction is applied at around 125 mmHg between dressing changes (see Ch. 16).

ANALGESIA

(From the Greek *an* = not + *algein* = to feel pain; hence, to not feel pain.)

1. Most wounds will be too painful to explore without attention to pain relief. Smaller wounds can be explored under local anaesthesia. Larger wounds will require the assistance of an anaesthetist.
2. Always have adrenaline (epinephrine) 1:1000 and hydrocortisone 100 mg available in case the patient develops an allergic or other reaction.
3. Lidocaine (lignocaine) and prilocaine in a concentration of 4% is effective when applied topically on mucous membranes but is largely ineffective on the skin. However, consider applying it topically into open wounds or serous cavities, joint spaces and fracture sites. Lidocaine 25 mg and prilocaine 25 mg in 1 g of cream (EMLA) applied 1.5–3 g/cm^2 for a minimum of 2 hours under an occlusive dressing is usually effective in producing skin analgesia.
4. Local infiltration anaesthesia is a simple and safe method of producing a limited area of analgesia. Lidocaine 0.5–2.0% can be injected up to a maximum of 3 mg/kg body weight and its effect lasts up to 90–120 minutes. A maximum of 7 mg/kg can be injected with 1:200,000 adrenaline to cause vasoconstriction, reducing bleeding and slowing absorption. Adrenaline should not be used in end organs such as fingers and toes. Bupivacaine injected in concentrations of up to 0.5% with a maximum dose of 2 mg/kg body weight produces up to 12 hours of analgesia. It takes several minutes to take effect; lidocaine 1% and bupivacaine 0.5% may be mixed in equal volumes to overcome this. Ropivacaine 0.75% is an alternative to bupivacaine.
5. First raise an intracutaneous bleb, using a fine needle, away from a sensitive or inflamed area. Mark or note the place because the bleb will be absorbed and disappear. Always withdraw on the syringe needle before each injection, to ensure that you are not in a blood vessel. Inadvertent intravenous or intraarterial injection of local anaesthetic may result in cardiac arrhythmia. Wait for it to take effect, then inject through the anaesthetised spot, along the line of the proposed incision. You may produce a raised ridge resembling orange peel. Now infiltrate deeper, using a longer and larger needle, keeping the point moving as you inject, to minimise the danger of injecting into a vein.
6. Do not inject under high pressure, especially in the presence of inflammation. It is painful and the pressure of fluid will restrict the blood supply, as will the addition of adrenaline. A notorious risk when infiltrating a ring of local anaesthetic around the base of a finger is to raise the circumferential pressure, which may result in finger necrosis. Always inject proximally at the level of the interphalangeal web.

Key points

- Do not begin the procedure until the anaesthetic has had time to act. Wait a minimum of 4–5 minutes.
- You undermine the confidence and trust of the patient if your initial act causes pain.

INCISION

1. Decide the line and depth of the incision, taking into account the primary purpose of the procedure but secondarily considering the cosmetic effects, including the direction of the tension lines. If the incision will be complicated, first mark matching points with a skin marker pen or 'Bonney's blue' dye (Victor Bonney, London gynaecologist, 1872–1953) so that you can accurately appose them during closure. Do not make an incision directly over permanent marker, or you will tattoo the patient.
2. Stretch and fix the skin at the starting point using your nondominant hand (Fig. 6.3).
3. Except when creating a short stab wound, use the belly of the knife and draw it along the line of the incision, rather than pressing it in statically. Cut to an even depth throughout so that you can use the whole length of the wound. Do not leave half-incised ends that add to the length of the scar and add nothing to the access. Use the full length of your incision.
4. When possible cut boldly with a single sweep of the knife. Tentative scratches detach pieces that will undergo necrosis and delay healing (Fig. 6.4). Scissors are

121

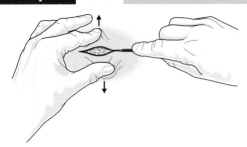

Fig. 6.3 Steady the skin using the fingers and thumb of your nondominant hand.

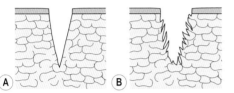

Fig. 6.4 Make smooth incisions, as illustrated in (A). Multiple cuts produce ragged incisions (B) with tags that will die and delay healing.

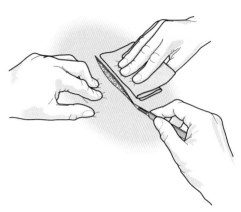

Fig. 6.5 Reduce oozing by compressing one edge with your nondominant fingers while your assistant compresses the other side. You may spread the pressure with a flattened swab.

occasionally preferable to a scalpel for cutting loose flaps, provided the blades are rigid and remain in contact; if they separate, the skin will be crushed and 'chewed'. Cut perpendicular to the surface to avoid slicing it. If you do not, you will have bevelled edges which will not oppose properly when you close the wound.

5. Control initial oozing from the cut edges by pressing with your fingertips along one edge while your assistant presses on the opposite side (Fig. 6.5). Use folded gauze swabs if necessary. Diminish severe oozing by applying haemostatic forceps at intervals of about 1 cm, to the dermal edges—not the epidermis—and lay the forceps handles onto the intact surface to evert the edges (Fig. 6.6). Never place haemostatic forceps on the epidermis. This crushes the skin and produces ugly scarring. The least damaging method is to retract the edges using fine skin hooks. You may identify and pick up individual vessels with fine artery forceps, twist them and release them. Avoid ligatures close to the skin surface. Use diathermy current sparingly since skin burns heal slowly; pick up the vessel with fine forceps and apply 'cutting' current at the lowest intensity for the minimal time. Bipolar diathermy is safer than monopolar diathermy since the current passes only between the two forceps tips and does not heat surrounding tissues.

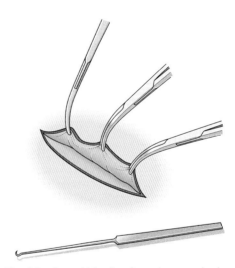

Fig. 6.6 Control bleeding from the wound edge, especially on the scalp, by attaching haemostatic forceps to the dermis and using them to evert the skin. However, handheld skin hooks are less damaging.

EXCISION

Skin lesions

1. Many lesions are amenable to excision under local anaesthesia. In the absence of infection, tend to use a dilute solution with added adrenaline, which can be infiltrated widely over the extent of the lesion to reduce oozing.

2. When excising skin that is diseased, scarred, traumatised, ischaemic or adherent to a lesion that must be completely excised, plan it carefully, if necessary marking the incision with a skin marker pen. Take into account the site; for example, facial skin has an excellent blood supply and heals well; palmar skin of the hands and plantar skin of the feet is specialised and cannot be replaced with skin of equal quality and nerve supply. Elderly patients often have mobile redundant skin.

3. When excising circular lesions plan an elliptical incision, aligned with the tension lines, with pointed ends (Fig. 6.7). The wider the ellipse, the longer it should be; otherwise the resulting scar will be ugly with a 'dog-ear' at each end. If you do find you have a 'dog-ear', this can be remedied by making a small incision at 90 degrees to the main incision from the apex of the 'dog-ear'. This raises a small triangular flap. As much of this flap as needs to be removed can then be excised to accommodate the skin of the other half of the 'dog-ear' (Fig. 6.8).

4. Excise benign lesions within the skin allowing minimal margins. There is no need to remove deep tissue.

5. Subcutaneous benign lesions attached to the skin may need to be excised with an ellipse of the involved skin. The specimen resembles a boat.

6. A malignant lesion should be totally excised with a margin of normal skin. In particular, *malignant melanoma* must be treated expertly. Its local invasiveness is measured by the Clark's level—the depth of infiltration. The most reliable prognostic measurement is the Breslow thickness from the granular layer of skin to the deepest growth. If the depth is less than 1 mm, a margin of normal skin of 1 cm appears to be safe but if it is greater than 2 mm a wider margin of at least 2 cm appears to be necessary. The incision should be carried vertically down to the deep fascia. Sentinel lymph node biopsy (SLNB) is now standard practice for skin melanomas providing both prognostic indication and a basis for further treatment. Whilst injection of blue dye may still be used for this, there has been much work on introducing new tracers such as radiotracers that can be picked up intraoperatively with a gamma probe, indocyanine green which is a near-infrared fluorescent dye, and single-photon emission computed tomography (SPECT CT).

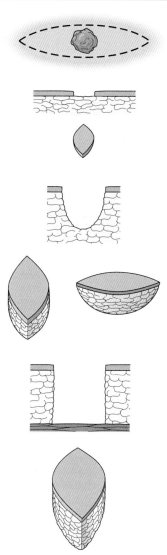

Fig. 6.7 Elliptical excision of lesions of the skin or attached to the skin. Above is shown the elliptical shape enclosing the lesion. It is preferably parallel to the skin tension lines. Below this is shown the horizontal defect resulting after removing a superficial skin lesion with the specimen below it. Below this is shown the defect resulting from the excision of a lesion extending into the subcutaneous tissues, and below that, the boat-shaped specimen. At the bottom is shown the defect following the excision of a possible or likely malignant melanoma, and the specimen with vertical walls extending down to the deep fascia.

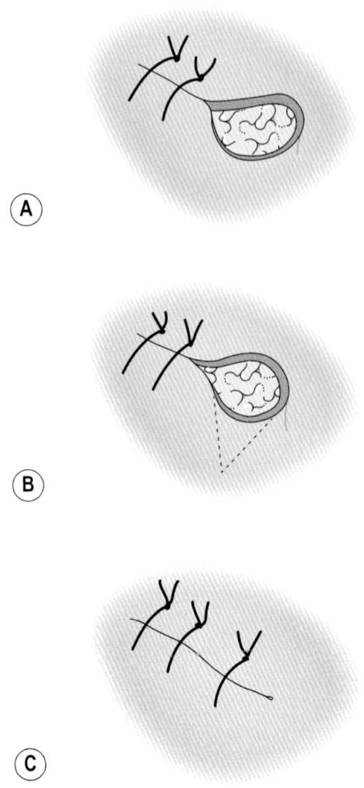

Fig. 6.8 Cutting out a 'dog ear' (A); the dog-ear (B) incision is made at 90 degrees to the end of the wound and an appropriate triangle is excised (C) so the skin edges come together without tension.

7. Make the incision while keeping the scalpel blade perpendicular to the skin surface to avoid slicing it. In some areas, such as the skin near the eyelids of young people, this may cause distortion and a local flap may provide a better cosmetic result.

Intradermal or subcutaneous cyst

1. This can be excised under local anaesthesia. You rarely need to shave the hair.
2. Carefully raise an intracutaneous bleb at the edge of the swelling. Through this inject dilute (0.5%) lidocaine intracutaneously over the top and around but not into the cyst. The volume of anaesthetic separates the cyst from the surrounding tissues.
3. Do not rush to make the incision. Allow about 5 minutes for the local anaesthetic to take effect.

4. Place the incision just off the centre of the punctum or summit of the swelling; otherwise, you risk entering the cyst.
5. Achieve haemostasis by identifying the small intradermal vessels and catching them with fine haemostats. The vessels lie in the subcuticular layer, not in the epithelium, so avoid catching this. As a rule, it is sufficient to leave on the haemostats until you are ready to close, but one or two vessels may need to be ligated with the finest absorbable material. If you intend to use diathermy coagulation, set it at the lowest effective setting and use it for the minimum time. If you burn the epithelium it will produce a visible scar. Prefer bipolar current diathermy.
6. Identify the cyst wall, work around it and gradually free it without rupturing it. Avoid grasping it with forceps. The last portion to free should be the punctum, attached to the skin surface; if necessary excise a small ellipse with it, to avoid puncturing it
7. If you rupture the cyst, carefully identify all the lining and excise it to prevent a recurrence.
8. After securing haemostasis, suture the skin.
9. As an alternative to a dressing, apply a varnish skin spray or tissue glue.

CLOSURE

Simple linear

1. Close a simple incision by accurately reapposing the living skin edges. To avoid any displacement of the edges of a straight incision, insert skin hooks at each end and have them gently distracted by an assistant while you insert the stitches.
2. Healing cannot take place if the dead, keratinised surface cells are apposed by inverting the edges. It is preferable to err on the side of slight eversion (Fig. 6.9).
3. For many small wounds, insert stitches 2–3 mm from the edges, 2–3 mm deep, and 2–3 mm apart. You may need to take larger or smaller bites depending on the site and the size of the wound closure.
4. Insert stitches on curved needles held in needle-holders. Use cutting needles mounted with fine thread. Use a monofilament polyamide and polypropylene suture. Use a 3/0 for the majority of skin wounds, but a finer gauge on the face, head, neck and digits.

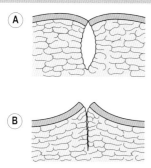

Fig. 6.9 (A) The skin edges are inverted, achieving contact only between the dead keratinised surfaces. (B) The edges are slightly everted; the living edges are in contact and can unite.

5. Grip the needle in the needle-holder on the swaged side of the middle. Fully pronate your hand so that the needle point enters perpendicular to the skin surface from the dominant side to emerge on the nondominant side, or from the far side to the near. As you progressively supinate your hand to drive the needle along the path of its curve, it emerges in the wound. Capture it and reinsert it into the other side exactly opposite. Progressively supinate your hand to drive the needle in a curved path through the tissues.

6. If the wound is in the sagittal plane in relation to you, insert the needle from your dominant to nondominant side. Start from far away and work towards you. If the wound lies transversely, insert the suture from far to near, placing the first stitches on your nondominant side, working towards your dominant side. This is not a firm rule. What is important is for you to feel comfortable and in control.

7. In some cases, you may pass the needle across the gap, to emerge on the opposite side. In other circumstances, you may need to pass through the needle on one side, capture it in the gap and reinsert it on the opposite side at a point in the same line. As the point emerges at the skin level, once more capture it, further supinating your hand to draw it through (Fig. 6.10). To aid the passage of the needle, gently apply counter pressure with closed dissecting forceps or use skin hooks to evert the skin edges.

8. If the skin tends to invert, use an everting mattress stitch (Fig. 6.11).

9. As important as the insertion of the suture is the tying and placing of the knot. Tie the

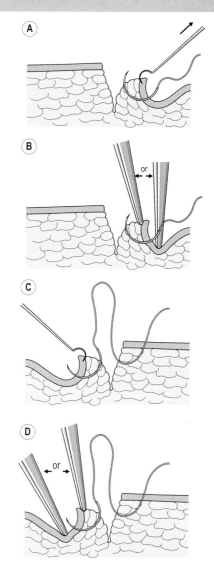

Fig. 6.10 Use a skin hook (A) or closed dissecting forceps (B) to evert the skin edges. Press closed forceps a short distance from the edge or use them to push back the edge to produce eversion. (C) Make sure that the needle crosses between the edges at exactly the same depth. (D) If you grab the skin with forceps you will crush it and cause scarring, so either grip the dermis with dissecting forceps or used closed forceps to deform it.

knot just tightly enough to appose the edges. The skin will swell slightly and if you tie it too tightly you will produce a ladder scar. Site the knot to one side of the closure, so the knot does not pressurise the healing wound.

125

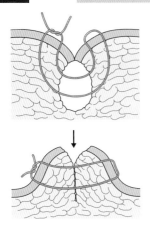

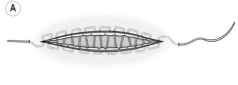

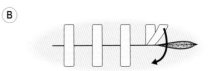

Fig. 6.11 An everting mattress suture will correct the tendency for the skin to invert.

Fig. 6.12 Skin closure. (A) Subcuticular stitch: when the stitch ends are distracted, the edges are drawn together. The stitch may be absorbable and can be left, or nonabsorbable and can be withdrawn. (B) Provided the wound is absolutely dry you may appose the edges using adherent strips of tape.

10. Remove sutures on the face after 3–4 days and after 7–10 days in abdominal and similar wound closures. In a wound area of reduced vascularization such as that following a limb amputation for ischaemia, you may need to leave the sutures for 2–3 weeks. When writing your operation note, you should specify when you wish the sutures to be removed.

Subcuticular stitch

1. An excellent alternative to conventional stitching is the subcuticular stitch, avoiding stitch marks on the skin. It is more difficult to ensure perfect apposition than when inserting conventional sutures. Use it only if there is no tension, or if you have overcome the tension by first inserting deeper stitches. Using an absorbable suture for this precludes the need to remove the sutures. Alternatively, a suitable smooth, nonabsorbable material is monofilament polyamide, polypropylene or polyethylene, though this will require an external mechanism such as a bead, a knot or skin tape at each end to ensure that the suture does not completely bury in the healing skin and can be removed. For small wounds, a rapidly absorbable braided suture such as Vicryl Rapide may be used.
2. Modern synthetic absorbable sutures can be inserted and do not need to be removed. Insert a subcuticular stitch at one end of the incision, pick up both sides and tie them together, burying the knot within the wound. Proceed from here along the wound, inserting subcuticular stitches on alternate sides until

you reach the far end. You may now tie a knot after taking a stitch through both sides. An Aberdeen knot is best suited to this. Alternatively, bring out the needle about 1 cm from the end of the wound to one side, and return the needle back through the same hole to emerge within the wound. Reinsert it into the wound to emerge about 1 cm from the end on the other side and back again. Finally, bring it to the surface and cut it off flush with the skin (Fig. 6.12). This offers sufficient fixation.

3. For a nonabsorbable suture, introduce the suture in the line of the wound about 1 cm from one end, into the extreme end of the wound. Insert stitches on alternate sides into the intradermal layer all at the same depth, each one crossing the gap at right angles to avoid distorting the skin (Fig. 6.12).
4. At the far end, drive the stitch to emerge on the skin about 1 cm beyond the end in the line of the incision.
5. The intradermal stitches lie parallel to the skin surfaces. It is necessary to have the needle-holder exactly perpendicular to the undisturbed skin surface in order to drive the curved needle in its jaws along a path parallel to the skin surface. Moreover, since you stitch alternately to one side, and then the other, you need to change the needle to point towards and away from you with each stitch. However, if you evert the skin using a skin hook or apply pressure with closed dissecting forceps, you can distort the skin edges, allowing you to insert the needle with

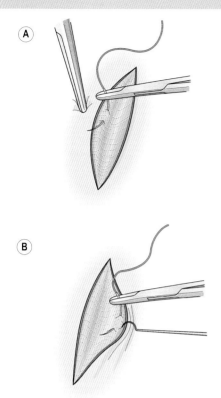

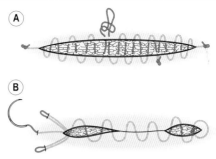

Fig. 6.14 Two tips when inserting subcuticular stitches. (A) When inserting a long nonabsorbable stitch, H. S. Tantawy of Cairo suggests coming to the surface every 5–6 cm, tying a slip knot, reinserting the needle into the same hole and tightening the knot down to the skin. A similar technique suffices to fix the ends. Withdraw the stitch in segments between the slip knots. (B) There are several choices for securing the ends of an absorbable subcuticular stitch. At the right end, an encircling subcuticular stitch has been inserted and tied within the wound. On the left, the needle has been brought out to the surface at an angle and returned through the same hole; repeat this at another angle and finally bring it out and cut it flush.

Fig. 6.13 Subcuticular stitch. By everting the skin edges, you can insert stitches that will be parallel to the skin surface when the eversion is relaxed. Produce eversion either by pressing with the closed tips of dissecting forceps as shown in (A), or by traction from a skin hook as shown in (B).

ease (Fig. 6.13). Do not use your fingers for fear of sustaining a needle prick.

6. Having inserted all the stitches, now distract the suture ends to straighten it, thus drawing the skin edges together. Tape the ends of sutures down to the skin. When the wound is healed, release the tethering, pull each end in turn to free the thread, then cut one end flush with the skin to avoid dragging it through the wound, and pull the remainder of the intact thread out from the other end. If the wound is long there is a danger that the incision will break when you try to pull it through in one piece; to avoid this, break it up into lengths of about 5–6 cm by bringing it to the surface and knotting it (Fig. 6.14).

7. Adhesive strips also offer an alternative to conventional stitches to appose skin edges (Fig. 6.12). Unless they adhere right up to the skin edges, they have an inverting effect, so ensure there is no oozing and that the skin is completely dry. If possible, first apply an adhesive such as a plastic spray or tincture of benzoin and allow it to dry.

8. Skin staples are sometimes used as an alternative to stitches (see Ch. 2). As a trainee take every opportunity to practise stitching. It is the most versatile method of joining soft tissues. Reserve staples for exceptional circumstances when these will be of benefit to the patient.

9. Tissue glue such as cyanoacrylate may be used for small wounds. This is highly adhesive and careful placement is imperative. It should not be placed within the wound. Firstly, you should ensure that the wound is clean and dry. The skin edges should then be manually apposed and a line of glue directed onto the line of the wound. The wound edges should remain apposed for 30–60 seconds to allow the glue to set. A further line of glue should then be applied with a thin line of glue on either side to increase the width of the glue application, giving it more skin to adhere to. Tissue glue should not be used on wounds where the skin cannot be closely apposed as it should not be allowed to seep into the wound.

Closing defects

1. Do not pull together skin edges under tension and expect them to heal.

2. In some cases, the skin edges fail to come together, not because there is a skin deficiency but because of a deficiency of the attached deep layers. You may transfer tension from the skin to the deeper layers by drawing them together first and then closing the skin without tension.

3. Close an elliptical incision (Fig. 6.15), if necessary after undermining the skin on either side. In order to appose the edges accurately, it may be convenient to start in the middle, working outwards. This tends to reveal the raised 'dog ears' that may mar the appearance of the scar. Mark out the base of the 'dog ears' and excise them so that you achieve a straight, flat scar.

4. Undercutting the skin is of value only if it is the deep attachments that prevent the edges from being drawn together (Fig. 6.16). If the skin is already tight, do not expect to succeed—the freed skin edges may merely retract further. Relatively avascular skin must retain its blood supply, so include the subdermal plexus within the subcutaneous fat. Evert the skin first with dissecting forceps or a skin hook, and later with the fingers (Fig. 6.17).

5. When the lengths of the edges of a defect are incongruous, insert guide stitches that will later be removed. Place the first of these into the middle of each of the edges, and place others halving the intervening space (Fig. 6.18), and so on. Now insert the definitive stitches and then remove the guide stitches; this way, you can spread the difference in length of the edges evenly.

6. If it is important to close a defect to provide skin cover, for example over a bony fracture, it may be necessary to create a relaxing incision over a parallel area with a good blood supply in the base, so that the adjacent skin can be slid across to close the defect (Fig. 6.19). Occasionally the defect you create to close the original one needs to be closed with a skin graft. Do not embark on such a procedure unless you have special training. Inexpert management will prejudice survival of the skin cover.

7. The most generally effective temporary measure is to apply a split-skin graft.

8. There are a variety of skin-harvesting mechanisms available. You should ensure that you are adequately trained in their mechanism before use.

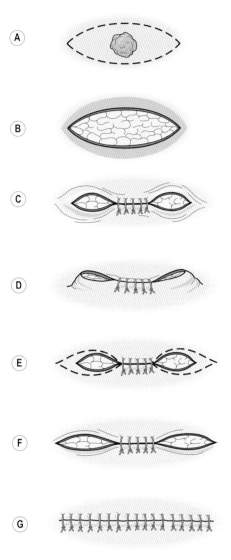

Fig. 6.15 (A) A circular lesion will be excised using an elliptical incision with pointed ends as in Fig. 6.7. (B) The resulting defect. The shading indicates possible undermining of the skin edges if this will facilitate closure. (C) Close the central part first. (D) This often produces raised 'dog ears' at each end. (E) Carefully outline the bases of the dog ears and excise them as in (F). (G) Finally, close the slightly longer but flat wound.

GRAFTS

1. The name is said to arise from the fact that shoots cut for grafting trees resembled a stylus or pen with which to write (derived from the

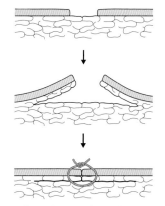

Fig. 6.16 If the skin is tethered but elastic, free it so that the edges can be apposed.

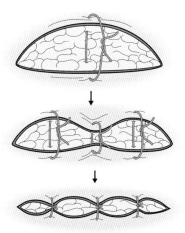

Fig. 6.17 While undercutting the skin, evert it to stay in the right plane.

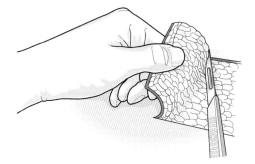

Fig. 6.18 If the length of the edges of the defect are incongruous, insert a stitch that joins the middle of each edge, then halve the space on each side, and so on. When you have inserted the definitive stitches, remove the guide stitches. This way you spread the difference in length evenly.

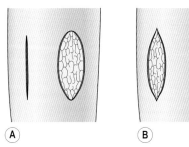

Fig. 6.19 (A) A defect that must be covered with good-quality skin; to the left of the defect a relaxing incision has been made. (B) The bridge of skin between the relaxing incision and the defect has been mobilised and slid across to cover the defect. The resulting gap could be closed with a split-skin graft.

Greek *graphein*). Its surgical use implies tissue that is totally freed and placed elsewhere, deriving its nourishment from the tissue bed in which it is placed.

2. Grafts can be cut under general or local anaesthesia. If you use local anaesthesia, consider first applying a cream containing lidocaine 25 mg and prilocaine 25 mg/g. Apply 1.5–3 g/cm^2 for a minimum of 2 hours beneath an occlusive dressing, over the donor area. Alternatively infiltrate the whole area with dilute (e.g., 0.25%) lidocaine with 1500 units of Hyalase.

3. Survival depends upon there being suitable conditions at the receptor site. These are:
   a. Adequate and stable contact between donor graft and recipient site. This implies that there is no separation because of graft movement, interposed necrotic or foreign material, slough, exudation, haematoma or seroma.
   b. Adequate blood supply to establish a source of nourishment. This implies no serious ischaemic or postradiation effects at the recipient site.
   c. Absence of certain types of microorganisms, in particular β-haemolytic *Streptococcus* type A, which produces fibrinolysin, thus prejudicing adherence of the graft.

Split-skin graft

1. This general-purpose graft, described by Karl Thiersch of Erlangen and Leipzig in 1874, includes some germinal layers but leaves behind the hair follicles, sebaceous glands

and sweat glands, which provide fresh epithelial cells to resurface the donor area usually within 1–2 weeks.

2. Split-skin grafts may be thin, requiring minimal nourishment and therefore surviving when the blood supply is relatively poor. They are fragile and not capable of withstanding heavy wear and tear. The donor site heals rapidly, allowing the taking of further grafts, which is useful if extensive skin replacement is required. Thick skin grafts demand a suitable base but once established are relatively robust. The donor site heals slowly.

3. The recipient site may be fresh, as following the excision of tissues including skin or preparation after skin loss resulting from burns, ulcers, pressure sores and other causes.

4. Following surgical excision or traumatic skin loss, immediate skin grafting can be carried out provided the base has an adequate blood supply; fat is poorly supplied with blood vessels and makes a poor recipient base, as does bone stripped of its periosteum. Before applying a skin graft achieve absolute haemostasis, since bleeding beneath the graft prevents it from adhering to the bed and gaining nutriments.

5. Healthy granulation tissue consisting of capillary loops and fibroblasts makes a suitable recipient base. It should be pink, fairly compact and not oedematous, with minimum exudation, and no slough. Take swabs for culture. Infection with many organisms does not preclude grafting, but group A β-haemolytic *Streptococcus* prevents successful graft take and releases hyaluronic acid, which prevents graft adhesion. If slough is present, be willing to excise it surgically. Ultrasound removal of slough is sometimes recommended. If granulation tissue does not form on a raw area, this suggests that a graft is unlikely to survive.

6. Cut the graft using a Watson modification of the Humby knife, which has an adjustable roller to control the thickness of the cut by adjusting the gap between the blade and the roller. As a rough guide, the no. 15 blade of a Swann-Morton disposable scalpel will just pass between the knife blade and the roller. A smaller instrument, the Silver knife, is valuable for cutting small grafts.

7. Grafts can be cut using powered dermatomes driven by electrical or compressed air motors. They reliably cut even grafts (Fig. 6.20).

8. Depending on the recipient site and the required extent of the graft, you may select the donor site. A common donor area is the

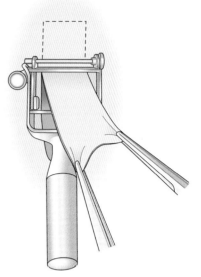

Fig. 6.20 Powered dermatome.

upper lateral front of the thigh. You need a flat skin surface and this is created by preceding the knife blade with a lubricated flat board held in your nondominant hand while your assistant holds a dry board, steadily applying counter pressure above the donor site to slightly stretch and flatten it (Fig. 6.21) with one hand, while supporting the undersurface of the limb with the other hand to create the largest, flattest area possible.

9. After adjusting the roller and lubricating the undersurface of the blade, hold the graft knife flat against the skin, concentrating on smoothly drawing it back and forth in a sawing motion, as you slowly draw the board just ahead of the knife, flattening and tensing the skin so that the knife blade does not drag it back and forth without cutting it.

Key points

- Closely watch an expert cut grafts and make sure you are supervised until you become competent at this procedure.
- Do not press hard or try to advance too quickly.
- Do not angle the knife or it will cut out.
- Try not to stop until you have completed the whole graft.

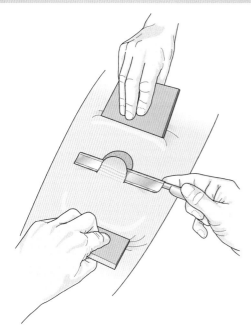

Fig. 6.21 Cutting a split-skin graft. Hold a lubricated flat board in your left hand and slowly draw it ahead of the knife held in the right hand, to flatten and stretch the skin as you cut the graft with a back-and-forth movement. Your assistant holds a dry, fixed board above the start of the cut to flatten, stretch and fix the skin. The assistant's other hand may lift up the soft tissues from below to expose a larger area on the upper surface.

10. The graft accumulates on the knife-like thin paper in folds. The donor site appears initially white, soon erupting with fine petechial haemorrhages if the graft is thin and with larger drops and more prolific bleeding following a deeper cut. Too thick a graft reveals subcutaneous fat. When you have completed the cut, raise the knife to lift the curtain-like graft and cut across with scissors.

Key points

- If you expose fat, do not continue; the donor site will not heal.
- Lay the graft back on the donor site; suture it in place and move to a different site.

11. Lay a large graft on tulle gras or paraffin gauze, outer side (dull, keratinised) down, living surface (shiny, pink) uppermost. Gently open

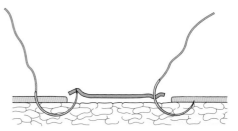

Fig. 6.22 On the left, the needle has passed first through the skin and as it pushes up through the graft it tends to lift and displace it. On the right, the needle first passes through the graft without displacing it.

out and spread the graft using closed dissecting forceps.

12. Pick up the tulle gras or paraffin gauze with the attached graft and lay it, graft side down, onto the recipient site, allowing it to overlap the edges of the defect. Make small incisions in the graft to allow for drainage.

13. A popular method of fixing the graft is inserting stitches around the periphery to fix it and use these to fix a compressing dressing over it. Insert the stitches through the graft and then through the skin; if you insert it first through the skin you lift off the graft (Fig. 6.22). Leave the suture long after tying it. If you cause bleeding under the graft carefully squeeze it out and maintain compression until it stops. When the graft has been encircled with sutures, place a carefully shaped cotton wool pad over the graft and tie the ends of the stitches over it to hold it in place. Plastic surgeons often use cotton wool impregnated with flavine emulsion or may alternatively use shaped polyurethane sponge. Depending on the site and your ability to attain fixation and create even compression, you may insert stitches only or compression only.

14. The donor site was formerly covered with tulle gras or paraffin gauze, but alginate dressings such as Kaltostat or an occlusive dressing are more comfortable. Silicone dressings are more expensive and less painful when removed. The donor site is more painful than the recipient site and takes 2–3 weeks to epithelialise.

15. Meshed grafts have several advantages. The skin is normally fed between rollers that cut it in a pattern that allows the sheet to be extended in a netlike pattern (Fig. 6.23). If a machine is not available, it is possible to create small mesh grafts using a scalpel. Meshing

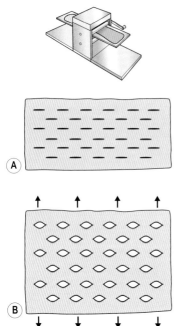

Fig. 6.23 The skin graft can be passed through a mesher, which produces small cuts. You can mesh it using a scalpel. (A) Make a series of cuts in the split-skin graft. (B) The graft can be stretched to increase its area.

increases the area of the graft, which is valuable if there is a large defect. Its other main advantage is that any exudates, blood or pus can pass through the holes in the mesh instead of gathering under the graft and lifting it off.

16. Store any spare skin graft in the refrigerator at approximately 4°C for up to 3 weeks after being wrapped in sterile saline-moistened gauze. Ensure that you comply with local tissue storage guidelines and that the specimen is properly labelled with the patient's name, identifying number and the date it was taken, as a minimum.

Full-thickness graft

1. This was described in 1873 by John Wolfe, an Austrian ophthalmologist who settled in Glasgow. It includes all layers of the skin freed of subcutaneous tissue. Because the whole thickness of the skin is used, the donor site will not heal spontaneously but may be closed after gently undermining the edges.
2. It is often used on the face because the cosmetic appearance is very good if the donor

site is carefully selected for thickness and colour. Favourite donor sites for replacement facial skin include postauricular, supraclavicular, antecubital and groin.
3. Because of its thickness the recipient site must be clean with a satisfactory vascular base and edges.
4. Make a pattern of the defect and draw it on the donor site with a skin marking pen.
5. Cut the graft with perpendicular edges, avoiding slicing them. Turn the graft and carefully cut off all the fat, since this will form a partition separating the graft from the base, depriving it of nutrition.
6. Carefully sew in the graft. As it is excised it shrinks and must be slightly stretched to normal tension to fit accurately into the new site.
7. The donor site can usually be closed as a linear scar.

FLAPS

A flap, unlike a graft, retains its blood supply through a pedicle instead of picking up a fresh supply at the recipient area like a free graft. These are mostly the domain of the plastic surgeon.

Random pattern flaps

Random pattern flaps have a haphazard blood supply. Because of this, the length of the base attachment is critical in relation to the length of the flap. Many such flaps survive better if they are raised but then returned to their base for 2 weeks before transfer.

Axial pattern flaps

Axial pattern flaps were identified when it was recognised that some flaps could be much longer in relation to the base and still survive. The reason proved to be that the blood vessels remained intact entering the base of the flap. These flaps may incorporate subcutaneous fat, fascia, muscle and bone.

Free flaps

Free flaps are axial pattern flaps in which the supplying blood vessels are divided and are then anastomosed to vessels at another site where the graft is needed (see later).

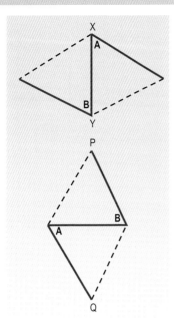

Fig. 6.24 Z-plasty. To extend the length of the line XY in the upper diagram, raise the triangular flaps marked A and B as far as the dotted lines. Transpose them and suture them in place as in the lower drawing so that the length PQ is longer than XY, at the cost of width.

Z-plasty

1. This overcomes the problem of linear shortening by taking advantage of the fact that skin is flexible and elastic; it may be shifted in from the side to increase the length of the contracture.
2. In Fig. 6.24, the diamond shape at the top is wider than its height. The line XY in the top diagram represents a linear contraction. Make an incision along it. At X, make an incision of the same length downwards and to the right at an angle of 60°; at Y, make an incision of the same length upwards and to the left at an angle of 60°.
3. Raise the flaps with tips marked A and B onto the bases marked with broken lines.
4. Now transpose A anticlockwise on its base and rotate B anticlockwise on its base so that they cross, as in the lower diagram. The diamond so formed is now taller than it is wide. The length PQ is greater than the height of the upper diamond, XY.
5. Increasing the angle of the side incisions increases the lengthening effect of the Z-plasty, decreasing the angle of the side incisions decreases the lengthening effect.

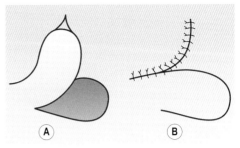

Fig. 6.25 Transposition flap. In (A), the excised area is shaded, and the flap is raised. In (B), the flap has been transposed into the defect and the gap left has been closed as a linear suture line.

6. A series of Z-plasties may be used to increase the length of a long contracture by incorporating width along its whole length.

Transposition flaps

1. When skin is lost or excised it may not be possible to draw the edges together, or to do so may cause distortion. A variety of flaps may be used.
2. A simple transposition flap can be used to close a defect (Fig. 6.25). If a defect has to be closed, a suitably shaped flap can be raised and sewn in to close it.
3. Close the defect left by the flap as a linear suture line.

Myocutaneous and compound flaps

1. As understanding of the blood supply has increased, advantage has been taken especially to close skin by bringing its blood supply with it.
2. An area of skin, nourished from the underlying muscle can be moved with the body of the muscle. Many muscles, such as the latissimus dorsi, have the neurovascular bundle enter them from one end. The other end, together with an area of overlying skin can be mobilised and swung a considerable distance to fill a defect (Fig. 6.26). The latissimus dorsi flap is frequently used to restore the contour following mastectomy. An alternative is the transverse rectus abdominis myocutaneous flap (TRAM) in which the lower rectus abdominis muscle and overlying skin are freed and swung up to the opposite breast.
3. Flaps may contain not only muscle but also fascia, cartilage and bone.

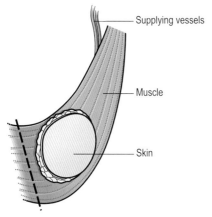

- Supplying vessels
- Muscle
- Skin

Fig. 6.26 Myocutaneous flap. The muscle has been transected along the broken line. The overlying area of skin, which derives its blood supply from the muscle, can be moved together with the muscle belly, hinging on its supplying blood vessels.

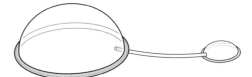

Fig. 6.27 Tissue expansion. The hemispherical expander is attached to a small reservoir. The expander is inserted subfascially or submuscularly. The subcutaneously sited reservoir can be injected transcutaneously with saline to gradually distend the expander and the overlying tissue.

FREE TISSUE TRANSFER

Since the blood supply can be identified and preserved in an axial pattern skin flap, or to a myocutaneous flap, the vessels can be detached and the whole can be transferred elsewhere. The blood vessels are joined into local vessels, usually two veins for each artery, employing microsurgical techniques (see Ch. 5). A popular reconstructive procedure following mastectomy is to free lower abdominal skin and fat, preserving the deep inferior epigastric perforating (DIEP) vessels and joining them to local vessels on the chest. As an alternative to the TRAM flap, this preserves the integrity of the abdominal muscles.

TISSUE EXPANSION

As an alternative to bringing in skin from elsewhere, local skin can often be obtained by expanding it. This is achieved by placing a plastic container under the fascia or muscle (Fig. 6.27). The container is connected through a tube. Over a period, saline can be injected into the reservoir to increase its bulk and expand the skin. When sufficient expansion has been achieved the plastic container can be removed and the spare skin is available to close a deficiency.

AESTHETIC PROCEDURES

Many procedures have been introduced to improve appearance, termed 'cosmetic' (from the Greek *kosmos* = order + *kosmein* = to adorn) or 'aesthetic' (from the Greek *aesthesthai* = feel or perceive; possessing or claiming to possess a sense of beauty).

Liposuction

Liposuction is the most frequently performed aesthetic procedure in the USA. A slim cannula is inserted into the subcutaneous tissue to remove excess fat. It is now usually power assisted with infiltration of fluid such as Ringer lactate, often containing lidocaine and adrenaline. Adjunctive ultrasonic cavitation of the fat cells facilitates the removal.

Lipoplasty

Autologous fat transfer is a method of increasing contour.

Clostridium botulinum

Clostridium botulinum type A neurotoxin complex injections into facial muscles paralyse them, reducing wrinkles. The effect typically occurs within 3–7 days and lasts up to 4 months.

Breast procedures

Following surgical operations for disease, repair and replacement may be achieved using skin grafts and flaps such as latissimus dorsi or transverse rectus abdominis myocutaneous (TRAM) (see also Ch. 7). A range of procedures are used to improve the contour. Implants are now usually of cohesive gel. Tissue expansion by, for example, a DIEP flap, is intended to replace or change the contour. Breast reduction may be performed to lessen the size and weight of excessively large breasts; also, following a partial mastectomy for disease on one side, the other breast may be reduced to match it.

FURTHER READING

Chang N, Goodson WH III, Gottrup F, Hunt TK. Direct measurement of wound and tissue oxygen tension in postoperative patients. *Ann Surg.* 1983;197:470–478.

Rutkowski P. Introduction to the special issue of European Journal of Surgical Oncology: New roads in melanoma management. *Eur J Surg Oncol.* 2017;43(3):513–516.

Grassetti L, et al. Aesthetic refinement of the dog ear correction: the 90 degree incision technique and review of the literature. *Arch Plast Surg.* 2013;40(3):268–269.

Moretti L, et al. The interplay of fibroblasts, the extracellular matrix, and inflammation in scar formation. *J Biol Chem.* 2022;298(2):101530.

Morrison S, Han D. Re-Evaluation of Sentinel Lymph Node Biopsy for Melanoma. *Curr Treat Options Oncol.* 2021;22:22.

Chapter | 7 |

Handling connective and soft tissues

Our bodies are composed of a wide variety of tissues. Some are homogeneous (from the Greek *homos* = same + *genos* = kind; made up of the same kind of cell) but most are a mixture of parenchymal cells, the soft active cells held together with connective tissue and permeated by vascular, neural and other structures. The connective tissue forms a scaffold or matrix supporting the parenchymal cells; the supportive cells are not merely passive or standardised but react with the parenchymal cells in health and disease.

> **Key points**
>
> - Familiarise yourself with the anatomy, structure, texture, surroundings, strength and fragility, at different ages and nutritional states, and in health and in various diseased states.
> - In addition, familiarise yourself with the tissue planes between the target structure and the surrounding tissues. Otherwise, you risk causing inadvertent damage.

PERCUTANEOUS DIAGNOSTIC PROCEDURES

Many procedures can be carried out under local anaesthesia. The availability of ultrasound and other imaging techniques, and advanced cytological techniques enables targeted diagnostic capture of fluid, microorganisms and cells, and the introduction of, for example, radio-opaque medium, into most places within the body. For example, breast, thyroid and prostate glands and superficial lymph nodes are commonly investigated in this way. For deep structures, fine 'skinny' needles of 0.7 mm external and 0.5 mm internal diameter can be introduced into many organs, especially the liver and lungs, while respiration is temporarily suspended.

Aspiration of fluid for cytology

1. Before you insert the needle, try to confirm the exact location of the fluid by eliciting fluctuation. If the fluid collection is superficial and large enough you may be able to transilluminate it by shining a pen torch light through it. If the fluid lies deep, you may use imaging methods such as ultrasound.
2. Carry out the procedure under sterile conditions. Use a needle that is long enough so you do not need to insert it to the Luer connection; otherwise, if it breaks off at the junction with the shaft, you may not be able to recapture the needle.
3. Attach a syringe and aspirate. If you obtain no fluid, try rotating the needle. Do not alter the direction of the needle except by first withdrawing it. It is best to begin aspiration slowly so that you have an idea of the viscosity of the fluid, and whether or not it is blood stained. Sudden high aspiration pressure may cause tissue trauma and iatrogenic blood staining.
4. Fine-needle aspiration cytology (FNAC) can often be carried out under local anaesthetic although even this may be unnecessary. Fix the target between the fingers of one hand while holding the syringe and needle (usually a 21-gauge) in the other.
5. When the tip is correctly sited apply suction by attempting to withdraw the piston of the syringe. Move the needle in and out in jerky

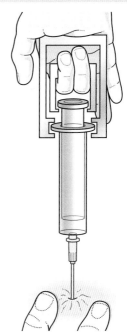

Fig. 7.1 The principle of fine-needle aspiration cytology. The action of a syringe holder allows the syringe and needle to be controlled with one hand while the other steadies the lump. Squeezing the handle of the syringe holder draws out the piston and exerts a suction effect through the attached needle.

reciprocal movements to detach cells, which will be drawn into the needle.
6. Simultaneous fixation of a lump, control of the needle position and aspiration of a standard syringe are difficult. A number of mechanical aids are available based on the principle shown in Fig. 7.1.
7. Cell harvesting is improved if the syringe and needle are first washed out with a mixture of physiological (0.9%) saline with 1000 units of heparin. After completing the procedure, withdraw the syringe and needle, eject the contents onto several prelabelled microscope slides and immediately apply fixative to them. Finally, draw up some fixative through the needle into the syringe from a specimen bottle and empty the syringe back into the bottle. The ejected cells will be recovered by centrifugation and stained along with those on the slides, for cytological examination. In some cases, the cells are immediately smeared onto a slide using a cover slip, air dried and then stained.

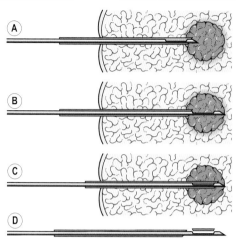

Fig. 7.2 Needle biopsy. (A) Insert the closed needle tip into the tissue that will be biopsied; (B) hold the needle still and advance the stylette into the tissue. Some of the tissue bulges against the thin shaft of the stylette; (C) hold the stylette still and advance the needle to cut off and enclose the core of tissue; (D) withdraw the needle and retrieve the core of tissue.

Needle biopsy

1. In order to confirm the histological diagnosis and grade, identify the receptor status, carry out a DNA analysis of a tumour, and obtain a core of tissue. Take advice beforehand from the pathologist about how the specimen should be preserved and sent for examination.
2. If the lesion is not palpable the needle may be guided with the aid of ultrasound or radiological imaging.
3. One method is with a hollow needle such as a Trucut (Travenol). From the end of a sharp hollow needle protrudes the bevelled cutting end of a stylette. The proximal part of the stylette does not fill the lumen of the needle (Fig. 7.2). After infiltrating the skin with local anaesthetic, make a small incision with a pointed scalpel, just large enough to accept the needle. Insert the closed needle through the incision and into the lump to be biopsied, while steadying a mobile lump with the fingers of the other hand.
4. Hold the needle still and advance the stylette further into the lump. Now hold the stylette still and advance the needle, which cuts off and encloses the tissue that bulged into the thinned section of the stylette. If the tissue is very hard, advance the closed needle into the lesion, hold the stylette still, withdraw, then advance the needle to close it.

5. Draw out the closed needle, then retract the needle to expose the specimen resting on the thinned section of the stylette. Place the specimen in the appropriate fixative and immediately label the container, fill out the request form and ensure that the specimen is sent promptly to the laboratory.
6. A spring-loaded wide-bore needle can be used, or a drill biopsy (a high-speed rotating hollow needle).
7. All forms of needle biopsy may cause severe bleeding, so apply steady pressure over the track for 3–5 minutes, timed by the clock.

Open biopsy

Excision biopsy implies removing the whole structure or lesion such as a discrete lump on its own or lying within more homogeneous tissue. This is intended to remove the lesion completely while providing material for histological examination. It is especially valuable if you think the lesion is (or could be) malignant; if this is a possibility, you must avoid transgressing into the lesion and potentially spreading tumour cells. In this case, assiduously keep the plane of dissection in healthy tissue. Some lesions appear to have a capsule and the dissection may be extracapsular, but the presence of a capsule does not preclude malignant penetration through it into the surrounding tissues.

Key points
• An apparent capsule may be merely compressed normal or abnormal tissues as a result of tumour expansion. • Even if there is a true capsule, it may have been infiltrated by malignant cells passing through to the surrounding tissues.

Incision biopsy involves the removal of a portion from a large structure. It provides material for study but is not intended to remove the whole of the diseased tissue.

1. Always try to include junctional tissue between diseased and normal tissues, where the architecture is recognizable.
2. If an edge is present, excise a wedge from it, leaving a defect that can usually be closed with sutures (Fig. 7.3). If there is no edge, excise an ellipse in the shape of a boat with the keel lying in the depths (Fig. 7.4).

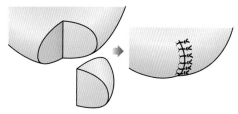

Fig. 7.3 Cut a wedge from the edge of a structure and appose the cut surfaces with stitches.

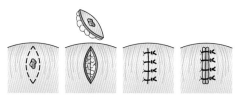

Fig. 7.4 Away from an edge, excise a boat-shaped specimen. If the tissue is supple you may be able to close the defect as a linear scar. If it is not, insert stitches and tie them, after drawing in nearby tissue to fill the defect, if possible. Alternatively, lay in gelatin foam or a similar haemostatic substance.

3. If you need to biopsy a deeply placed lump, make sure you can reach it safely without injuring nearby structures. You may have imaging views at 90° to each other as a guide. Be willing to make an adequate incision so you can identify structures you may encounter.
4. A *hooked wire marker* is used especially in the breast when a suspicious area such as a small mass or collection of microcalcification is identified on mammography or another imaging technique. As a rule, the radiologist inserts a hollow needle into the suspicious area, introducing through this a hooked or curved wire before withdrawing the needle (Fig. 7.5). You should now approach the suspicious area by the most direct route. Cut through the outer part of the wire, leaving the hook marker in place. Excise the suspicious area and marker, if necessary taking X-rays of the specimen to confirm that the correct tissue has been excised.

CONNECTIVE TISSUE

This varies from flimsy areolar tissue to tough ligaments, tendons and aponeuroses (from the Greek *apo* = from + *neuron* = nerve or tendon), which are flattened tendons attached to muscles.

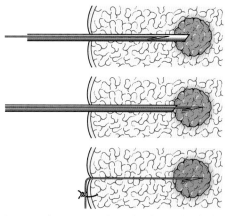

Fig. 7.5 The suspicious lesion has been identified by surface measurement, stereotactic measurement or ultrasound. After inserting a needle into it, pass through the needle a hooked or bent wire and then remove the needle. You may bend the wire and suture it flush with the skin to prevent it from being dislodged.

The vascularity of stable connective tissue is minimal, but blood vessels may cross connective tissue spaces, bound for other tissues and organs.

Tendons and aponeuroses have most of the fibres running in one direction along the line of the attached muscle contraction.

Areolar tissue

Areolar tissue (from the Latin *areola*, diminutive of *area* = an open, empty place) occupies the space between structures that move relative to each other; for example, between muscles and around tendons. It is an important guide to tissue planes and often has slack vessels crossing it to supply a moving structure such as a tendon or muscle, and from deep structures to supply mobile skin.

Cut it with a scalpel or scissors, preferably after sealing any fine vessels with a diathermy or harmonic scalpel. Occasionally it can be gently stripped with your fingers. Repair it using very fine absorbable stitches mounted on a round-bodied needle.

Aponeuroses

Because these transmit the pull of muscles the fibres tend to run parallel, although cross-fibres bind the parallel fibres together.

1. Whenever possible split them parallel to the fibres. If this is done they require minimal or no repair, since returning muscle tone pulls all the fibres straight, closing the constructed gap (see later: gridiron incision).

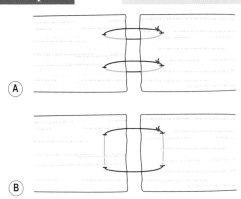

Fig. 7.6 The aponeurosis has been cut across the fibres. (A) Simple stitches tend to cut out. (B) Horizontal mattress sutures hold better.

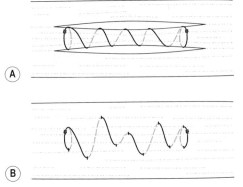

Fig. 7.7 The aponeurosis has been split between the fibres. (A) Stitches inserted all at the same distance from the edges tend to drag away a strip of fibres. (B) Stitches hold better if they are inserted at varying intervals from the edges.

2. The cross-link fibres in aponeuroses that have been cut across the fibres are weak and single stitches may cut out. The tendency is reduced if you use horizontal mattress stitches (Fig. 7.6). For the same reason, when the fibres have been split and you repair it with sutures inserted at the same distance from the edge, they will separate off a strip if the aponeurosis is subjected to tension across the fibres. In this case, insert the sutures at varying distances from the edges (Fig. 7.7). Healing of aponeuroses is slow. If they are subjected to strain at an early stage, the repair will give way or stretch. The ability to stretch is increased during pregnancy, in nutritional deficiency and in old age. In some diseases, there are molecular defects in collagen or elastic fibres.

3. Attempts to appose weak or stretched aponeuroses, especially if they are likely to come under tension, are usually doomed to fail. For many years surgeons attempted bridging of congenital and acquired parietal (from the Latin *parietum* = a wall) defects. Sutures and darns inserted under tension swiftly or gradually give way. In the past biological and artificial materials were inserted, intended to create an inflammatory reaction, in the hope that fibrous tissue would be laid down. Nonabsorbable synthetic meshes, usually of polypropylene or polyester, evoke little inflammatory reaction but are incorporated into the tissues. Cut a piece larger than the defect, so that it overlaps the edges, extending all round onto robust tissues without any tension, and suture or staple it in place (see later: hernia).

> **Key points**
>
> - Pulling edges of aponeurotic defects together with stitches has a high failure rate.
> - Bridge the gap with tension-free plastic mesh.

Tendons

Tendons (from the Greek *teinein* = to stretch) are composed of aligned collagen and elastic fibres to transmit the pull of muscles. They have the highest tensile strength of any connective tissue. If they are split in the line of the fibres they often eventually heal without loss of strength. If they are transected across the fibres, the ends retract. Following repair, the join is weak and stitches tend to cut out.

1. Stainless steel sutures were previously used but synthetic polyamide, polyester or polypropylene have improved the results. Polyethylene terephthalate (Ethibond) is commonly used, though newer hybrid sutures combining a core of high molecular weight polyethylene surrounded by polyester are being introduced (e.g., FiberWire). Monofilament sutures are better for flexor tendons as they cause less abrasion in the tendon sheaths. The larger the area of the repair the greater the chance of satisfactory union; consider cutting the ends obliquely or stepwise.

2. Tendon repairs are sometimes performed after applying a tourniquet to ensure that the field is not obscured with blood.

3. Be particularly careful where a close-fitting tendon changes direction over a fibro-osseous pulley-like smooth ridge or under an aponeurotic band to prevent bow-stringing of the tendon, encased in a synovial sheath to reduce the friction. Do not injure the fine, mesentery-like connections (vinculae) or the delicate mesothelial cells lining the synovium when bringing the blood supply from the deep surface. If you leave an irregularity at such sites, adhesions develop between the tendon and the sheath, limiting or preventing movement.

4. If two tendons lying together have been divided, there is a danger that following repair of them both, they will adhere to each other or abrade each other. Less bulky repairs can reduce friction, and early physiotherapy may retain movement. Furthermore, there is much research into hydrogels to wrap around the tendons reducing adhesion. If necessary, one of the tendons may be sacrificed. When the flexor digitorum profundus and superficialis of a finger are both divided, the superficialis tendon might not be repaired.

5. Do not grasp the tendon ends with forceps; this will have a crushing effect, damaging and roughening the surface. Manipulate them with needles. One method is to transfix each of them with a straight needle about 2–2.5 cm from the cut ends. The needles can be drawn together and rotated as necessary to align the ends but protect the needle points to prevent needle-stick injury. Make sure that the clean-cut ends come together, if necessary by flexing the join across which the tendon acts. The ends should fit together without any twist, angulation or step.

6. Repair the tendon with a mattress stitch. Insert a stitch, emerging 1.5 cm from the end. Now reinsert the needle close to where it emerged, to cross the diameter of the tendon transversely, immediately opposite the point of insertion. Reinsert the needle close to the point of emergence, to reappear at the cut end. Bridge the gap between the cut ends and enter the other end, emerging 1.5 cm from the end, crossing the diameter of the tendon, back to the cut end (Fig. 7.8). It is often convenient to employ a straight needle but hold it with a needle-holder. Draw the two ends together, ensuring they fit without twisting. Tie a perfect knot that will lie between the ends, holding the ends in perfect apposition, without bunching. Finally insert a fine

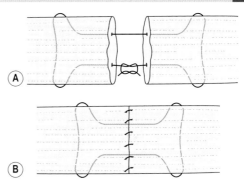

Fig. 7.8 Repair of a tendon. (A) Insert stitches bridging the tendons. Draw the ends together and tie a knot that will be buried between the apposed ends. (B) Insert very fine continuous stitches to repair the paratenon.

monofilament circumferential stitch to draw into continuity the paratenon, producing the smoothest possible surface.

7. Reduce tension to a minimum following repair by immobilizing joints in a position that brings the muscle origin and insertion as close as possible. Collagen laid down during healing stretches if it is strained, so unless the muscle pull is restrained, the tendon will be lengthened and muscle action subsequently restricted.

8. When a tendon ruptures as it joins the bone, unite the ends provided the distal stump has retained its blood supply. Otherwise, unite the proximal end into the bone. This is usually achieved by resecting a patch of cortical bone and drawing the tendon into contact with the underlying cancellous bone using nonabsorbable stitches inserted through the tendon and through holes drilled through the bone.

Ligaments

These are bands or sheets of fibrous tissue connecting bones, cartilages and other structures (from the Latin *ligare* = to bind or tie), or acting as supports for fascia, joints or muscles.

1. Torn supporting ligaments can often be repaired in a similar manner to aponeuroses or tendons.

2. Ligaments that stabilise joints such as collateral and cruciate ligaments of the knee are challenging to repair and demand specialist expertise. Unless they retain their length and strength, the joint becomes unstable. Some can be repaired like tendons. Cruciate ligaments

of the knee can be repaired using either the tendons of hamstrings or the central portion of the patellar tendon with a piece of the tibia and the patella at each end, which can be anchored in tunnels within the femur and tibia. Allografts (from the Greek *allos* = other) such as bovine collateral ligament have been used, as well as a number of artificial materials such as carbon fibre, polyester and polytetrafluoroethylene.

NERVES

Nerve fibres are enclosed within and protected by the endoneurium; the perineurium encloses bundles or fasciculi of nerve fibres, and around the whole nerve is the epineurium (Fig. 7.9).

Neurapraxia (from the Greek *a* = not + *prassein* = to do) is a temporary physiological block.

Axonotmesis (from the Greek *temnein* = to cut) results from disruption of the axon but the endoneurium remains intact. Wallerian degeneration (Augustus Waller, 1816–1870, English physiologist) occurs in the distal axon. The proximal axon sprouts distally along the intact endoneurial tube, eventually connecting with the end organ.

Neurotmesis results from division of the nerve. If the ends are coapted, axon sprouts enter the distal endoneurial tubes, but the result is invariably less than perfect. Recovery of function is proportional to the perfection with which the original orientation is achieved so that axons enter the correct distal endoneurial tubes.

Key point

- The sooner you perform the repair and the more expertly you repair it, the better the result.

1. You may first need to eliminate infection and bleeding, achieve skeletal stability and assure primary skin closure. If you cannot fulfil these conditions, join the ends with a single stitch, close the skin or cover the nerve with well-vascularised tissue, elevate the part to prevent oedema and delay repair until the conditions are suitable.
2. Repair is usually carried out after applying a tourniquet to ensure there is adequate, bloodless exposure. Ensure that you have good light,

available magnification with fine, microsurgical instruments and a loupe or operating microscope (see Ch. 5).
3. If the nerve ends are ragged, trim them with a scalpel blade so you can appose them in perfect orientation.
4. Carefully unite the epineurial sheaths using monofilament 8/0–10/0 nylon. Fascicular repair is possible in some cases.
5. If a segment of the nerve is lost, or the ends have retracted, you may interpose a graft, usually taken from the sural (from the Latin *sura* = calf of the leg) nerve. This does, however, prejudice the final result. During parotidectomy for a tumour, a branch of the facial nerve may be transacted or resected accidentally or deliberately because of tumour involvement. It is usual to bridge the gap with a segment of the great auricular nerve.
6. Following repair and closure in a limb, immobilise it in a position that avoids traction on the repair.

SKELETAL MUSCLE

Relaxed muscle is remarkably fragile and easily crushed. In contrast healthy contracted muscle is remarkably resistant to injury. If the motor nerve supply is lost the muscle is paralysed and atrophies (from the Greek *a* = not + *trephein* = to feed). If a muscle is transected, the muscle fibres do not reunite but they are connected by intervening fibrosis. The single muscle becomes double-bellied at best, but the ends frequently distract, become attached to the muscle sheath and so lose their contractility.

It is a remarkable phenomenon, that haematogenous metastases of neoplasms are rarely seen in skeletal muscle. It has been suggested that the high metabolic requirements and repeated repair cycles in skeletal muscle result in sustained oxidative stress such that the malignant cells cannot proliferate.[1]

1. Apart from operating on muscles for local trauma or disease you frequently need to pass between or through them to reach your deeper surgical target. The muscles are often layered. Respect the fine external investing fascia which allows them to glide over each other without friction. The nerves and vessels usually enter from the deep surface (an exception is the serratus anterior muscle).

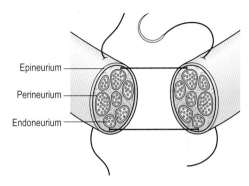

Epineurium

Perineurium

Endoneurium

Fig. 7.9 Repairing a cut nerve. Groups of fibres are encased in an endoneurial sheath (endoneurium), the fasciculi have a perineurium and the nerve has an epineurium. Ensure that the ends are brought into perfect alignment with the bundles correctly orientated, without tension or rotation. In some cases, you need to use epineurial stitches only; in others, you can connect the perineurial sheaths.

Excessive displacement may prejudice the nerve and blood supply.

2. Reappose muscle fibres running parallel to each other and separate using absorbable sutures mounted on round-bodied needles, but do not tie the sutures tightly or they will strangulate the muscle fibres and cut out. Indeed, it is unnecessary in many situations to insert sutures since the fibres realign once muscle tone returns. Horizontal mattress stitches inserted to reappose the ends of transected muscles tend to cut out.

3. *Volkmann's ischaemic contracture*, described in 1872 by Richard Volkmann of Halle in Germany, results from muscle ischaemia. This can be caused by too-tight encircling plaster, by swelling of muscle within inelastic fascia as in the anterior compartment of the lower leg, or by pressure on, for example, the brachial artery following supracondylar fracture of the humerus. A too-tight plaster can be split; a supracondylar fracture can be manipulated to relieve pressure on the artery. If the ischaemia is not relieved the muscle atrophies and is replaced with fibrous tissue; as this matures it shortens, causing contractures.

4. Encircling full-thickness burns of a limb have a similar effect to a tight plaster and usually the skin and often the deep fascia may need to be fully split longitudinally; such burns of the upper trunk cause restricted respiratory movement.

They both demand immediate release by longitudinally splitting the eschar—the dry, hard scab-like burned skin. This is the original meaning of debridement (from the French *débrider* = unbridle, release).

5. *Compartment syndrome*, for example in the lower leg, from swelling of the muscle within the inelastic fascia, causes severe unremitting pain. If the pressure rises above 30 mmHg or differs less than 30 mmHg from diastolic pressure, severe necrosis is likely. It can be relieved by slitting the fascia and skin (open fasciotomy) to allow the muscle to bulge through. In the lower leg, it is important that you release all four muscle compartments. Traditionally, two incisions are made under general anaesthesia; an anterolateral and a medial. In some cases, this can be carried out subcutaneously if the fascia alone is causing the compression and the overlying skin is sufficiently slack. However, if in doubt, make the full-thickness incision. The thigh and arms may also develop compartment syndrome. In abdominal compartment syndrome, the intraabdominal contents swell, respiration and circulation are prejudiced, and the urine output may reduce. A useful indicator that this may be occurring would be increased bladder pressure and increased ventilatory requirements. This must be relieved by performing a laparostomy.

CARTILAGE

1. Pure cartilage covers the ends of bones in contact at joints, or as menisci are interposed between bone ends. It has limited ability to regenerate because it has no intrinsic blood supply, usually obtaining it through peripheral attachments. It usually heals with the deposition of fibrocartilage.

2. Fibrocartilage can be cut, sutured and stitched after drilling stitch holes and transplanted from one site to another as part of a composite graft.

3. The management of cartilaginous defects is in a state of flux as efforts are made to repair, renovate and regenerate it. Tears and dislocations that were formerly treated through open approaches, often involving total removal of intraarticular menisci of joints such as the knee, can now be repaired and smoothed using arthroscopic techniques.

MUCOPERIOSTEUM

This is a strong conjoint double layer with a good blood supply, covering among other areas the hard palate and bony nasal walls. It can be elevated from the bone as a flap to cover bony defects to close palatal defects in congenital cleft palate.

1. Choose the suture material depending on the feasibility of removing them. If they can be removed, use 3/0 black silk which is easy to see, or monofilament nylon which evokes minimal reaction, mounted on half-curved, reverse-cutting, eyeless needles.
2. If it is difficult or impossible to remove stitches, insert 4/0 synthetic absorbable stitches.

BREAST

Breasts are glandular skin derivatives and supernumerary breasts may develop anywhere along the 'milk line' extending from the axilla to the groin. The consistency varies depending on the proportions of glandular and adipose tissue. The upper, outer quadrant and axillary tail tend to have denser glandular tissue than elsewhere. This variation makes it difficult to differentiate lumpiness from lump.

1. Cysts can be aspirated and the fluid sent for cytological examination. Deeply placed cysts may be reached guided by ultrasound imaging.
2. During lactation retained milk may produce galactoceles (from the Greek *galaktos* = milk + *kele* = a swelling) and infection of the breast can result in cellulitis and abscess formation. At an early stage, antibiotics may thwart abscess formation but if an abscess forms, the pus can often be aspirated as an alternative to open drainage.
3. Palpable lumps should have a radiological assessment. Image-guided needle core biopsy should be done in patients who are 25 years or older. If the imaging shows a benign lesion in a patient under 25 years then a biopsy may not be indicated. If the lump is radiologically occult, a clinical needle core biopsy may be necessary.
4. Impalpable doubtful lumps detected by imaging can be marked with a clip and when the open biopsy is done it can be localised with a hooked wire aiding accurate removal of the lesion.
5. *Open biopsy* is rarely required when the diagnosis is in doubt. Carry out an excision biopsy unless the lump is very large, in which case you should remove a thin slice for histological examination. Place the incision so that it can be incorporated within a wider incision if this proves necessary. Avoid damaging the architecture. Hold on to the attached connective tissue, not the lump itself. Do not try to close the gap but obtain perfect haemostasis before carefully closing the skin.
6. When operating on the breast constantly bear in mind the radial distribution of the lobules which drain centrally to reach the nipple. Plan incisions to consider the cosmetic result. Skin tension lines are mainly transverse before the breast develops but change as the breast fills and eventually sags.
7. Avoid the development of a haematoma by achieving perfect haemostasis.
8. For a palpable or localised carcinoma employ a wider excision, keeping well clear of the lump. As a safeguard against local recurrence, the cavity walls may be resected when the lump has been removed. If there is proven lymph node metastasis preoperatively, this may be combined with a limited or complete axillary lymph node clearance. If the lymph nodes appear normal on preoperative imaging, then it is combined with a sentinel lymph node biopsy (see below).
9. A more certain procedure is *quadrantectomy* which removes a quarter of the breast down to the pectoral muscles like a quarter of a round cake, from nipple to periphery. A plastic or oncoplastic breast surgeon will routinely assist with mobilization of the parenchyma of the breast tissue to minimise the volume deficiency. This is termed a therapeutic mammoplasty. Close the skin after attaining perfect haemostasis.
10. *Modified radical mastectomy* is the total removal of the whole breast including the axillary tail down to the chest wall but preserving the pectoral muscles and chest wall, including clearance of the axillary glands, described by David Patey of the Middlesex Hospital London in 1948. It is a modification of the operation devised by William Halsted of Baltimore (1852–1922), which included resecting the pectoral muscles.

LYMPH NODES

Enlargement of lymph nodes indicates local inflammation, infection, or malignant or other disease; alternatively, it may be a local manifestation of generalised disease.

Enlarged nodes may be singular, multiple, discrete, matted, mobile or fixed. Superficial enlarged nodes are usually palpable although the physical signs may be misleading. Infected subfascial nodes may rupture, forming an abscess which may then burst through the fascia to present subcutaneously; this is a 'collar-stud' abscess.

Deeply placed nodes can be demonstrated by various methods of imaging or displayed at operation.

1. Before operation discuss with the pathologist how to prepare the specimen and identify which receptacles are needed.
2. Carry out fine-needle aspiration cytology and needle core biopsy only if you are confident of the anatomy; otherwise, recruit the aid of a radiologist who can use ultrasound or other imaging methods for guidance.
3. Lymph nodes are fragile and, if crushed, the accuracy of the diagnosis is prejudiced.

Key points

- Lymph node biopsy is not a minor or casual procedure; most nodes are in close proximity to important structures.
- Never attempt to remove a node without studying the anatomy and obtaining adequate exposure. Many surgical disasters result from a cavalier attitude to removing what appears to be a solitary, mobile lymph node.

---

4. Place the incision in a skin crease if possible and approach the node with caution. Lymph nodes may be very fragile, especially if they are diseased. Having reached the surface of the node, work around the sides but do not grasp it with forceps because you may damage it; if possible leave a little connective tissue attached to it so that you can grasp this.
5. As you reach the deeper aspects, move the mobilised gland from side to side so that you can examine its attachments from different aspects. Remember that the vessels usually enter from the undersurface and that there may be an adherent important structure. The majority of complications arise because we are tempted to lift the gland, put the resulting pedicle under tension, then cut it—and often regret it.
6. Carefully check the field and ensure total haemostasis.
7. On occasion you must remove one or a few glands from a matted mass of glands. Do not damage glands you do not intend to remove.

8. In widespread lymphadenopathy, the groin nodes are least likely to give a tissue diagnosis and are more likely to be reactionary.
9. Divide up the node, without crushing it, into the required number of specimens and place them in the appropriate receptacles.
10. Close the wound to give the best possible cosmetic result.

Sentinel node biopsy

1. Before operation for diagnosed breast carcinoma, a peritumoral or periareolar injection of a radioactive substance such as ^{99m}Tc-labelled nanocolloid may be injected. To improve the accuracy of sentinel node localization a dual-modality method may be applied; patent blue V dye is injected in addition to the radioactive tracer.
2. It is taken up by lymphatics and carried to the lymph nodes where it can be detected using a gamma probe. This first draining node can be removed and examined to detect cancer cells. The sentinel node is seen as 'hot' to the radioactive tracer and blue dye. Both can be seen to track within the lymphatics to the glands (Fig. 7.10). If the removed gland is free of tumour cells, it is unlikely—though still possible—that the cancer has spread more widely in the lymphatic system.
3. Intraoperative assessment of tumour cells within the sentinel node is a routine procedure. Frozen section or touch-print cytology may be utilised to achieve this. In the latter, the node is halved and the dissected surface is imprinted to a histological slide to be reviewed by an experienced cytologist. A recent advancement is to subject the sentinel node to one-step nucleic acid amplification (ONSA) for the CK19 gene. This is a PCR amplification for the CK19 gene which is indicative of metastatic cancer.
4. The technique may be used to determine the extent of the spread of other neoplasms such as malignant melanoma (Ch. 6) and oesophageal adenocarcinoma.

Fat transfer

Where there is a defect in fatty tissue fat cells can be transferred from elsewhere in the body.

1. It is used to correct volume deficiency following wide local excision of a breast lump, and in plastic surgery for defect lesions elsewhere in the body.

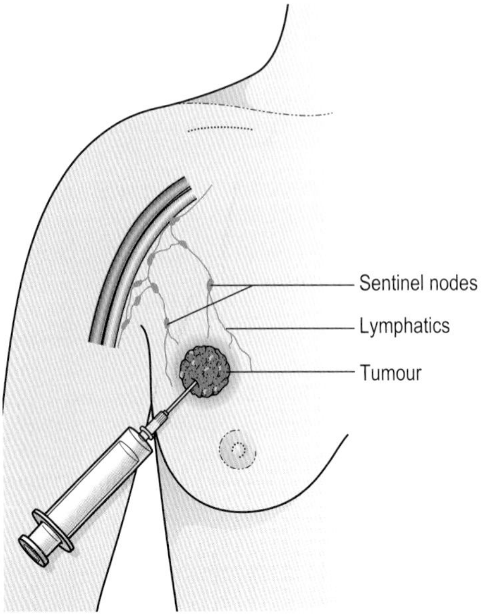

Fig. 7.10 Sentinel node biopsy is an aid in determining the extent of breast cancer dissemination and deciding on the extent of the resection. A radioactive substance is injected around the tumour and tracked to the sentinel nodes using a gamma probe. Alternatively, or in addition, vital blue dye may be injected and identified in the lymphatics passing to the glands. Histology of the excised glands offers guidance on the extent of tumour spread.

2. The cells are harvested by wet or dry liposuction from the donor site (often the abdominal wall).
3. The harvested fat cells are purified and then injected directly into the recipient site.
4. It should be remembered that the site of fat transfer can result in suspicious lesions on subsequent breast imaging, but this is commonly due to the appearance of fat necrosis.

ABDOMINAL WALL

The usual purpose of incisions in the abdomen is to achieve the best possible access to structures within the cavity. The descriptions are intended merely to outline the steps of the frequently performed procedures. Whenever possible, avoid cutting through muscle. This can be achieved in two standard incisions, a midline vertical and a 'gridiron' incision for appendicectomy.

Midline abdominal incision

1. As a rule, stand on the supine patient's right side if you are right-handed.
2. The incision divides the skin, linea alba and peritoneum in the upper or lower abdomen, or central abdomen by skirting the umbilicus. Divide the skin with the belly of the scalpel, holding the knife so that it cuts vertically without slicing. Start at the upper end, cutting from your left to right. Alternatively, after cutting through the skin layer, you may divide the subcutaneous fat with a cutting diathermy.
3. If you are making a midline incision that includes the umbilicus, the majority of surgeons will skirt around it. This is best achieved by tilting the scalpel slightly more towards the point and continuing your incision as a semicircle around the umbilicus leaving approximately a 2–3 mm margin. An alternative method is to grasp the edge of the umbilicus with an Alliss tissue forcep and, holding it in your nondominant hand, pull the umbilicus towards you out of the way of the straight-line incision; then make the incision in a straight line staying in the midline. Once the incision is made you may remove the Alliss and you will see that the incision skirts around the umbilicus.
4. After achieving haemostasis, continue in the same line through the white, firm, fibrous linea alba and then stop as you reach a variable layer of fat overlying the fused fascia transversalis and peritoneum. Once through the skin, you may wish to switch to cutting diathermy instead of a scalpel blade.
5. Pick up the final layer with the tips of a haemostat to tent it, allowing you to grasp it again, alongside the first grip. Remove and then replace the first forceps while holding up the peritoneum with the second forceps, to allow any viscus inadvertently picked up by the first forceps to slip clear. Now have both haemostats held up, tenting the peritoneum while you make a small incision between them. This allows air to enter the abdomen so that viscera can fall clear (Fig. 7.11). Insert a finger into the peritoneal cavity and move it in a complete circle to confirm that there is no viscus in danger. Having assured yourself, insert one blade of Mayo's scissors and carefully slit the peritoneum in the line of the initial incision.

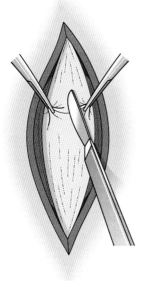

Fig. 7.11 Incising the peritoneum after tenting it between two forceps.

6. To close the incision, grasp the peritoneum at each end with strong, straight haemostatic forceps and have them lifted clear of the underlying viscera by your assistant. You may also apply similar forceps in the middle of each edge, allowing the handles to lie outwards, everting the edges. Insert a nonabsorbable suture such as 1 monofilament nylon mounted on a round-bodied curved needle. This may be a single suture or a double-looped suture. Alternatively, the sutures can be mounted on blunt taper-point needles that will penetrate the tissues but do not easily penetrate surgical gloves or the skin. Absorbable synthetic sutures are popular with many surgeons because their strength is reliably retained for a period before they are absorbed.

7. It is usually most convenient to suture from the upper end to the lower, from your non-dominant to your dominant side, as the incision lies transversely in front of you. Take a bite through all layers, except the skin and subcutaneous tissues, from out to in on the far side, in to out on the near side, and tie the suture securely. Ensure that the bristly short end is well buried. Alternatively, for a looped suture

insert your first stitch, then pass the needle through the loop; this produces a less bulky means of securing the start of the suture line.

8. Insert a continuous, over-and-over stitch until you reach the other end. This is an 'en masse' closure. Drive the needle from without in on the far side, from within out on the near side, approximately every 1 cm, placed 1 cm from the edge, forming a spiral within the tissues, and using a suture that is at least four times the length of the incision This is Jenkins' rule. This allows the stitches to adjust so that the tension is equalised between them and reduces the chances of a burst abdomen.

9. Carefully avoid over-tightening the stitches. Once you have apposed the edges, have your assistant steady the emerging thread so you can avoid the sawing action of tightening, slackening and retightening the stitches.

10. Take care to avoid injuring structures with the last few stitches by inserting them slackly, with the edges separated, then tightening them seriatim.

11. At the end, hold on to the final loop on one side and the single thread on the other. You may either tie the loop to the single thread or employ an Aberdeen knot (see Ch. 3).

12. As a rule do not insert subcutaneous stitches.

13. Now carefully close the skin. If this has been a clean procedure, subcuticular works well. If there has been contamination, then interrupted sutures or skin staples are preferable in case a couple or more need to be removed at a later date to release superficial infection.

Key points

- Ceaselessly and vigilantly protect the abdominal contents from injury.
- Place every stitch carefully, through all the intended layers.
- Do not damage the suture material or you will weaken it.
- Over-tightened stitches strangle the tissues and are likely to cut out, risking a burst abdomen.
- Tie knots securely and turn the bristly ends under, so they do not project under the skin.

Gridiron incision

1. Whilst the majority of appendicectomies in the Western world are now performed laparoscopically, there may still be a place for an

open procedure via this approach. The incision is named after the crossed iron bars laid over a fire on which to grill food, resembling the crossed lateral abdominal muscle layers. It is associated with the New York surgeon Charles McBurney (1845–1913), who established the diagnosis and surgical treatment of appendicitis. He described a point in the right iliac fossa at the junction of the middle and outer thirds of a line between the umbilicus and anterior superior iliac spine where the maximal tenderness is felt in the disease and on which the incision is centred.

2. Make the skin incision centred on the point. McBurney's skin incision was at right angles to the spinoumbilical line with one-third above and two-thirds below his point. Otto Lanz of Amsterdam (1865–1935) described an incision along the skin crease which results in a more cosmetically acceptable scar. Incise the subcutaneous tissue in the same line.

3. You expose the shining aponeurosis of external oblique muscle. Split the fibres without cutting them, to reveal the fibres of internal oblique muscle, at right angles to the external oblique. Split these to reveal the fibres of transversus abdominis muscle. For each layer, make a small incision with a scalpel, then gently insert the tips of Mayo's scissors into the gap and open them in the line of the fibres. Split these to reveal the conjoint transversalis fascia and peritoneum (Fig. 7.12).

4. Pick up the peritoneum with artery forceps to tent it, grasp the raised tented portion, release and regrasp the peritoneum with the first forceps. Have the two forceps held up while you make a small scalpel incision between them to let in air and allow the viscera to fall away. Insert a finger to ensure that there is no adherent structure before introducing one blade of a pair of scissors to enlarge the opening fully within the muscle boundaries.

5. Close the incision in layers. First, hold up the ends of the peritoneal incision and insert a continuous suture of 2/0 or 3/0 absorbable synthetic suture to close it, ensuring you do not injure any intraabdominal structure. Using the same material, insert interrupted stitches to appose each of the muscle layers, taking care not to pull the stitches tight. Finally, close the skin using interrupted or continuous sutures. To achieve a good cosmetic result, you may wish to insert a subcuticular stitch (see Ch. 6).

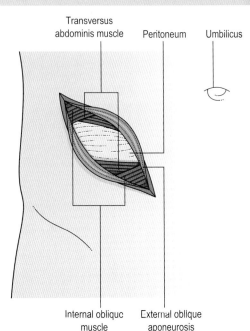

Fig. 7.12 The gridiron incision for appendicectomy. Split but do not cut the fibres of the aponeurosis and muscles to reach the peritoneum.

Hernia

Defects in aponeuroses congenitally acquired or from trauma, atrophy or paralysis may allow deep structures to bulge. Such a protrusion is a hernia. Plastic mesh repair has transformed the repair, notably in the groin and incisional hernias following failed repairs of abdominal incisions. Whilst most developed countries now repair many hernias using a laparoscope, open repair is still in use.

1. Expose the superficial layer of the bulge, which is the peritoneum in abdominal hernias, and define the margins of the defect. You may be able to invaginate the bulge and, if necessary, plicate it to keep it out of the way of the repair.

2. If the hernia bulges into an elongated sac you must first reduce the contents, if necessary after opening the sac, then close the neck of the sac and excise the excess.

3. Lay the mesh, with generous overlap of the defect edges, superficial to the defect, or under the deep surface from within the underlying cavity. In the groin, an appropriate slit is made to encircle the spermatic cord, with the two resulting 'fish-tails' stitched together around it.

4. Fix the mesh using simple sutures or staples (Fig. 7.13).

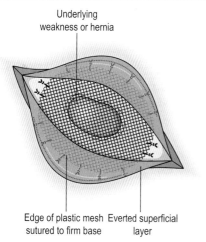

Underlying
weakness or hernia

Edge of plastic mesh   Everted superficial
sutured to firm base   layer

Fig. 7.13   Plastic mesh tension-free repair of a hernia. The superficial tissues have been undermined and the mesh laid in, generously overlapping the margins. It is now sutured or stapled in place and then covered over and the wound is closed.

5. An abdominal wall hernia may be repaired transperitoneally using laparoscopic methods from within the abdominal cavity (TAPP). Alternatively, it can be approached extraperitoneally after creating a space between the abdominal wall and peritoneum, then expanding it with an inflatable balloon (TEPP).
6. This tension-free technique is highly successful. The mesh is well tolerated. Fibroblasts lay down collagen fibres that embed it securely in the tissues.

ABDOMINAL CONTENTS

Bowel

Provided the normally rich blood supply is intact and edges are carefully apposed, bowel (from the Latin *botellus* = a sausage) heals well (see Ch. 4). Although the contents of the small bowel are normally almost sterile, as soon as there is any stagnation, microorganisms flourish here, as they normally do in the colon.

Key point

- Repaired bowel must have a good blood supply, perfect apposition of the edges and an absence of tension.

Liver

1. Liver is honeycombed with blood vessels and bile ducts so that it bleeds and oozes bile when cut. The capsule, described by Francis Glisson of Bristol about 1677, encloses the liver, extending into the porta hepatis, and is of variable strength.
2. Liver is amenable to fine-needle aspiration or to needle biopsy. Ultrasound or other imaging methods may be used to guide the needle to lesions. A long, fine 'skinny' needle can be inserted percutaneously into the intrahepatic bile ducts and contrast media injected into them to produce a cholangiogram (from the Greek *chole* = bile + *angeion* = vessel + *graphe in* = to write). By using the Seldinger technique (see Ch. 5), the biliary system can be entered, and a guidewire passed through the common bile duct and into the duodenum. Following the passage of dilators over the guidewire, stents can be placed across a stenotic section.
3. In the presence of bleeding oesophageal varices secondary to cirrhosis and portal venous hypertension, a number of procedures can be performed. The anastomotic channels draining the hypertensive portal venous system into the systemically drained oesophageal veins can be disconnected, or the portal vein can be drained directly into the inferior vena cava–portacaval shunt. This can now be achieved percutaneously by creating a transhepatic intrajugular portal-systemic shunt (TIPS) within the liver. A guidewire is passed down the right internal jugular vein, superior vena cava, right atrium, inferior vena cava, right hepatic vein, then through liver substance and via a tributary, into the portal vein. A stent is placed across as a bridge, creating a portal/systemic conduit.
4. At operations on the liver, bleeding and bile leakage can be controlled using diathermy current and employing blunt dissection. 'Finger fracture' consists of compressing a portion of liver between finger and thumb, crushing the liver cells but not dividing the vessels and ducts; these can then be identified, doubly ligated and divided. Ultrasound, electrosurgical, high-pressure water jet, laser, and radiofrequency methods are used to facilitate liver resection without causing excessive blood loss (see Ch. 9). Oozing surfaces can be sealed using a variety of applied haemostatic materials, and an argon beam can be used to carry an electrosurgical

149

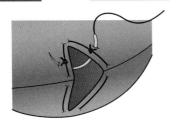

Fig. 7.14 Suture the liver using a large, round-bodied needle. It may be an advantage to insert an encircling stitch close to the edges before bringing the edges together with apposing stitches placed outside these.

high-frequency current to the surface, coagulating the vessels with minimal penetration.
5. After achieving haemostasis, absorbable synthetic sutures mounted on large round-bodied curved needles can be inserted to appose the cut surfaces. Take bites well away from the cut edges and tighten them only just sufficient to appose the surfaces or they will cut out. In some cases it is beneficial to insert stitches parallel with the edges to slightly constrict and support them before placing stitches to appose the cut edges (Fig. 7.14).

Spleen

In the past, splenectomy was carried out with little concern as part of other procedures, even if the spleen was only slightly damaged. This aggressive attitude stemmed from the propensity of the damaged spleen to continue to bleed or develop recurrent bleeding.

The dangers of postsplenectomy infection are now recognised, especially in children, so that it is preserved whenever possible.
1. A capsular tear may seal if you apply haemostatic agents such as fibrin glue, gelatin sponge, polyglycolic mesh, microfibrillar collagen or crushed muscle.
2. If there is a tear in the pulp, consider inserting stitches to close it, if necessary tying the stitches over a gelatin sponge or a tongue of omentum.
3. If you need to remove the spleen, consider placing slices of the spleen into pockets constructed in the greater omentum.
4. Determine whether or not to give an antipneumococcal vaccine postoperatively. Advise adults to seek treatment at the first sign of infection and give children prophylactic penicillin for 2 years.

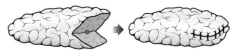

Fig. 7.15 Repairing the pancreas. Cut the stump end like a fish tail and suture together the two flaps you have created.

Pancreas

The pancreas (from the Greek *pas* = all + *kreas* = flesh) is well protected from injury but is very fragile. The enzymes are extremely erosive if released and activated.
1. The gland does not hold stitches well, so repair is difficult to achieve.
2. The body or the tail can be removed, followed by closure of the main duct.
3. Close the parenchyma. This may be conveniently achieved by cutting the stump in the shape of a fishtail (Fig. 7.15) and suturing the edges.

UROLOGICAL SYSTEM

Kidney

1. This has a rich blood supply; it is a firm capsule which holds stitches well and is amenable to repair provided the drainage system is intact. The vessels are end arteries, so partial nephrectomy must reflect the distribution. Control the bleeding, insert fine absorbable sutures to close collecting system defects and insert absorbable stitches through the capsule, crossing the parenchyma tied just tightly enough to appose the tissues without them cutting out.
2. The majority of partial nephrectomies are now carried out laparoscopically or robotically. Sutures may damage vessels and compress parenchyma all of which impact residual renal function. Therefore, the options relating to renorrhaphy (renal closure techniques) have been adapted accordingly and reflect some of the challenges associated with a minimally invasive approach.
3. The potential cheese-wire effect alluded to above (where sutures under tension effectively lacerate the parenchyma) is a particular concern in robotic surgery where there is a lack of haptic feedback. A V-Loc suture is a unidirectional self-locking barbed suture that evenly distributes tension along a wound. The sutures 'lock' after

each pass thus avoiding the need for multiple knots. Laparoscopic and robotic renorrhaphy generally incorporate the use of V-Loc sutures and Hem-o-lok clips in a 'sliding clip' technique. The barbed suture is passed through the outer renal capsule after which a Hem-o-lok clip is placed on the exiting loose end of the suture and is subsequently slid down to provide a degree of tension before the next suture pass.

Ureter

1. This must be sutured with fine absorbable stitches to avoid obstructing the narrow channel (see Ch. 4). Where a direct end-to-end anastomosis is required the risks of luminal stenosis are minimised by spatulating the ends of each ureter prior to suturing. Alternatives to a direct end-to-end ureteric anastomosis to restore continuity include intestinal interposition (where the distance between the two ends of a ureter can only be bridged by interposing a segment of bowel), transureteroureterostomy, cutaneous ureterostomy and kidney autotransplantation.

2. If it must be repaired in the lower third, it may be preferable to join it directly to the bladder by raising a flap of bladder harvested from (but remaining in continuity with) its dome and which is fashioned into a tube to bridge the gap, described by Achille Boari in 1894 (though not performed in humans until 1936).

3. Alternatively (and occasionally in combination with) a Psoas-Hitch procedure (so-named by Richard Turner-Warwick and Peter Worth) may be used to bridge the deficit. The bladder is mobilised from the surrounding peritoneum and opened lateral to the bladder dome on the side of the ureteric injury. The psoas minor tendon is identified (and distinguished from the genitofemoral nerve) above the level of the iliac vessels. The bladder is then advanced in the direction of the ureter and sutured (hitched) to the tendon. The ureter is attached using a tunnelled approach (which serves as an antireflux mechanism) before the bladder defect is closed longitudinally. A JJ stent is positioned into the ureteric lumen prior to bladder closure and effectively serves as a splint for the healing of anastomosis.

Bladder

1. The wall is robust and holds sutures well. Many urologists exclude the lining epithelium from the stitches, which catch all the other layers.

Bladder repairs are undertaken using absorbable sutures, generally in two layers.

2. Closures can be 'leak-tested' at the time of the repair by direct vision after distending the bladder with saline via an appropriately positioned urinary catheter (and occasionally aided by the addition of methylene blue to the saline instillation).

Testis

Torsion of the testis is treated whenever possible by untwisting it and fixing it, and its twin, to the scrotum to prevent recurrence.

1. Following the manual derotation of the testis, a Jaboulay repair (eversion of the surrounding tunica vaginalis) is generally performed prior to a three-point fixation using nonabsorbable sutures (such as Prolene) which are used to attach the newly exposed tunica albuginea to the adjacent scrotum. In a paediatric population, a sutureless dartos pouch fixation technique is increasingly preferred because of unresolved concerns relating to microabscesses and nonabsorbable sutures as well as the placement of sutures through the testis and the disruption of the blood-testis barrier given experimental evidence which suggests this could generate an autoimmune response which may impact on fertility.

2. Following a standard Jaboulay procedure, a 1-cm incision is made over a finger positioned in a dependent portion of the scrotum and a pledget or haemostat is inserted under the skin and used to fashion a space or pouch between the overlying skin and the underlying dartos muscle and into which the derotated testis can be placed. A clamp is then passed through the skin incision and the underlying dartos and used to grasp adventitial tissue around the testis. The testis is then drawn back into the appropriately fashioned pouch without the need for additional 'fixation' sutures.

3. The contralateral testis is only explored in the event of ipsilateral testicular torsion or the demonstration of a bell-clapper deformity (high insertion of the tunica vaginalis) in an otherwise normally positioned (unrotated) testis which had presented acutely and may have untwisted by the time of exploration. Whenever possible, undescended testis is freed and brought down into the scrotum.

4. For the treatment of malignant disease, the testis is removed with ligation of the vas deferens and blood vessels. All surgery for malignant disease of the testis requires a radical orchidectomy for which an inguinal approach is mandatory. The external oblique is exposed, incised and cremasteric fibres dissected free from the cord structures before its mobilization in the inguinal canal. The cord is clamped and divided at the level of the internal ring after which the stump is suture ligated.

5. In order to perform male sterilization, the spermatic cord is identified and under local anaesthesia, incised to expose the vas deferens. A section is excised, both ends closed, and the upper end is buried to avoid the possibility of reconnection. If both free ends are folded back on themselves and tied it may reduce the possibility of reconnection.

Penis

Apart from cultural reasons *circumcision* needs to be performed only for phimosis (from the Greek word for muzzling). It needs to be performed expertly. As a rule, the foreskin is first incised dorsally to enable the adhesions between it and the glans to be gently separated. The prepuce is excised circumferentially while preserving the frenulum (from the Latin *frenum* = bridle) on the undersurface. After achieving perfect haemostasis, the two layers are joined together with interrupted, fine absorbable sutures.

GYNAECOLOGICAL SYSTEM

Uterus

The thick muscle is tough and holds stitches well, following for example caesarean section to deliver a child when vaginal delivery fails or sometimes for other reasons. However, the suture line leaves a scar that is relatively weak compared with the remainder of the wall. The uterine tubes have a narrow lumen. If they are to be repaired, use the finest sutures inserted with great care, preferably with magnification (see Ch. 4). Fibroids can usually be dissected free. Very large ones can sometimes be reduced in size by thermoablation or diathermy. Hysterectomy (from the Greek *hystera* = womb) may be necessary for large, multiple fibroids or uterine cancer.

Ovaries

Formerly, the only common procedure carried out on the ovaries was removal, but they are treated by conservative surgery whenever possible and may be preserved in part or whole by freezing.

CARDIORESPIRATORY SYSTEM

Lung

The lung remains expanded because it fills the intermittently subatmospheric pleural cavity. It collapses if air enters the potential space through either a breach in the chest wall or a damaged lung.

1. A leak usually reseals if you insert a chest drain connected to an underwater seal (see Ch. 11).
2. Suture large tears in the lung using absorbable synthetic sutures.
3. Each area is supplied with arteries, veins and bronchi allowing resection of a lung, lobe or segment.

Heart

Heart muscle holds stitches well and they can be inserted while the heart continues to beat. It is possible to stop the heart and bypass its pump action in order to perform delicate procedures on it such as valve replacement within the lumen. Some aortic valve replacements are now performed percutaneously by specialists (transcatheter aortic valve replacement; TAVI). Pericardiocentesis should now be performed with the aid of two-dimensional echocardiography to avoid complications.

ENDOCRINE SYSTEM

Glandular tissue is relatively soft but the connective tissue usually provides good support. The thyroid gland is vascular, especially in thyrotoxic states. Surgery of the thyroid gland demands intimate knowledge of the anatomy. At risk are major blood vessels, the recurrent laryngeal nerves and the parathyroid glands (see also Ch. 8, Tissue planes). The adrenal gland is fragile and has small veins that are easily torn. It is now usually operated upon by minimal access techniques.

BRAIN AND SPINAL CORD

These are extremely fragile. If they are damaged, healing is by the deposition of connective glial (from the Greek word for glue) tissue. The unmyelinated nerve fibres cannot reunite, although the brain is 'plastic', in that it appears to be able to use alternative connections in response to lost tracts.

A further difficulty with some tumours is in differentiating them from normal brain. Modern imaging aids such as computerised tomography (CT) display brain abnormalities including displacements. Magnetic resonance imaging following intravenous gadolinium-DPTA highlights tumour vascularity and is valuable in outlining the margins of tumours.

1. Nerve tracts can be approached within the brain and in the spinal cord by direct approach or by stereotactic (from the Greek *stereos* = solid, three-dimensional + *tassein* = to arrange) techniques.

2. The brain is richly supplied with blood vessels which may become blocked or bleed. These may be treatable by interventional radiographic techniques. Extradural vessels such as the middle meningeal vessels may bleed following a cranial fracture, lifting the periosteum and dura and reducing the intracranial space. Sudden impacts or rotations may tear the veins crossing from the brain to the intracranial venous sinuses, resulting in subdural haemorrhage. Aneurysms in the circle of Willis may rupture, causing subarachnoid haemorrhage. Vessels within the brain may rupture, causing intracerebral bleeding, or they may clot; intracerebral thrombosis produces a 'stroke' which may manifest as a transient ischaemic attack (TIA) with neurological deficit lasting less than 24 hours or a cerebrovascular accident (CVA) lasting more than 24 hours.

3. Operations on the brain present special difficulties because in most areas the brain tissue of obvious functional areas, and what were in the past considered 'silent' areas, do not differ in appearance. The cortex was mapped by surgeons, such as Wilder Penfield (1891–1976) in Montreal, using an electrical probe while operating under local anaesthesia on conscious patients. In order to detect incipient functional damage when operating close to vital areas, neurosurgeons often carry out intracranial operations with the patient conscious and monitored.

4. Some intracranial operations are undertaken with the patient awake so that any neurological deficit can be instantly monitored. Intraoperative neurophysiological monitoring has also advanced precise localization of brain lesions.

5. Advanced three-dimensional imaging methods allow tumours to be accurately located. A stereotactic frame can be positioned and used as a guide to locate lesions, including in outpatient stereotactic brain biopsy. As an alternative to open surgery, many can be treated in a single session using Gamma Knife radiosurgery, particularly for small tumours or vascular malformations. Multiple narrow intersecting beams are focused on the tumour with minimal damage to the surrounding normal brain.

REFERENCE

1. Crist SB, et al. Unchecked oxidative stress in skeletal muscle prevents outgrowth of disseminated tumour cells. *Nat Cell Biol.* 2022;24(4):538–553.

FURTHER READING

Jenkins TPN. The burst abdominal wound: a mechanical approach. *Br J Surg.* 1976; 63(11):873–876.

Kaoutzanis C, et al. Autologous fat grafting after breast reconstruction in post mastectomy patients–complications, biopsy rates and locoregional cancer recurrence rates. *Ann Plast Surg.* 2016;76:270–275.

Chapter | **8** |

Handling bone and joints

BONE

Physical characteristics

1. Although it appears rigid and static, bone is a complex, flexible, dynamic and highly specialised connective tissue. There are four types of bone: long bone (long thin shape, e.g., femur), short bone (cube shape with a squat, e.g., carpal bones), flat bones (flattened with broad surface, e.g., skull bones) and irregular bone (shape does not conform to other types of bone, e.g., vertebrae). Long bones must grow as a child develops towards adult size. At one end (usually at both ends) of the main central section, the diaphysis (from the Greek *dia* = between + *phyein* = to bring forth; to grow), is a growing bone, a hyaline cartilage growth plate, the physis, beyond which are the ends, the epiphyses (from the Greek *epi* = upon). The epiphyses commonly participate in joints. The part of the diaphysis beneath the physis continuing to grow until maturity is the metaphysis (from the Greek *meta* = apart). The perichondrial ring of Lacroix (Pierre LaCroix, 1910–1971, Professor of Anatomy and Chief of Orthopaedics, Louvain, Belgium) is a circumferential ring in the periphery of the epiphyseal cartilage, at the chondro-osseous junction. Deep to this is the groove of Ranvier (Louis Antoine Ranvier, 1835–1922, French histologist) which contains the cells that induce chondrogenesis and osteogenesis. Make every effort to protect the growth plates—the perichondrial ring—from damage. Recognise and allow for this in growing children.

2. The architectural structure of a long bone is complex. The outer cortex is compact with a porosity of only 5–10%. Successive layers of collagen fibrils, orientated at right angles to each other like plywood, form an elastic matrix with great tensile (from the Latin *tendere* = to stretch) strength. On this are deposited crystals of calcium phosphate, providing rigidity and high compression strength but low tensile strength. The medulla is cancellous; a latticework, with a porosity of over 50%. The distribution is not haphazard—trabeculae (small beams, in Latin) carry the weight to the cortex, especially near joint surfaces.

3. Bone is absorbed or deposited in response to the imposed stresses of gravity and activity; this is theorised to be mediated by a piezo-electric (from the Greek *piezein* = to press; electricity generated by strain on certain crystals) effect and streaming potential changes in the bone fluids. The bone undergoes demineralization during inactivity but in the presence of continued high stress the compact cortex increases; osteoclasts first create space in which osteoblasts form mineralised tubular Haversian canals (Clopton Havers, 1657–1702, London anatomist and physician). The bone surface is covered with periosteum, consisting of an outer durable connective tissue layer covering an inner cambium layer rich in osteoblasts; these form the primary source of cells uniting a fracture or osteotomy, so avoid crushing or unnecessary stripping. Be aware of and preserve the bone blood supply. Apart from the nutrient artery which pierces the diaphysis giving ascending and descending medullary arteries, vessels enter at muscle, tendon, ligament and capsular insertions, especially around the metaphysis.

4. Infection of bone results from pathogens that reach the bone by haematogenous spread, direct trauma or direct extension from a focus of infection. Persistent bone infection may result in a cycle of inflammation, increased pressure, local ischaemia and bone necrosis which may further result in chronic infection and respond poorly to antibiotics. During operations sedulously avoid contamination by adhering to a 'no touch' technique, using instruments rather than fingers to manipulate bone whenever possible, and wearing two pairs of gloves. A compound, or open, fracture is potentially more serious than a closed fracture and needs to be addressed more urgently.

5. Bony union, following fracture or osteotomy, occurs only if the surfaces are brought into fairly close contact or if the gap is filled with bone graft. Perfect apposition, absence of movement and compression of the fragments achieves primary union. This is known as absolute stability resulting in primary bone healing. A haematoma develops if there is movement or separation of the fragments; this is invaded in turn by granulation tissue, cartilage and osteoid tissue, called 'callus', which later ossifies. Rigid fixation allows early return of function and weight-bearing, avoiding joint stiffness and muscle wasting. It is, though, recognised that a slight degree of movement encourages healing. This is known as relative stability resulting in secondary bone healing.

6. Consider your patient's age; physiological age may be more important than chronological age. Furthermore, consider their gender, nutritional status and any comorbidities; their reaction to operation and subsequent healing is markedly influenced by all of these factors.

EXPOSURE

1. Many approaches are standardised. Learn and apply them to avoid damaging overlying structures. Important things to note with surgical approaches include anatomical landmarks, incisions, muscular planes, nervous planes, local anatomy and structures at risk. Equally important is avoidance of unnecessary periosteal stripping, and damage to the perichondrial ring around the physis in children.

2. This is no excuse for failing to revise the anatomy of the whole area because missiles, trauma and invasive diseases do not respect anatomical planes. You may need to explore beyond the intended limits.

Steadying

1. Do not work on unfixed and unsteadied bone with sharp, and especially powered sharp, tools. Your tools will inevitably slip and damage the bone and vital soft tissues. Stable control of the bone and tools is essential. This can be achieved manually or with the aid of instruments such as clamps or percutaneous wires.

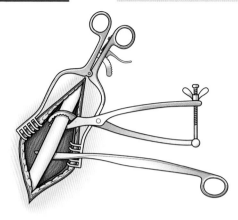

Fig. 8.1 Use a self-retaining retractor and a bone lever to expose a long bone. Have your assistant steady the bone with bone-holding forceps.

2. Make use of retractors, levers, forceps, guard plates, swabs and your assistants to protect the tissues from inadvertent damage (Fig. 8.1).
3. If you change your point of attack, reassess your safeguards (e.g., retractor position) and if necessary rearrange them.

BIOPSY

1. Although radiological imaging methods have developed, histological diagnosis, by bone biopsy, may still be required to obtain definitive diagnosis of general and bone disease.
2. If the area is soft, diagnostic cells can be recovered using fine-needle aspiration cytology or Tru-Cut needle biopsy, introduced percutaneously and guided by imaging methods if necessary.
3. Under local anaesthesia, through a small skin incision you may obtain a bone marrow specimen using a Jamshidi type needle (Khosrow Jamshidi, Iranian haematologist); a hollow needle with a cutting edge. This is rotated in a reciprocal fashion to pierce the cortex. Larger amounts can be obtained by multiple punctures, especially from the posterior iliac crests. The needle is used in an emergency to infuse fluids into the bone marrow when venous access is difficult. The most suitable site is the tibia, 1 cm medial and 1 cm below the tuberosity. They can be used in children in an emergency trauma situation. A circular trephine cuts by rotating

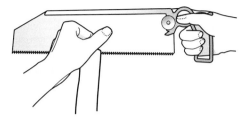

Fig. 8.2 Start the saw cut by drawing the blade towards you, steadying the blade with the nondominant thumb placed high up on the blade.

it like a circular pastry cutter. Guided biopsy may be performed under imaging control.
4. Open biopsy, usually under general anaesthesia, requires exposure of the bone. Use cutting tools to remove bone; soft tissues can be removed with a knife or curette.

CUTTING OF BONE (OSTEOTOMY)

Hand saw

1. Hand saws are infrequently used now, even for major amputations.
2. Decide the line of the cut and expose it fully, clear of other structures.
3. Protect the soft tissues in the line of the cut and those that might be damaged if the saw blade slips. If you cover them, you also protect them from bone dust.
4. Hand saws are designed to make straight cuts. Do not attempt to change the line of the cut or you risk jamming the blade. Start a fresh line.
5. First create a starter groove by drawing the blade towards you, while steadying it against your nondominant thumb placed well above the teeth (Fig. 8.2).

> **Key point**
>
> • Remember that saws remove a wider thickness of bone than the thickness of the blade, because of the 'set' of the teeth.

6. In some cases, you can use a saw guide.
7. Use a steady, rhythmic, to-and-fro movement, the full length of the blade, putting no downward pressure on the saw. The teeth cut as you push the saw away from you.

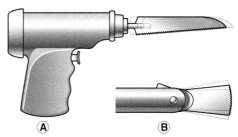

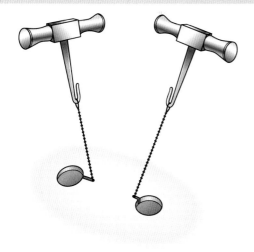

Fig. 8.4 Powered saws are of two types. (A) A reciprocating saw moves the blade back and forth in the same manner as a hand saw (see Fig. 8.2). (B) A powered oscillating saw blade moves in a limited segment of a circle.

Fig. 8.3 The Gigli wire saw can be passed under the bone, handles attached and drawn on in turn, to cut up to the surface.

8. At the end of the cut avoid putting a strain on the bone or you will fracture it. Prefer to lighten the movement so that the last section does not suddenly give way. In some cases, you can make a counter-cut from the opposite side, so the break occurs away from the edge and avoids leaving a sharp projecting splinter.

Gigli saw

The cutting wire can be passed under a bone, or a portion of bone demarcated with access through holes. Attach handles at each end and draw the saw, using a reciprocal motion, towards the surface, sawing within the bone. This reduces the risk of damaging deep structures (Fig. 8.3).

Powered saws (Fig. 8.4)

1. Power is by electricity or compressed air. Circular rotation is potentially dangerous because the unengaged portion of the blade is liable to damage other tissues–or you. A reciprocating (from the Latin *re* = backwards + *pro* = forwards; hence, back-and-forth; reciprocating) saw is less dangerous.
2. Radially oscillating (from the Latin *oscillare* = to swing) blades, sawing in a small segment of arc only, at approximately 15,000 cycles/second, reduce the cutting areas.
3. High-speed saws produce a fine cloud of bone particles. Protect surrounding tissues or they

will be covered with bone swarf, which is a potential contaminant.

4. The saw blade heats up during long cuts, overheating bone in contact with it, which will die. Continually cool the blade with a sterile saline solution.
5. Do not use blunt blades in powered saws; they cut unreliably.

Key points
• Protect the tissues from inadvertent damage and bone swarf.   • Wear eye protection to avoid getting 'splatter' into your own eyes.   • Avoid overheating bone or it will subsequently die. Use saline irrigation.   • Be doubly careful when nearing the end of the cut in case the saw rapidly over-runs the desired course.

Osteotome

1. This is thin, has bevels on both sides and is designed to make only straight cuts (Fig. 8.5A) rather than destroy bone, as opposed to a chisel that has a bevel on one side.
2. Plan the cut carefully to avoid deviation, which would strain the thin metal shaft.
3. Hold the osteotome in your nondominant hand and drive it using a short-handed mallet to limit the striking force (Fig. 8.6).
4. To prevent shattering any brittle cortical bone, either first drill holes in the line of the cut or first cut chips out of the cortex so it can accommodate the thickness of the blade (Fig. 8.7).

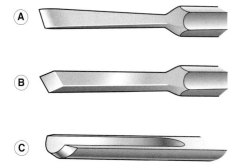

Fig. 8.5 (A) Osteotome. (B) Chisel. (C) Gouge.

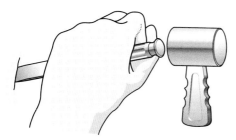

Fig. 8.6 Cutting with an osteotome or chisel. Steady the hand holding the tool to prevent it from slipping to one side or cutting right through the bone and damaging soft tissues beyond.

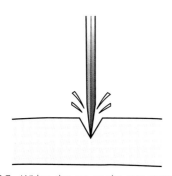

Fig. 8.7 Widen the cut as the osteotome bites deeper by successively chipping flakes from each side so that the thickness of the instrument can be accommodated to prevent splitting.

Key point

- Steady the hand, holding the osteotome in such a way that you prevent the tool from slipping to one side or cutting through the bone into the soft tissues beyond.

Chisel

1. The bevel (Fig. 8.5B) on the chisel (from the Old French *cisel*, derived from the Latin *caedere* = to cut), also driven by a short-handled mallet, resists cutting along a straight path.
2. If you place the chisel on a bony surface, bevel uppermost and tap it, it may chip off a flake of superficial bone (Fig. 8.8). As it bites, the bevel makes it angle deeper so that the handle swings more vertically. There is a danger that the thickness of the chisel may fracture the bone.
3. If the bevel is on the undersurface, you need to start the cut with the tool held more vertically or it will fail to bite and will slide along the surface. As soon as the bevel enters the bone, the chisel tends to lift the edge on the unbevelled side and the handle is angled downwards. When you drive the chisel further, the effect of the bevel is to guide the cutting edge towards the surface, lifting off a sliver (from Old English, *slifan* = to cleave) of superficial bone, as the chisel lies almost parallel with the surface.
4. A gouge (Fig. 8.5C) has a hollow blade to scoop out. The bevel is on the outside so that it does not bite deeply. It is useful for harvesting cancellous bone.

Cutting forceps

1. These act as scissors (Fig. 8.9) so you can make small cuts through bone that is not too thick or brittle, such as a rib, although a special guillotine type of tool is available for this purpose.
2. It inevitably has a crushing effect on the bone. In case of doubt, therefore, prefer to use a saw when this is appropriate.

Rongeurs

1. There are several versions of these (Fig. 8.9) and as the name implies (from the French *ronger* = to gnaw), they nibble away bone, especially in difficult corners or cavities.
2. They are valuable where a power tool or an osteotome may endanger vital tissues as in spinal laminectomy.
3. Rongeurs are useful for obtaining specimens for histology from bone or other hard tissues. Because the jaws are hollowed out, they do not excessively crush and destroy the architecture of the specimens.

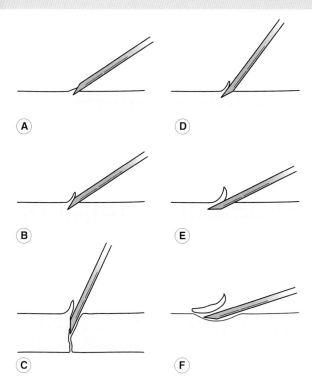

Fig. 8.8 Driving a chisel into bone. (A) Bevel uppermost. (B) It tends to angle vertically as it bites more deeply. (C) It becomes even more vertical and may split the bone. (D) Bevel on the underside. (E) The chisel tip lifts a sliver of bone and tends to flatten. (F) The chisel has cut out and lies almost parallel with the bone surface.

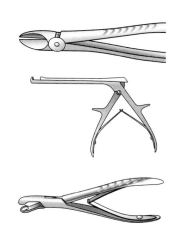

Fig. 8.9 Bone cutting forceps at top. Rongeurs at centre and bottom; these have cupped blades so fragments of detached bone are grasped but not crushed and can be removed.

File

As bone is not homogeneous like metal and wood, files tend to be used only for rasping sharp edges from angular cuts made with saws and other instruments, for example following an amputation.

DRILLING OF BONE

1. Hand drills (Fig. 8.10) are not now used routinely for drilling bone. It may be difficult to start the hole, especially on rounded, hard, cortical bone, without first making a preliminary notch with an awl or sharp punch. Otherwise, the drill point tends to 'walk' away from the intended point of penetration.
2. Because both hands are fully occupied with holding and turning the drill it is difficult to control. Limit the penetration of the cutting bit by ensuring that only the required length protrudes from the chuck or fix a clamp to the bit to act as a buffer when it hits the bone surface.
3. A hand brace (Fig. 8.11) can be used when trephining the skull; in this case, the bit is

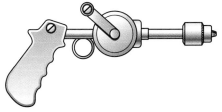

Fig. 8.10 Hand drill.

159

Fig. 8.11 Brace and tools for opening the skull. At the top is a perforator and below are two types of burrs.

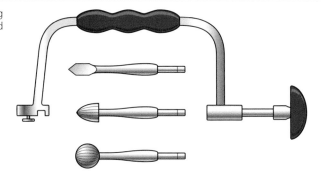

not a drill but a shaped cutting perforator that prevents sudden uncontrolled penetration. The opening in the skull can then be enlarged using burrs, which act like circular rasps.

4. Powered drills (Fig. 8.12) are now routinely employed. Properly controlled, they allow you to concentrate on the process of drilling without the need to turn the bit yourself. Since they rotate at a higher speed than manual drills, they may easily 'run away'. Identify and carefully protect vulnerable soft tissues from damage and from the spray of bone dust.

5. Powered drills that are run continuously may heat the bone to 50°C, causing irreversible necrosis and reabsorption.

Key points

- When overheated bone dies and is reabsorbed, inserted screws loosen.
- Drill intermittently for short periods.
- Cool the bit with cold, sterile, physiological saline.

---

6. Once a hole is drilled it may be enlarged using a reamer (the Old English term meaning 'to make room'). Various shaping bits can be used, as when preparing a joint socket for replacement.

7. The availability of accurately made prostheses (from the Greek pros = to + thesis = a putting; hence an addition to or substitution of, for example, lost parts) demands that they are accurately fitted. When fixing bones by screwing on metal plates and similar devices, you must drill the holes accurately both for perfect alignment and also to avoid excessively weakening the bone. Whenever possible make use of drill guides (Fig. 8.13). For many standardised procedures special drill guides form part of the kit to enable you to drill screw holes accurately.

8. Clear away bone chips after drilling a hole.

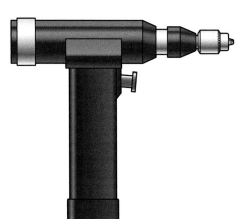

Fig. 8.12 Powered drill.

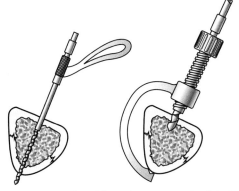

Fig. 8.13 Drill guides. The one on the left is handheld; the one on the right can be firmly attached to the bone, leaving you two hands to control the drill.

Key points

- Protect the soft tissues using drill guides or retractors.
- Avoid damage to soft tissue beyond the opposite cortex from emerging drill bit by controlled drilling.
- Protect your eyes.
- Repeatedly check that the exit is free from tissues that could be damaged or caught up.
- Do not bend drills; the bits are brittle and will break.
- Do not exert excessive pressure or you will jam the bit.

FIXING

Screws

1. Properly used, screws are very versatile and provide a valuable method of fixing bones, and for fixing plates and prostheses to bone.
2. Screws are made from a variety of metals including stainless steel or titanium alloys. Pure titanium provokes almost no tissue reaction and does not interfere with magnetic resonance imaging (MRI). Biodegradable screws, usually of long-chain polymers, can also be used in specific cases.
3. When using metals, ensure that they are compatible. If screws of one metal hold plates of another metal they generate electrolytic action, weakening the metal and provoking bone absorption. This process is known as galvanic corrosion.

Key points

- Do not screw cortical bone as you screw cancellous bone or wood, which accepts the extra volume of a screw by compacting.
- Cortical bone is already compact and brittle. Provide an adequate hole or it will split.

4. Screws differ according to the function they are intended to perform (Fig. 8.14). Those that need a firm grip of the dense cortex have a thicker stem and short, strong threads. Those inserted into the less dense cancellous bone have a slimmer stem and wider, thinner

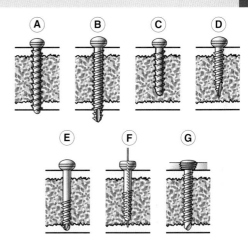

Fig. 8.14 (A) Cortical screws are usually inserted through both the near and far cortices of, for example, a long bone. For this reason, the hole is normally drilled and tapped so it grips at both ends. The screw end is rounded so that its projecting tip does not potentially damage soft tissue beyond. A cortical screw cannot be self-drilling because the sharp edge of the tip is blunted by the first cortex and cannot penetrate the second one. (B) Cortical screws may be self-tapping, but the bevelled tapping tip must project far enough for the full succeeding thread to engage within the distal cortex. (C) Cancellous screws have narrower shafts but wider threads in order to compact and grip the looser cancellous bone. They are self-tapping and are not intended to enter and grip the distal cortex. (D) A self-drilling and self-tapping cancellous screw has a sharp-edged tip that cuts a thread as the screw is inserted. This facilitates percutaneous insertion, increasingly valuable with modern techniques. (E) Cancellous screws may have a thread formed only at the distal end of a screw while the proximal shaft remains smooth. This is a lag screw. If it crosses a gap before reentering the cancellous bone and is then tightened, it closes the gap. (F) When it is difficult to align a screw correctly, insert a guidewire, check that it is correctly positioned and pass a cannulated screw over it and screw it in before withdrawing the guidewire. (G) A screw fixing a plate to bone may then be solidly fixed to the plate. The screw head is threaded and engages with an internal thread on the inside of the hole. The screw is cancellous, self-tapping. It does not penetrate the far cortex because the cutting edge is lost on the near cortex.

threads since they can compact and grip the medullary inner bone. It was conventional to drill a hole, tap the hole and finally insert the screw for cortical screws, but cancellous screws are able to cut their own threads through the softer bone. Self-tapping cortical screws are

161

now used in most units. Self-drilling and self-tapping screws exist. These are used with extreme caution if the screw is intended to grip the far cortex since the cutting edges can be damaged as they pass through the near cortex.

5. Lag screws have smooth shafts near the head and screw threads only on the distal portion. The intention is that the thread draws whatever it enters tightly up against the material near the proximal part (see later). Screws can be used in a lag mode. This means drilling a larger diameter proximal hole and a smaller diameter distal hole, so the screw grips the distal portion of bone hole.

6. It may be difficult to place a screw correctly. One method of avoiding an error is to insert guidewires until one proves to be correct. A cannulated screw can be fed over the guidewire and screwed in, after which the guidewire is withdrawn. Screws holding bone plates can be locked to the plate by having a threaded screw head which engages with an internal thread in the plate hole (see later).

7. If a cortical screw is inserted across a longitudinally split long bone and tightened, it will not close the gap (Fig. 8.15). If the proximal cortex is drilled oversize so that the threads in the proximal cortex do not engage, the threads in the distal cortex draw the separated bones together. This is known as lag screw mode, as previously mentioned. Do not attempt to employ a cancellous screw with a smooth proximal shaft for this because the distal cancellous screw threads will not grip the dense distal cortex.

8. When fixing long bones, the specialised screws must pierce and grip the dense outer bone, usually of both cortices; these are cortical screws and are threaded along their whole length. First, drill a hole of the same bore as the shank of the screw from which the thread flanges project. Measure the length of the hole so you can select the correct length of screw. Now use a tap of the correct size to cut the thread. Unscrew the tap, remove the loose bony fragments and insert the screw (Fig. 8.16).

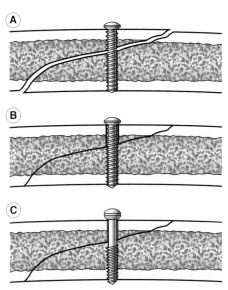

Fig. 8.15 (A) A fully threaded screw inserted in a fully tapped track created while the bones remain apart will have no compression effect on the gap. (B) If the proximal cortex is drilled oversize, the screw acts as a lag screw, compressing the bones. (C) Do not use a cancellous screw, with an unthreaded part of the shank, as an alternative to drilling the proximal fragment oversised and using a cortical screw. The cancellous screw will not grip the far cortex sufficiently securely.

Key points

- Do not over-tighten screws; if you do, you will strip the threads.
- Perform the final tightening with finger and thumb pressure on the screwdriver.

9. If you place a screw perpendicular to the bone surface to unite oblique surfaces in a long bone, such as a fracture line, it will slip when longitudinal stresses are applied. Instead, insert the screw perpendicular to the fracture line (Fig. 8.17). In practice, the single screw will not stabilise the fracture, so it will usually be supported by a plate and screws; these plate-holding screws are inserted at right angles to the bone and do not cross the fracture (see later).

10. If there is a spiral fracture, insert the screws through the middle of the fragments along the bone, so they also form a spiral (Fig. 8.18).

11. If a screw head protrudes and will interfere with function, cause pain or be unsightly, use a countersink drill bit to create a depression into which the screw head fits.

12. Sometimes retained screws and other metal inserts, such as plates, cause problems after they have served their purpose and may need to be removed. The short- and long-term

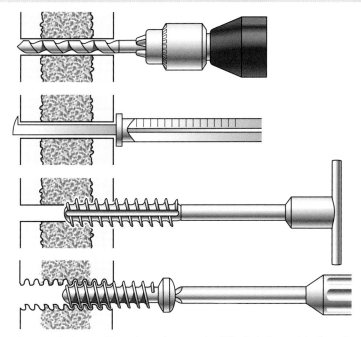

Fig. 8.16 Inserting a cortical screw. From above downwards: drill a hole through both cortices. Use a depth gauge to measure the required screw length; tap the hole to cut the screw thread; insert and drive home the screw.

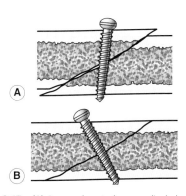

Fig. 8.17 (A) A screw inserted perpendicularly across the bone will not hold an oblique fracture, which will slip. (B) The screw must be perpendicular to the fracture and oblique to the shaft. Of course, a single screw would not suffice. If the fracture needs plating, the plate screws are inserted perpendicular to the bone.

results of both glass ceramic and biodegradable screws are under trial.

Suturing

Surgical sutures (or stitches) hold connective tissue together; they can be inserted into the periosteum or ligaments. Alternatively, you may drill holes

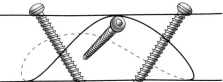

Fig. 8.18 Insert screws through the middle of the fragments to stabilise a spiral fracture, so they also form a spiral.

into which you can insert sutures. Special small screws can be inserted into bone, which carry a thread. The thread can be used to attach a structure to the bone.

Wiring

1. The commonest use of wires in surgical practice is to maintain bone fragment alignment by transfixation or blocking technique usually using Kirschner wires (K-wires) (Martin Kirschner, 1879–1942, German surgeon). Bone can also be fixed by encircling it with wire (Fig. 8.19). This may prejudice the blood supply, so it is infrequently used for normal circumstances and the wire is often removed later.

2. Tension band wiring can be achieved by twisting the wire ends evenly. If you keep

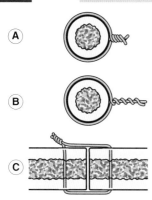

Fig. 8.19 Wiring bone. (A) The ends of the encircling wire are evenly twisted. (B) One wire has been wound around the other wire, which is straight. This is insecure. (C) Drill the bone and pass wire through the holes in the manner of a stitch.

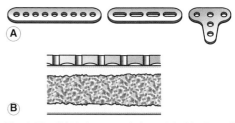

Fig. 8.20 (A) Various metal plates. (B) Side view of low contact plate designed to reduce pressure on the periosteum.

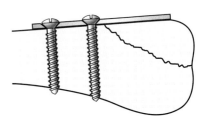

Fig. 8.21 Plate used as a buttress to hold a fragment in place.

one end straight and wrap the other around it, it has no holding power. If you over-tighten the wire it will fracture. Turn the ends of the twisted wire so they do not protrude under the skin or press upon vulnerable structures.

3. As an alternative to encircling wire, drill holes through the bone and use wire like a stitch.
4. In some situations, the bone can be stapled, especially if it is cancellous. Tap in the staple in an introducer, then remove the introducer so the staple can be driven fully home.
5. Use of encircling wire fixation is increasing as patients with longstanding prosthetic joints develop peri-prosthetic fractures. Screw fixation of plates may not be possible but special screws with eyed heads can be screwed into plate holes so that encircling wires can be attached to the eyes and tightened to fix the plate.

Plates

1. Metal plates are manufactured of stainless steel, vitallium and titanium (Fig. 8.20). They may be straight, angled flat, tubular, with round or oval holes, holes arranged in rows or staggered. It is now recognised that the pressure of the plate tends to crush the delicate periosteum and occlude the blood supply to the underlying bone. Whenever possible, use low contact plates which are undercut between the screw holes.
2. Plates may be used as struts to maintain mechanical support or as buttresses pushing in a fragment (Fig. 8.21).

3. During surgery, place the bones in correct alignment, select a suitable-sized plate and if necessary bend it to fit accurately. Make sure that at least two holes lie over each fragment (the number of holes required will depend on several factors, e.g., size of bone, degree of instability, mode of fixation).
4. Clamp the plate in place while drilling through the centre of each hole towards the opposite cortex using a drill guide.

Key points

- Do not overstrip the peritoneum or crush it. When possible, use low-contact plates.
- Be very careful not to splinter the bone as the drill emerges at the opposite cortex and so prejudice the grip of the screw on the cortex.

5. Estimate the required screw lengths using a depth gauge. Create threads in the hole by a process called tapping. Screws are inserted into the tapped holes (Fig. 8.22). Do not over-tighten them.
6. You may not have access to the ends of the bone on the opposite side from the fracture. If they are not in contact, the plate bridging the break becomes a fulcrum when the bone comes under tension; the bone ends are

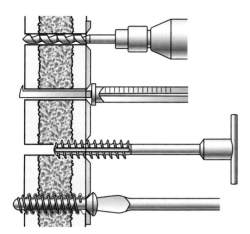

Fig. 8.22 Plating and screwing long bone. Ensure that the plate lies in contact along its length. From top to bottom, drill a hole through both cortices; measure the required screw length using a depth gauge; tap the hole; insert the screw, which should grip the opposite cortex as well as the near one.

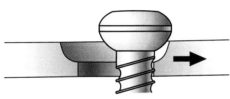

Fig. 8.23 As the round-headed screw head is tightened into the oval hole in the plate, it produces distraction.

alternatively compressed and retracted on the side opposite the plate, causing reabsorption and preventing union. Make sure to check for a gap with an intraoperative image intensifier.

7. *Compressing* the separated ends of the bone facilitates primary union. A simple method of achieving this is to use compression plates with longitudinally oriented oval holes. As the round-headed screw is tightened into the hole, it distracts the plate, effectively shortening it (Fig. 8.23). If the other end of the plate has been firmly fixed to the other fragment, the result is to draw the bones together.

8. A special compression plate can be used. First securely anchor one end on one side of the break. Apply the other component, crossing over the break (Fig. 8.24), so that the hook on the fully opened anchored section can engage in the nearest screw hole. Fix the second

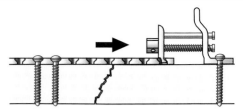

Fig. 8.24 Compression plate. Firmly fix the compression device on the right. Place the plate, crossing the break, so the hook on the fully opened compression device fits into the last screw hole. Fix the opposite end of the plate. Tighten the compression device. Place intermediate screws on both sides of the break. Slacken off and remove the compression device before inserting the last screw in the hole formerly occupied by the hook of the compression device.

plate at its far end from the compression device. Now tighten the screw to draw the two parts together. Insert intermediate screws on both sides of the break. Finally, release the compression device, unscrew it and insert the final screw in the plate that had been engaged with the compression device hook.

9. *Locking plate* fixation is a major advance offering some of the advantages of external fixation. The plate does not need to be in close contact with bone throughout the whole length and can bridge partial gaps, reducing the need for muscular and periosteal stripping. Unicortical screws suffice since they have threads on their heads which engage with screw threads cut into the plate holes; when fully engaged, they grip the bone and are also locked to the plate (Fig. 8.25). The procedure can be partly accomplished by sliding the plate down through an incision under imaging control. Some of the locking screws can be inserted percutaneously through small incisions. The effect is similar to that of external fixators, with pins locking the bones on each side of the break and holding them in a firm relationship with each other.

External fixators

1. Many of these are complex and require advanced skills in order to employ them. Consequently, they are described only to outline the principles on which they work. An important advantage is that the site of a break in continuity can be left undisturbed, fixation being undertaken at a distance on each side.

2. Two or more threaded pins are inserted percutaneously, through small local incisions, into

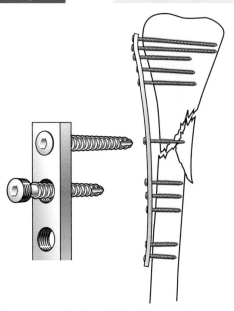

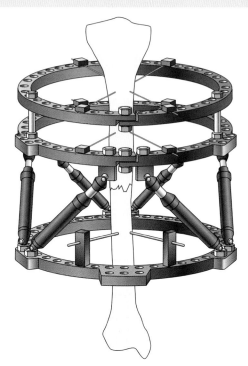

Fig. 8.25 Mechanism of locked plate. As the screws are driven through the plate and into bone, the screw thread on the head of the screws engages with the threaded hole in the plate, locking it and fixing the bone and plate. Note that the plate does not need to be in contact with bone everywhere along its length.

Fig. 8.27 The Taylor Spatial Frame is a versatile development of the Ilizarov method of fixation of fractures. Tensed cross wires within the upper two rings form a stable base for the proximal bone and the lower single ring can be adjusted to align the distal bone correctly by changing the lengths of the adjustable struts.

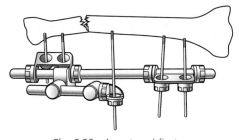

Fig. 8.26 An external fixator.

the bone on either side of the break, and at a distance from it. The pins can then be fixed with clamps at each site. After ensuring, usually with radiological confirmation, that the fragments are perfectly aligned, the clamps are locked onto a common external linkage (Fig. 8.26). The fixators can be adjusted and then relocked if necessary, and the distance between the two groups of fixing pins can be reduced or increased to compress or distract the ends. A more stable arrangement is for the pins to pass right through the limb so the projecting ends can be attached to a second fixator.

3. During the 1950s, G. A. Ilizarov in Kurgan, Siberia, developed a system of transfixing the bones above

and below a break, using wires crossed at right angles to each other, attached under tension across external metal rings. The rings are linked across the break by rods and can be adjusted with turnbuckles to compress or distract the ends. The versatility of the method was further extended by the spatial frame developed by Taylor, allowing realignment by finely adjusting the turnbuckles on the six oblique struts to alter the relation of the rings (Fig. 8.27).

Intramedullary fixation

1. Smooth, double-pointed wires of various lengths and diameters were invented by Martin Kirschner, Professor of Surgery in Heidelberg, in 1909. They can be driven through bone with a T-handled chuck or a powered drill (Fig. 8.28) and inserted percutaneously or introduced at operation. Use a single wire to fix small bones such as phalanges by impaling them as though on a skewer. A number of

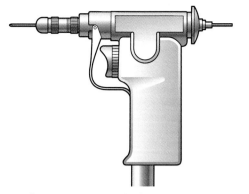

Fig. 8.28 A powered drill to insert wires.

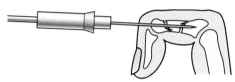

Fig. 8.29 Impaled fragments of a phalanx on a Kirschner wire.

fragments can be threaded on the wire like a kebab (Fig. 8.29). Use the largest size you can insert without splitting the fragments. Insert several wires in order to prevent rotation of the fragments (Fig. 8.30). Kirschner wires offer a valuable method of stabilizing fragments while you apply permanent fixation.

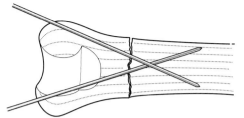

Fig. 8.30 Insert Kirschner wires to prevent rotation of the fragments.

2. An early intramedullary fracture fixation was the trifin nail for femoral neck fractures developed in 1931 by the Norwegian-American Marius Smith-Peterson. The femoral neck and intertrochanteric region are now usually treated using a large cancellous lag screw which engages with the cancellous bone of the femoral head. The smooth proximal shaft of the screw slides within a tube fixed to a plate screwed to the femoral shaft. As the screw is tightened it compresses the neck but as weight-bearing further compresses the fracture the screw can slide within the tube. It is thus dynamic (from the Greek *dynasthai* = to be able) as opposed to static (Fig. 8.31), producing a stabilizing compression effect.

3. In 1940, Gerhard Küntscher of Kiel developed the intramedullary nail for femoral shaft fractures. In many long bones intramedullary nails can be inserted, often through the

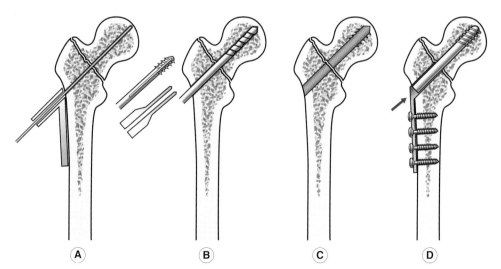

Fig. 8.31 The principle of the lag screw is to compress and stabilise a fractured neck of femur. (A) A guidewire is passed and the correct depth is calculated. (B) The track is drilled out. (C) The section external to the break is reamed out, while the section internal to the break is tapped. (D) A lag screw type of pin is screwed into the inner fragment, and a plate is fixed to the shaft of the femur, carrying a tube within which the shaft of the lag screw can slide and rotate, producing a dynamic hip screw.

167

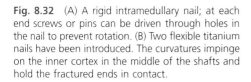

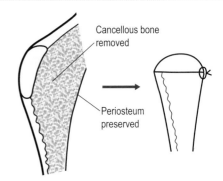

Fig. 8.33 Harvesting cancellous bone. Elevate the iliac crest like the lid of a box, remove cancellous bone, then replace and suture the crest.

Fig. 8.32 (A) A rigid intramedullary nail; at each end screws or pins can be driven through holes in the nail to prevent rotation. (B) Two flexible titanium nails have been introduced. The curvatures impinge on the inner cortex in the middle of the shafts and hold the fractured ends in contact.

metaphysis and with minimal exposure, then locked with screws or pins introduced percutaneously through the bone and holes at each end of the nail, to prevent rotation. Especially for children, flexible titanium nails can be inserted, usually avoiding damage to the metaphysis (Fig. 8.32).

Bone grafts

1. Cancellous (from the Latin *cancelli* = latticework; hence, spongy, porous) bone has little strength but has osteogenic potential. A convenient site is the iliac crest. Expose it, detach the external muscles and cut across the crest with an osteotome, leaving it still attached to the internal muscles. Cut thin slices from the exposed edge. Remove the exposed cancellous bone using a gouge, leaving the inner cortex intact. Finally, replace the iliac crest and secure it by suturing the muscles over it (Fig. 8.33).
2. Cortical bone is strong and can be fixed in place. It is, though, slowly vascularised, may be reabsorbed and has little osteogenic potential. It can be used as a support or strut, to fill a gap.
3. Autografts (from the Greek *autos* = self) are usually used. Allografts (from the Greek *allos* = other; from other humans, usually by donation) that are free from viral infection can be used intact or morselised (chopped), obtained from bone banks, or stimulated by bone morphogenetic proteins.

AMPUTATION

1. Plan amputation (from the Latin *ambi* = around + *putare* + to prune) distal to a joint in order to preserve joint function if possible. Aim to retain the muscle insertions into the distal stump. Preserve a sufficient length of stump if you wish to fit a prosthesis onto it.
2. As a rule, fashion flaps of healthy skin with underlying tissue retracted to expose the bone. Single or double flaps are used depending on the vitality and vascularity of the tissues. Divide the fully exposed bone with a saw after protecting all the soft tissues. Establish perfect haemostasis. Smooth the bone stump using a rasp.

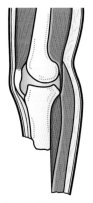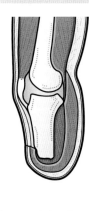

Fig. 8.34 Amputation. This shows a below-knee amputation. Leave the tibia sufficiently long so that a prosthesis can be fitted to it and the knee can be controlled by the descending muscles. The posterior flap has been kept long so that it can be brought over the bone end and stitched to the short anterior flap. Note the rounding of the anterior edge of the tibia.

3. Close the flaps over the stump (Fig. 8.34). Monitor the stump vitality carefully until it is fully healed.
4. Amputation can often be avoided when a length of long bone must be removed for some tumours. After excising the diseased bone, the defect can sometimes be bridged with a graft or metal prosthesis, leaving the limb intact.
5. A method of attaching a prosthesis to an amputated limb has been developed after studying the annual growth and shedding of antlers in deer. A metal terminal prosthesis implanted into the distal end of the transacted bone carries a screw end that protrudes through the skin. A porous ring lying just beneath the skin allows a natural seal to form, preventing bacterial invasion. A prosthesis can be attached to the protruding screw.

JOINTS

1. Many operations are now carried out on joints using arthroscopy. An intraarticular space is created by distending the joint with normal saline. Different parts of the joint may be made accessible by moving the joint during examination or operative procedure.
2. The hyaline cartilage covering the bone ends engaging in synovial joints is avascular and nourished by diffusion, so it has a limited ability to repair itself if diseased or damaged.

On the other hand, the meniscus has a peripheral blood supply with variable vascularity from the inner third to the outer third. Intraarticular tears of the meniscal cartilage (e.g., in the knee), can be treated nonoperatively or operatively. Nonoperative management may involve spontaneous healing while operative management includes repair, partial/total meniscectomy or transplant. Total meniscectomy is avoided because of the risk of eventual arthritis. There have been significant strides in improving surgical techniques for meniscal transplants.

3. The capsule surrounding synovial joints is composed of tough fibrous tissue and this is in places thickened into ligaments which stabilise the joint and limit its movements. Unlike tendons, ligaments are elastic and will stretch if subjected to continuous tension exerted accidentally as following an uncorrected dislocation, or deliberately, to increase joint mobility.
4. A torn intraarticular ligament such as the anterior cruciate ligament of the knee may be removed and replaced. Prosthetic synthetic materials may be used or allografts (from the Greek *allos* = other; from another species). Autografts (from the Greek *autos* = self) are commonly used of two types (see later).
5. Certain joints or joint elements can be replaced when they are diseased or damaged.
6. For some fractures of the hip the best treatment may be replacement of the femoral head and neck with a metal prosthesis. The new head and neck are fixed into the femoral medullary cavity by means of a metal stem (Fig. 8.35). Stem fixation may be achieved using polymethylmethacrylate cement or the stem surface can be coated, for example with sintered metal beads to encourage direct bonding with the tissues, which grow around the beads, providing a solid fix.
7. For complete hip replacement, the acetabulum (from the Latin phrase for vinegar cup) is reamed out to enlarge it and a cup is inserted to receive the replacement femoral head. The head may be of metal, plastic material or ceramic; this has a low wear rate, and its former brittleness has now been overcome. Ultra high molecular weight polyethylene (UHMWPE) articulating with metal may be a successful combination.
8. Other joints can be successfully replaced, or the contacting surfaces can be replaced. Small joints, such as those in the fingers, can be replaced using one-piece flexible, usually Silastic, prostheses.

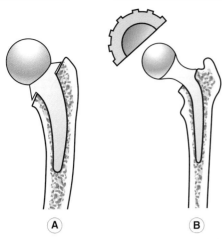

Fig. 8.35 (A) Replacement femoral head which fits into the acetabulum. (B) Total hip replacement. The replacement head fits into a socket fixed into the reamed-out acetabulum.

CARTILAGE

1. The articulating ends of bones are covered with hyaline cartilage. Articular cartilage is avascular and intraarticular with an indirect blood supply in the subchondral region. When damaged, it has limited ability to regenerate and usually repairs by the formation of fibrocartilage. Healing is more certain, the nearer the damage lies in relation to the blood supply. In some joints, notably the knee, there are cartilaginous menisci between the bone ends. The contacting surfaces can be smoothed. This is usually achieved arthroscopically.
2. Various techniques are used in the hope of replacing deficient articular cartilage, such as creating multiple perforations in the bone, with the hope that the underlying bone marrow contains pluripotent cells that can reproduce the cartilage; alternatively, periosteum contains pluripotent cells. Multiple cartilage-covered bone grafts may be laid down.

LIGAMENTS

1. These unite bone to bone, preventing or restricting movement. In many joints, they may form part of the surrounding capsule.
2. When subjected to increased tension over a period, ligaments stretch, especially in youth, permitting an increased range of movement.
3. Ligaments around the knee are particularly at risk of damage. Lateral trauma tends to open the knee joint medially and tear the medial collateral ligament and vice versa.
4. A twisting motion, especially when the foot is firmly on the ground, may rupture the anterior cruciate ligament (ACL). Women are more at risk than men. Operative management is not always necessary. In some cases, the ACL tear can be repaired with different techniques which are of great research interest. More commonly, in clinical practice, the completely ruptured ACL is reconstructed. In one method, braided hamstring tendons are led between the tibia and the femur. Alternatively, the central section of the patellar ligament, with attached bone from the patella and the tibia, may be used since the bone fragments at each end will fuse with the femur above and the tibia below.

TENDONS

1. Tendons unite bone to muscle and are stiffer than muscle.
2. If a tendon ruptures at its insertion into bone it is usual practice to cut out a cortical panel so that it can be inserted into cancellous bone and sutured in after drilling stitch holes through which can be passed nonabsorbable stitches.
3. If a distal stump of well-vascularised tendon remains, unite the ends. The latter can be achieved nonoperatively by splinting the limb until the tendon heals or operatively by repairing the tendon ends.

Chapter | 9 |

Handling dissection

Dissection (from the Latin *dis* = apart + *secare* = to cut; hence to cut apart) may be necessary to approach a structure to identify, display, examine, repair or resect it. It demands an intimate knowledge of the anatomy and the differential makeup of tissues in health and disease. One of the hallmarks of surgical competence is the ability to carry out dissection in the presence of unusual conditions. For this reason, patients with complications from previous operations, those with difficult and extensive diseases and those with comorbidity tend to be referred to surgeons who are recognised to have exceptional competence. They did not acquire the competence by chance but by outstanding concentration and effort.

ORGANISE

1. Ensure that the patient is in a position that facilitates exposure: supine, prone, level, flexed or tilted.
2. If the operating table is tilted, ensure that the patient is properly secured.
3. Make use of gravity; for example, when operating on the pelvis, to empty it of bowel, place the patient with their head down (the position named after the German surgeon Friedrich

Trendelenburg, 1844–1925). Alternatively, place the patient head up to ensure that the neck veins are not congested when operating on the neck (often called 'reversed Trendelenburg'). Raise the limbs to reduce congestion. However, remember that prolonged positioning with the legs up can cause compartment syndrome.

4. Place pillows or sandbags to elevate a part or retain the patient in the required posture.

5. In some cases, ensure that you can turn the patient or limb during the procedure and drape up accordingly.

6. Ensure that you have good, shadowless, glare-free light. When appropriate, make use of light-carrying retractors or a headlight.

7. Ensure that pressure areas are protected (see Ch. 14)

8. Ensure that measures are in place to prevent deep venous thrombosis (see Ch. 14).

EXPOSE

1. Plan the incision carefully. Do not compromise on attaining safe access but consider the cosmetic and functional effects. Many generations of surgeons have accumulated a wealth of standardised safe approaches. Use a standard approach whenever possible but remember that there are anatomical anomalies and also that disease processes or recurrent surgery may change the anatomy. In addition, many standard approaches have caveats (from the Latin *cavere* = to take care), such as the need to avoid entering the brachial artery when giving an intravenous injection at the elbow, and to avoid injury to the facial nerve when operating on the parotid gland. If you need to use a novel method, study the anatomy carefully, asking yourself why your approach is not normally used. In the skin, keeping to Langer's lines (after the anatomist Karl Langer, 1819–1887) where possible will produce a better cosmetic and functional result. Remember to avoid skin incisions that cross the flexor surface of joints at 90 degrees to the skin crease as this may result in contractures.

2. In some cases, you cannot predict the findings and may need to extend the incision, so adjust your incision to accommodate this. For limb surgery, A. K. Henry, Professor of Anatomy in Cairo, used the term 'extensile exposure' in his book on limb surgery,[1] meaning approaches that can be enlarged.

3. Make sure you are in the correct tissue layer; failure to do so may lead you to error.

4. When possible gently split muscle and aponeurotic fibres rather than cut them. You may be able to displace nerves, blood vessels, tendons and ligaments rather than transect them. If you need to keep such delicate neurovascular structures out of the way a slim silicon vessel loop can be used to gently retract.

5. Make use of the full length of the incision and if necessary, have the wound edges retracted. Prefer dynamic retraction by an assistant, which can be adjusted as necessary and relaxed at intervals, to fixed self-retaining retraction, where possible. Your assistant can gently displace intervening structures with fingers, after covering slippery tissues with a gauze swab (Fig. 9.1), though this technique should be avoided if you are dissecting with a scalpel, to avoid injury to your assistant. Apply tissue forceps to tough structures to retract them (Fig. 9.2).

6. Make use of gravity by moving the patient or a part to displace an obstructing, intervening

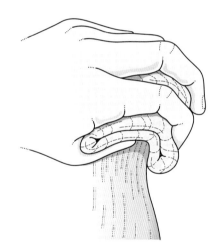

Fig. 9.1 Retracting with fingers over a gauze swab to improve the grip on slippery tissues.

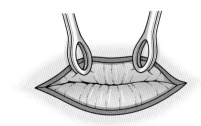

Fig. 9.2 Use tissue forceps to retract tough tissues.

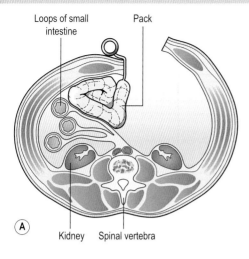

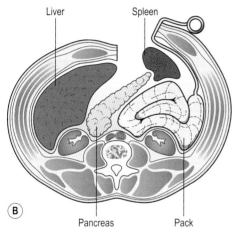

Fig. 9.3 Large packs. (A) The pack holds aside a structure to prevent it from intruding into the wound—in this case, small bowel loops. (B) A large pack placed behind a structure lifts it up into the mouth of the wound. Note the tape attached to large metal rings left outside the wound.

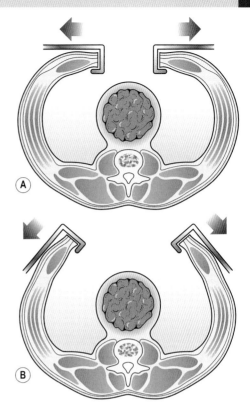

Fig. 9.4 Displaying a fixed deep structure. As an alternative to retracting the wound edges, as in (A), is it possible to depress them as in (B)?

delicate procedure in the depths where the lighting and access are limited. Sometimes a pack can be placed beneath a structure to raise it (Fig. 9.3); alternatively try depressing the edges of the incision (Fig. 9.4).

Key points

- Exposure is prejudiced by poor haemostasis. Blood staining obscures the distinctive appearance of differing tissues.
- If you wish to see what you are doing, first stop the bleeding.

DISSECTION METHODS

Sharp

structure. Alternatively, use large packs with tapes attached to substantial metal rings kept outside the wound or clipped to the external towels, to guard against leaving them inside (Fig. 9.3). Sometimes a structure cannot be removed but can be rotated on its anchoring tissues; for example, the left lobe of the liver can be gently folded to give access to the oesophageal hiatus, and the column of the trachea, larynx, oesophagus and thyroid gland can be rotated to bring the posterior aspect of the pharynx into view.

7. Prefer to bring a mobile structure to the surface of the wound in preference to carrying out a

1. The scalpel divides tissues with the minimum damage. If the tissues move under the drag

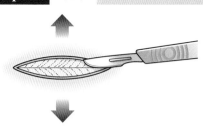

Fig. 9.5 If you apply tension to separate the margins of the incision when cutting with a scalpel, you display the depths of the wound, so you do not inadvertently cut too deeply.

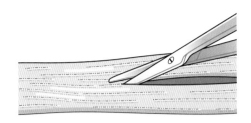

Fig. 9.7 Splitting parallel fibres with scissors. Almost close the scissors and push the small 'V' between the blade tips into the tissues, along the line of the fibres.

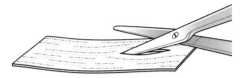

Fig. 9.6 When cutting with scissors, protect the underlying structures from inadvertent damage by the deep blade.

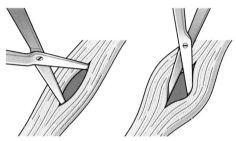

Fig. 9.8 Splitting parallel fibres with scissors. Push the closed tips into the sheet of tissue and open them parallel to the fibres. If there are underlying structures with side branches, open the scissors at a right angle to the line of the intended split.

of the scalpel steady them with your fingers, if necessary separating your fingers to open up the incision, displaying the deeper structures (Fig. 9.5).

2. Expertly performed scissors dissection produces minimal damage especially when floppy tissue is difficult to stabilise for cutting with a scalpel. Do not use blunt or loosely hinged scissors. The blades must remain in contact, or they tend to chew through the tissues. Scissors have the advantage that they can be used for blunt or sharp dissection. Insert the closed blades and gently open them to define a plane of cleavage or cut the tissues to separate them. A potential danger is that the deep blade is hidden in some circumstances (Fig. 9.6), so first carefully inspect and palpate the deep surface.

Blunt

1. Splitting is a valuable method of dissecting muscle and aponeuroses or opening up tissues along the direction of linear structures such as vessels, nerves and tendons. It is a method that allows you to follow a natural path rather than creating one by sharp dissection. The line of cleavage is parallel to the strong fibres, which are held together by weaker interconnecting fibres. Scissors can be used to split a sheet after it has been penetrated in one place

and separated from deep structures. Insert one blade of almost fully closed scissors into the hole and push them in the direction of the fibres (Fig. 9.7).

2. A different splitting action can be achieved with scissors by holding them perpendicular to the plane of the tissues. Push the closed tips between the fibres and gently open the blades (Fig. 9.8). Alternatively, use artery forceps instead of scissors since the tips have gently rounded backs. Even more gentle splitting can be achieved by inserting closed dissecting forceps and allowing them to open; the force is limited by the spring of the blades. The handle of a scalpel makes a convenient splitting instrument in some situations, but it would be wise to use one without a blade attached.

3. Tearing may seem to be a traumatic method, and so it can be if employed inappropriately or roughly. Used judiciously it allows you to find the line of weakness, perhaps when two structures are adherent, and you do not wish to risk sharp dissection in case you inadvertently cut into one of them. Try inserting two

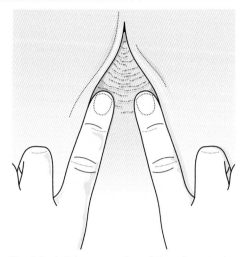

Fig. 9.9 Judicious separation of tissue by a tearing action, trying to sense the correct line of separation.

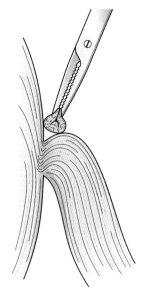

Fig. 9.10 Using a pledget of gauze held in forceps to peel an adhesion.

fingers and gently separate them (Fig. 9.9); you have a very accurate feel of the force you are exerting. As you pull the tissues apart, feel and watch carefully to ensure the path of the separation does not deviate.

> **Key point**
>
> - Always apply distraction force as closely as possible to the line of separation.

4. Peeling is valuable when a flexible structure must be detached from another along an adherent tissue plane. Depending on the shape of the attachment, you may use a gauze pledget held in forceps (Fig. 9.10), a fingertip (Fig. 9.11), a fingertip wrapped with a gauze swab (Fig. 9.12), or a swab held in the fingers (Fig. 9.13). Peeling is not wiping, which traumatises the tissues. If you need to wipe your way through the tissues, you do not know your anatomy. Occasionally you need to use a wiping action to grip by friction something you wish to wipe away from a surface provided this does not abrade the surface.
5. Pinching is sometimes valuable when you cannot obtain a view of an attachment in the depths of the wound. You may not be able to view the line of cleavage but by gently pinching the union you can assess the line of fusion (Fig. 9.14) and may be able to pinch it off (Fig. 9.15). The manoeuvre enables you, for example, to detach a benign gastric ulcer

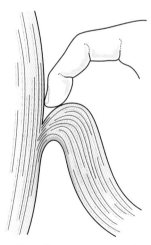

Fig. 9.11 Peeling off a structure using the tip of a finger.

that is adherent to or penetrating another structure.

6. Finger fracture of solid organs sounds crude but when expertly performed it is an effective and safe method of splitting a bulky organ such as the liver. The split must be through healthy tissue because the consequences of compressing diseased tissues are unknown and could be disastrous. The scaffold matrix of connective tissues, vessels and ducts remains

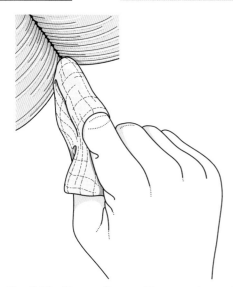

Fig. 9.12 Wrap a finger with gauze to peel structures.

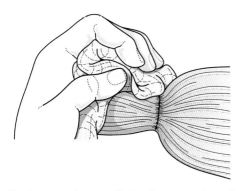

Fig. 9.13 To give you a frictional grip in peeling off a larger structure, hold a gauze swab in your hand.

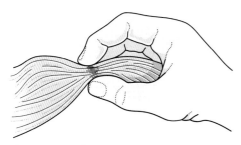

Fig. 9.14 Gently pinch the junction to assess it if you cannot easily visualise it.

intact while the parenchymal cells are dislodged and disrupted (from the Greek *para* = beside + *enchyma* = an inpouring; from an ancient belief that the essential tissue cells

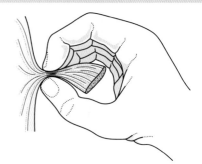

Fig. 9.15 By a combined pinching and peeling action from both sides simultaneously, you may be able to separate the tissues safely.

were poured in and congealed). The vessels and ducts remain intact, crossing the created gap, and can be identified, isolated, sealed electrosurgically or ultrasonically, clipped, sutured or double ligated with division between the ties. Because no heat has been applied with the finger compression, their structure is not weakened.

Instrumental (see also Ch. 2)

1. A long-established electrosurgical method of dissection is cutting diathermy, usually applied through a unipolar needle. A mixed cutting and coagulation current may be used to seal blood vessels as they are cut. Bipolar diathermy forceps allow small bites to be taken and sealed.
2. A Kelly haemostatic clamp used in gynaecology can be placed along the line of dissection, crushing and disrupting parenchymal cells but preserving vessels and ducts so they can be clipped and ligated or sealed with diathermy, in a similar method to finger fracture.
3. Ultrasound dissection usually at 20–30 kHz acts mainly by cellular cavitation and disruption of parenchymal cells. It can be applied by a rod or hook, leaving the vessels and ducts intact. The CUSA system incorporates an irrigation and suction facility to wash out and remove the dislodged debris. It is a valuable method of dissection in fragile tissue, as in ocular cataract phacoemulsification and also in the brain. At higher frequencies such as 55.5 kHz, small bites of tissue can be compressed within a clamp, such as the Harmonic Scalpel, so that vessels within it are flattened, coapting and coagulating the intima to seal them, before dividing them.

4. Tissue can be grasped, cauterised and then divided using the LigaSure electrosurgical system. It is activated on the tissue enclosed and compressed in the jaws, to melt the collagen and elastin to form a seal, then automatically switched off, when the tissues can be transected. It is claimed to seal vessels up to 7 mm in diameter.
5. A high-pressure water jet also dislodges parenchymal cells while preserving other structures.
6. Lasers of different types are used to incise or destroy a variety of tissues, but this requires special training and careful regulation of the depth of penetration.
7. Cryosurgery is accomplished using liquid nitrogen to create an ice ball which eventually separates.
8. An argon plasma (ionised) beam created between an electrosurgical generator and the tissue surface allows the high-frequency electric current to flow, to coagulate and seal small vessels.
9. Radiofrequency thermal ablation can be carried out by implanting an electrode that produces ionic agitation and heating with destruction before dissection.

LAYERED OR SOLID TISSUES?

The difference between dissecting within layers of tissue and sectioning a solid structure, such as a large organ, a large mass or an agglomeration of tissue forming a mass, is often unrecognised.

1. Layers can be separated into planes and each dealt with sequentially. By keeping in the correct plane at all times, the risk of inadvertent damage is minimised. You have access to the undersurface of each layer as well as the presenting surface.
2. When you enter a solid mass you have only the presenting surface available to examine directly. You must, from your anatomical, pathological, imaging and experiential knowledge, make a judgement of the underlying tissues within the mass.
3. Appreciate the difference between dissecting in layered and solid tissues. Layered tissues can be separated and identified by feel, often by folding, to examine the deep surface. A light can be placed beneath successive layers to transilluminate them so that vessels can be identified and ligated or sealed before dividing

them. Solid tissue of an indeterminate nature may be impossible to deal with by creating artificial layers and must be divided from the surface while attempting to anticipate vital structures ahead.

Key points

- Anticipate, identify and react to the type of dissection required.
- Dissection of diseased solid structures demands a surgeon with exceptional skill and experience. Do not be afraid to ask for supervision or senior assistance if needed.

The need for constant awareness of danger and supreme operative skill applies especially to dissections within structures like the brain and liver. It is particularly demanding during the extracapsular removal of a potentially invasive tumour, keeping it outside the apparent plane of cleavage.

TISSUE PLANES

Key points

- This is, perhaps, the most neglected aspect of dissecting. Intimate knowledge of the correct plane distinguishes the master from the ordinary surgeon.
- When the anatomy is distorted, once you confidently reach the surface of an identified structure, do not lightly wander from it, because you are then entering an unknown area.

1. For example, when operating on the thyroid gland you need to pick up sequential diaphanous layers of fascia with two pairs of fine forceps and incise between them, until you see the veins on the gland fill up as the last restraint is removed, confirming that you have entered the correct plane. Similarly, when exposing the abdominal oesophagus at the hiatus you need to incise the peritoneum and then the phreno-oesophageal ligament. Dissecting in the limbs requires you to know and follow the structures in relation to each other so you can reach your target site with minimal damage to others; A. K. Henry, who was a

professor of anatomy in Cairo, beautifully described classic limb exposures.[1]

2. When you are dissecting near the liver, for example, do not lightly wander from it. It is a valuable marker; its surface is a tissue plane you can follow to reach contiguous structures safely.

3. When opening up an obliterated tissue plane you may know the structure and the strength of the structure on one surface, but do not assume the strength of the tissues that you are separating from it, so take great care until you have confirmed its nature.

4. When dissecting along a structure such as a nerve or blood vessel, proceed carefully to avoid damaging any branches, tributaries or other structures. Nerves, arteries, veins and lymphatics often run in parallel. You will cause less damage if you dissect longitudinally along such structures to avoid transecting them.

5. The greatest challenge is to leave the safe plane in order to encompass tissues, such as an infiltrating malignant tumour, which must be excised together with a surrounding layer of healthy tissue. The difficulty is two-fold: you must know the normal anatomy and the possible results of distortion, and you must be able to distinguish normal tissue from potentially malignant tissue.

Key points

- If disease has distorted the anatomy, do not inexorably persist in your intended approach. Try approaching it from different aspects.
- Also, try starting your dissection from a short distance away in normal tissue and work towards the diseased area. You are more likely to find expected planes in this way.

6. Membranous layers often overlie important structures, and you may find it impossible to be sure if the underlying structures are attached until you have breached the layer. If the membrane is sufficiently lax, pinch up a fold with your fingers to estimate its thickness and mobility on underlying structures by rolling it between your fingers. Now pick up a fold with dissecting forceps to tent it. Apply a second forceps close by on the tented portion, and release and reapply the first forceps to allow anything caught in its initial grasp of

untented membrane to fall away. Have the two forceps held up to create a raised ridge. Make a small scalpel incision on the crest of the ridge to let air enter and allow any structure to fall away (Fig. 9.16). This is a standard technique when opening the peritoneum in abdominal operations.

7. Enlarge the incision so you can insinuate your finger and explore the undersurface of the membrane to ensure it is clear. Through the entry hole insert the blades of dissecting forceps, or two separated fingers, under the membrane and cut between them (Fig. 9.17). As you proceed it becomes progressively easier to inspect the deep aspect of the membrane.

8. When it is critically important to avoid cutting more than the membrane, infiltrate the layer with sterile physiological saline to expand the tissues and render them more translucent.

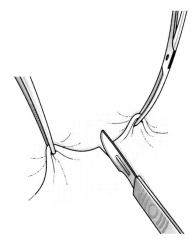

Fig. 9.16 Make an initial incision through a membrane after lifting a ridge with forceps.

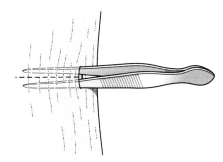

Fig. 9.17 To enlarge a hole through a membranous layer, insert dissecting forceps through the hole and incise the membrane between the blades of the forceps, as indicated in the dotted line.

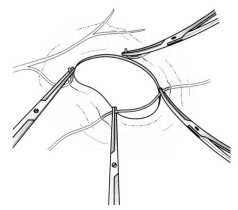

Fig. 9.18 Dividing a sheet of vascular connective tissue. Isolate and doubly clamp the vessels before incising the sheet.

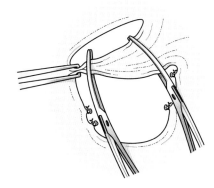

Fig. 9.19 Dividing a vascular membrane between haemostatic clips. The forceps on the right will not grip the full width of the flattened ribbon. On the left, the portion of membrane has been bunched with dissecting forceps before clamping it. Note that the left-hand forceps have the tips projecting beyond the clamped membrane, to facilitate the application of a ligature.

9. If the membrane is the peritoneum and it has been opened previously, always start the new incision just beyond the end of the previous closure where you can tent it and also reduce the risk of cutting an adherent structure. If it is too tense to be tented, infiltrate it with saline to thicken it and allow you to estimate the residual thickness.

10. To divide a sheet of vascular tissue first doubly clamp major vessels before incising the membrane. The less tissue that is included in the ligatures, the less likely are they to be dislodged (Fig. 9.18). If there are few major vessels you may double clamp, divide and ligate sections (Fig. 9.19). Do not attempt to gather too large clumps within the forceps. Artery forceps grip well only near the tips. In addition, if vessels lie within bunched-up tissue within a ligature, they can retract from the constricting ligature and rebleed.

11. If the sheet is very vascular, use cutting and coagulating diathermy, or ultrasonic dissection. Alternatively, consider infiltrating it with isotonic saline containing adrenaline (epinephrine) in a concentration of 1:400,000 to produce vasoconstriction and reduce oozing.

SOLID TISSUES

The difficulty of such dissection is variable depending on the degree of homogeneity and the disease process necessitating the intervention.

Imaging

Modern imaging methods that help delineate deep-seated tumours are invaluable. Preoperative ultrasound (US) may now be studied in three dimensions in some units; intraoperative imaging partially compensates for the lack of the sense of touch, especially in minimal access techniques. Computerised tomography (CT) can produce three-dimensional views. Magnetic resonance imaging (MRI) with gadolinium contrast provides accurate information about the increased vascular network that results from the development of blood vessels within actively growing neoplasms. 3-D printing is increasingly used for complex tumours or reconstructions.

Dissecting

1. Within large masses of lipomatous connective tissue, avoid overconfidence. Vital structures at risk may not be evident and are often also infiltrated with fat which both disguises and weakens them. Blood vessels may be torn and subsequently bleed.

2. Dissection is often necessary within a mainly healthy solid organ to reach a diseased area and is facilitated if the anatomy is well understood and conforms to expectations. The approach to the objective is sometimes

signalled by slight changes resulting from reaction to the disease, including an apparent capsular effect because of expansion and resulting pressure. The presence of such a lesion may additionally distort the otherwise normal placement of ducts and blood vessels.

3. A particular difficulty is identifying the margins of a lesion within a solid organ when it has the same appearance and consistency as the normal tissues. The margin between the normal and abnormal may be indistinct, or, in some cases, what appears to be a margin or a capsule is not the real margin of the lesion; it may be compressed normal tissue resulting from expansion of the lesion or a capsule, but neoplastic microscopic disease has passed through it.

4. Knowledge of segmental anatomy of some organs such as the liver and the lungs provides a means of resecting less of the healthy functioning organs than in the past. In the case of the lung, a single segment may be dissected from the hilar artery, vein and bronchus. In the case of the liver, the hilar vessels can be controlled by gently occluding them with a noncrushing clamp for up to 60 minutes at a time, known as 'Pringle's manoeuvre' (as described by James Hogarth Pringle in 1908). By freeing and rotating the liver, the hepatic veins can also be secured. The method of dissection can be finger fracture, crushing clamp, ultrasonic dissection using the Cavitron Ultrasonic Surgical Aspirator (CUSA), electrosurgical, high-pressure water jet or other methods. Haemostasis may be achieved using conventional methods, argon beam diathermy and a fibrin glue such as Tisseel before apposing the raw surfaces.

5. If a mass consists of adherent structures that you must separate, it is likely that both the structures and the adhesions vary in strength. The force required to separate adhesions may cause tearing of important tissues, often requiring critically important selection and flexible choice of methods. It is in such circumstances that extremely delicate, controlled separation is required. You must be instantly aware of exactly where you are applying distraction and be ready to stop instantly if there is any incipient tissue rupture.

6. The difficulty and danger are greatly increased if you need to encompass a lesion without encroaching on diseased tissues, as when performing a radical resection of a possible or confirmed malignant tumour. The presence of the tumour may distort the anatomy. You are creating a tissue plane through normal tissue, without inadvertently encroaching on the diseased tissues.

7. In the brain it may be difficult to differentiate between functionally vital and 'silent' areas of the cortex and in such cases it is usual to perform the operation under local anaesthesia so that functional or sensory loss can be anticipated. As you attempt to free the tumour, you may distort and tear vital areas or tracts. The pia mater is usually first sealed with bipolar diathermy before using a combination of bipolar diathermy and gentle suction to dissect into the brain, often using magnification. The CUSA is frequently employed as a dissecting instrument. If a plane of cleavage can be identified between normal and abnormal brain, a gentle water jet may extend it in the same plane. Occasionally a tumour cannot be removed completely for fear of causing damage to a vital structure or to a major blood vessel, including the superior sagittal sinus. Following accurate stereotactic (three-dimensional location) imaging, the residual tumour may respond to accurately focused radiotherapy or gamma knife surgery in which beams of radiation, each insufficient alone, intersect at one point and destroy the residual tumour.

8. When reoperating be wary of scar tissue, which is often white in appearance but may still be oozy when cut. Furthermore, you may find blood vessels and nerves encased within the scar tissue, so blind diathermy cutting should be avoided without careful consideration. Slow and careful dissection is imperative in such a situation. If reoperating early (within a few weeks) soft tissues are often more friable.

9. A severe challenge is to reexplore a patient following a previous procedure of which you have no record, but which has failed or developed complications, or when the disease has recurred following a previous operation.

10. The ultimate challenge is to reoperate on patients who may have had a series of previous operations, perhaps when it is not clear what was found, what was attempted, what may or may not have been achieved, and what the nature of the deterioration that necessitates reexploration is.

Key points

- Surgeons who specialise in reoperations that have failed or been followed by complications are at the pinnacle of professional competence.
- They appear to have a sixth sense in anticipating nearby important structures. It is not magic. It is supreme familiarity with the appearance and feel of normal and diseased tissues.
- You will not yet be called upon to repeat their accomplishments but try to acquire their sensitivity to incipient tissue changes and their expertise in dealing with them.
- It will stand you in good stead.

11. Be flexible in the use of instruments for dividing the tissues. If you use a scalpel, scissors, diathermy, ultrasonic or other dissector, in the depths, you must try to detect in advance what you will uncover with each attempt to deepen the dissection and choose the appropriate instrument. Remember that electrosurgical and ultrasonic dissectors may cause heating effects in the tissues beyond the division, although the manufacturers claim that this is localised.

12. If possible separate the sides following an incision, to open it out and allow you to estimate the depth and quality of the remaining tissue. Make each successive cut along the line of the preceding one in the deepest part of the wound. Tentative, scratch-like cuts create ragged, oozing tags. The fibres are sometimes aligned predominantly in one direction. Try to split, rather than transect the fibres. If you are likely to encounter an important structure, prefer to dissect parallel to it rather than across it.

13. In some cases, you may be able to take the full thickness in successive thin layers so you can identify important structures within each layer. As each successive layer is confirmed to be free from important structures you can then safely divide it. Create the layers by inserting the closed blades of scissors, artery forceps or dissecting forceps, then open the blades, or allow them to open, to create a space.

14. When seeking a structure within homogeneous tissue, it is often convenient to use a combined technique of cutting and blunt dissection. Remember, if you insert the closed blades of scissors or artery forceps and open

them, the force at the tips of the blades is very high. Proceed slowly, inserting your finger to feel what is ahead.

15. Some structures vary in texture in different parts, especially in granularity. The breast often feels denser in the axillary tail, the pancreas may feel more granular and solid in different areas. As a result, it becomes difficult to differentiate lumpiness from lump. Fat also varies in texture in different areas.

Key points

- Whatever method you use to dissect, make sure you do not damage healthy tissues that will remain at the limit of your separation.
- Damaged tissues are likely to break down, bleed, prejudice healing or become infected.
- The last connection you cut to free the base of a tumour is the most likely to bring disaster unless you are very cautious.

DISEASED TISSUES

1. Take note of the changes as you approach an area of active inflammation. Watch out for increased vascularity, oedema, tissue tension and fragility. Palpate the tissues as you proceed because the heat is immediately evident, even through your glove, especially on the dorsal surface of the second phalanx of your fingers. If the blood vessels are congested there is increased fluid filtration with high protein, thus raising the extracellular colloid osmotic pressure and causing appreciable turgidity. Deliberately sniff in case you can detect a distinctive smell.

2. As you approach chronically inflamed tissues you may detect increasing fibrosis. You may also anticipate increased vascularity, but this is not always evident.

3. Remember that it is not only infection that increases local vascularity; the vascular growth factors released by fast-growing neoplasms also generate increased vascularity and remarkable vasodilatation occurs in acute noninfective inflammatory diseases.

4. In chronic disease the fibrous tissue laid down in response to many disease processes is often irregular and opaque, so there is no warning of impending disaster. The connective tissue that normally encloses many important

structures may be destroyed by disease. You may suddenly expose the structure and inadvertently damage it.

5. Disease often alters the character of the tissues so that they are not easily recognised. The anatomical features may be distorted, sometimes as a result of contraction of the fibrous tissue that has been laid down, as it matures. This effect is multiplied if the disease is chronic or recurrent, when there is successive deposition and reabsorption of fibrous tissue. Fibrous attachments sometimes draw out diverticula from hollow organs and ducts, which are in danger during dissection.

6. Remember that the differential strengths of tissues may be changed by disease processes. Tearing, splitting or pinching require you to anticipate which structure will give way. Be very cautious and sensitive to incipient tearing in an unexpected area. Structures that are normally swept aside confidently may be adherent, thickened and resistant to blunt dissection, so you may prefer sharp dissection.

7. Whenever possible, start the dissection in normal tissue away from the worst of the disease and work towards the diseased area, maintaining exposure and identification of important structures throughout.

8. Tissues that have previously been subjected to radiotherapy may be unforgiving, friable and poorly healing. Be cognizant of this before you start the operation. If you are uncertain look for the little tattoo dot on the overlying skin indicating where radiotherapy might have been directed.

NEOPLASMS

Key points

- Do your 'homework' beforehand. Do not hope for the best. Read, and reread, standard texts; your predecessors have recorded best approaches, likely and less likely findings, dangers, as well as advice on avoiding errors and recovering from errors.
- The basis of good management of neoplasms is built on the two pillars of anatomy and pathology.
- Make sure you know the up-to-date guidelines for the extent of tissue margins for individual tumour types. Some tumours require wider margins to be clear than others.

1. If the tumour is a type known to be benign, or if a biopsy or cytology has demonstrated this, you do not need to carry out wide excision. If it is encapsulated, you can dissect close to the capsule and avoid damaging the surrounding structures.

2. Resection of a malignant neoplasm often demands dissection outside the normal planes in order to excise the tumour totally, along with associated channels of likely spread, for example along lymph channels and tissue planes. A significant margin of surrounding normal tissue is usually required. Check the current guidelines for the particular tumour you are resecting. Become acutely sensitive to detect warning signs of impending encroachment on the neoplasm or of inadvertently damaging an important structure that should have been preserved. This can be extremely difficult but anticipate increasing vascularity, turgidity, fragility, fixation, fibrosis or prominent lymph nodes.

3. Some malignant neoplasms appear to be limited and perhaps encapsulated but tumour cells penetrate and extend outside the apparent tumour margins, so you need to carry out an extracapsular excision, dissecting through normal tissues. Be aware that the surrounding structures may be displaced and infiltrated by the growth. In some cases, the extent of the growth may be indefinite either on preoperative imaging or at operation. Neurosurgeons may find it impossible to detect the junction with surrounding normal tissue that can be excised and vital brain tissue that must be preserved.

4. Bulky tumours may be reduced using electrosurgery, laser, ultrasound and radiofrequency. Gynaecologists may destroy large fibroids in this manner to diminish their size, and neurosurgeons reduce the bulk of, for example, posterior fossa tumours. Neurosurgeons occasionally debulk a tumour from within rather than try to dissect around a large mass that may be overlying a major structure such as a blood vessel.

5. Do not squeeze the specimen as you gradually free it—you may be squeezing malignant cells into the bloodstream. If you are removing it for diagnosis, crushing it will distort the specimen. Steady it by controlling contiguous and adventitious tissues.

6. If you think you may have encroached on unsuspected malignant tissue, immediately stop and call in expert help and advice. If you carry on, your gloves and instruments may carry, and implant, malignant cells elsewhere.

AIDS TO DISSECTION

Anatomy

Learn the anatomy of the part. You must know the normal appearance and situation of the structures and the appearance, texture and relative strengths. It is disappointing that many trainee surgeons do not take the opportunity to revise the anatomy before every operation, whether they are performing it or assisting with it.

Palpation

If an important structure is likely to be palpable, feel for it before starting. It is valuable to make a habit of feeling the abdomen before starting an operation when the abdominal wall is relaxed.

During the operation feel for arterial pulsations, but remember that tension may obliterate the pulse.

> **Key points**
>
> - Take every opportunity to feel normal and abnormal structures.
> - Until you know the range of what is normal, you cannot confidently identify the abnormal.

Haemostasis

Keep the operative field clear of blood, which obscures the view and stains every structure the same colour. Bleeding is inimical to safe, effective dissection. Prevent potential bleeding, control it when it occurs and remove any blood that collects as a result of bleeding. Do not attempt to work in the depths, in a pool of blood, with continuing uncontrolled bleeding. This is a recipe for disaster. When you are operating on limbs you may use elevation and a tourniquet to produce a bloodless field (see Ch. 10), and you may position the patient to raise the operative field and prevent congestion of the veins.

Find a safe starting point

In some circumstances, you can identify an initial structure that remains your guide.
1. When excising a parotid tumour, first identify the facial nerve emerging from the styloid

foramen by developing the space just anterior to the tragus of the external ear. You can then follow it as it divides, and preserve it, and its branches.
2. Some vessels and nerves have reliable relationships to fixed structures and you can follow them from here. A well-known relationship is that of the long saphenous vein, which can be found reliably 5 cm (1½ inches) above the tip of the medial malleolus of the tibia.
3. In the abdomen, find a structure such as the liver edge, that you can follow. In the right iliac fossa, you can find the base of the appendix by identifying the right paracolic gutter, the caecum and the ileocecal junction.

Tension

1. The ability to put tissues under tension is a valuable aid as a preliminary to dissection. It can be exerted by drawing structures apart with tapes, your hands or fingers, dissecting forceps, retractors, packs or tissue forceps (Fig. 9.20).

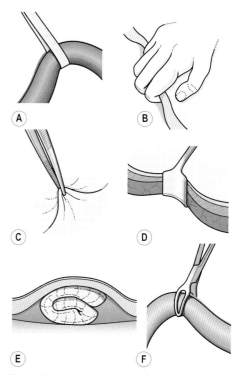

Fig. 9.20 Some methods of exerting traction. (A) Tape. (B) Fingers or hand. (C) Dissecting forceps. (D) Retractor. (E) Packs. (F) Tissue forceps.

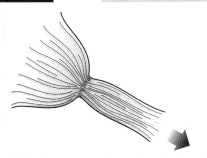

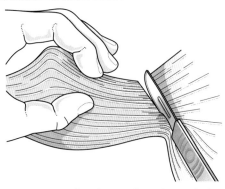

Fig. 9.21 Use gentle traction to test the strength and view the line of attachment.

Fig. 9.24 Combined use of tension and sharp dissection with a scalpel is very effective when the attachment is strong.

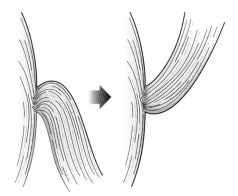

Fig. 9.22 Tension on the attachment is greatest at the point opposite the direction of traction, so you can observe the attachment around the whole circumference and plan the best site for attack.

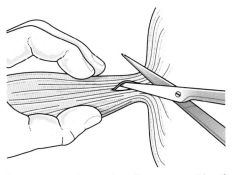

Fig. 9.25 Gentle traction allows you to identify strong bands, which may be isolated and divided with scissors.

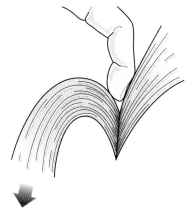

Fig. 9.23 Combined gentle traction and fingertip peeling will separate the two structures safely.

2. Judicious use of tension aids the identification of attachments, and the safest line of separation (Fig. 9.21). By varying the angle of traction, you can judge the whole extent of the attachment and test the strength in different areas, since most force is exerted at the edge opposite to the direction of angled traction (Fig. 9.22). As soon as an edge begins to separate, change the angle, so that you are constantly working around the attachment, aiming that the last separation takes place at the centre of the union. Use your assistant wisely but remember that you are in charge of the operation and must give clear instruction.

3. Be willing to combine techniques. If you apply tension to one structure, it may present an edge that you can peel down (Fig. 9.23). A combination of traction and sharp dissection is very effective (Fig. 9.24 and Fig. 9.25); as you draw one tissue from another, the connections can be examined and selectively divided. Keep changing your line of approach if you encounter difficulty.

Key point

- If you are applying tension to separate two structures, apply it as close as possible to the intended point of cleavage; the further the distance of your fingers from this, the less your control (see Ch. 1; p. 5 and Fig. 1.4).

Dissecting around structures

1. You may need to dissect behind a large structure, either to secure the blood vessels entering and leaving it before excising it, or to carry out a procedure on another structure hidden behind the mass.
2. Ask yourself if you can avoid the problem by using another approach or reducing the size of the mass; for example, deflating distended bowel or aspirating fluid from a cystic mass.
3. If you encounter difficulty, do not proceed doggedly. Stop and reassess the problem. Can you approach it from a different aspect, lengthen the incision, improve the retraction, improve the light, and further mobilise the intervening structure?
4. Remember that the difficulty is usually greatest at the beginning. As you mobilise the target structure, exposure improves. However, do not forget that the other danger point is when you divide the final attachment; you may become too casual and spoil a previously painstaking dissection. Furthermore, you may find that the final attachment is affording you traction that is giving you appropriate vision or haemostasis, so it is worth assessing this before making that final cut.
5. Choose to start where you get the best view, where you are most confident about the anatomy, where you can best control blood vessels, and where a minor division of the tissues is likely to reap the highest rewards in facilitating further dissection. Of course, not all these aims are fulfilled at a single point, so choose the best compromise.

Key point

- Do not cut blindly. Try not to burrow beneath the visible field when you can more clearly dissect superficial tissues. Failure to see is an indication for reassessment, not obsessive continuation.

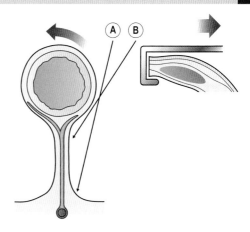

Fig. 9.26 The base of the pedicle is most easily seen at (A), but the vessels can be better controlled if they are first sought at (B).

6. Make sure that you have good control of potential bleeding. When trying to locate blood vessels, remember that applying tension is likely to obliterate arterial pulsations and empty veins so that you cannot identify them.
7. When transecting a pedicle underneath an overlying structure, it may be initially easier to transect it as far as possible from the mass, but this may leave the remaining pedicle short and more difficult to secure (Fig. 9.26).

Needles

If a sought-after structure is hard—as a stone, for example—try locating it with the point of a sharp needle. Search for a cavity, duct or vessel containing fluid with a fine-bore hollow needle attached to a syringe to detect if you can aspirate identifiable fluid.

Fluid infiltration

In case of difficulty do not hesitate to infiltrate the tissues with isotonic saline to facilitate the separation of the structures. Fluid renders the tissues translucent, making it easier to see approaching structures. In some circumstances, it is valuable to infiltrate the tissues with saline containing adrenaline (epinephrine) in a dilution of 1:200,000 in order to reduce oozing.

Transillumination

Sometimes the structures can be lifted and viewed against a light, or a light can be placed behind them.

This allows you to view the vessels, but remember that compressed and emptied veins transilluminate. Always relax the tissues during transillumination. This method is very valuable when you are resecting or joining bowel, since it allows you to identify the supplying vessels in the mesentery.

Probes and catheters

Place a probe or catheter in a track or duct that you wish to excise or preserve, as a marker. The technique is valuable during the excision of a thyroglossal fistula. On occasion, it is helpful to insert a ureteric catheter before excising an extensive and adherent tumour nearby. You can then often preserve the ureter from inadvertent damage. If you need to resect a portion of it, you can take the appropriate steps to deal with the problem. If you have not marked it, you may be unaware of it and therefore unprepared for the consequences.

Dyes

Some surgeons inject a coloured dye, such as vital blue dye, into a complicated fistulous track as a marker It is not always very helpful because the dye tends to leak widely and stain all the tissues.

When operating on some cancers a vital blue dye may be injected around the lesion. This is taken up by the lymphatics and carried to the nearest lymph nodes, which are labelled 'sentinel' since they stand guard over the lymphatic pathways of spread. If the local sentinel nodes are excised and shown to be free of malignant cells it is likely that more distant nodes are also free of growth (see Fig. 7.10). There are various other types of dye and marker.

Marker stitch

You may wish to come back to a structure later in the operation or at a subsequent operation. You may have unexpectedly found a small doubtful lesion in the bowel and wish to complete the intended procedure and come back to it. Place a marker stitch (such as PDS or silk, or a metal clip) close to it so it is easy to find. When performing Hartmann's operation for obstructive carcinoma of the rectosigmoid colon, you bring out a terminal colostomy and close off the rectum. You may intend to return after an interval and establish colorectal continuity, but the closed rectal stump may be difficult to identify. Mark it with a marker stitch or metal clip. An alternative, in an open operation, is to form a mucous fistula bringing the stump out at the bottom end of the laparotomy wound.

Intraoperative ultrasound scanning

Small probes can be used to help in locating important structures and also to indicate the substance. The combination of ultrasound with Doppler analysis (duplex scanning) allows you to detect blood flow in vessels.

Flexibility

1. Do not invariably display structures from only one direction. From time to time look from other aspects, especially if you are in difficulty or uncertain. If you are using tension or distortion of the tissues to facilitate the procedure, relax it from time to time and review the situation with the tissues returned to their normal state.
2. Do not be limited in your technique. Make use of the whole range of possible skills to carry out the procedure safely. For this reason, see as many other surgeons as possible across different specialities–you may find you can adapt some of their techniques and instruments to your own practice.

Priorities

Worry about problems in the correct order. Do not become obsessed with one problem at the expense of other considerations. Do not concentrate on details at the expense of important principles. If you encounter difficulty do not obsessively continue along the path of your original decision; review the possibilities and decide if you should change your priorities. Good surgeons incorporate all their findings into their decisions. Call for senior help if needed; the safety of the patient should be prioritised above your surgical pride.

REFERENCE

1. Henry AK. *Extensile exposure applied to limb surgery*. Edinburgh: E & S Livingstone; 1945.

Chapter | **10**

Handling bleeding

Full discussion of prevention and control of bleeding demands a major textbook. In a monograph on basic techniques, it is possible only to outline the practical management in the operating theatre. You should prepare yourself by studying the background science of bleeding and clotting.

HAEMORRHAGE

(From the Greek *haima* = blood + *rhegnynai* = to burst.)

Arteries bleed bright red blood in spurts when cut. They usually constrict and seal if they are transected, provided they are healthy. Diseased, calcified arteries and those with side holes cannot contract efficiently.

Veins ooze dark blood. They can constrict—but do not trust them! Remember the peripheral valved veins bleed from distally, but if proximal valves are defective, they may bleed from proximal sources. Venous sinuses are held open; for example, intracranial sinuses do not constrict when they are breached.

Capillary bleeding stops following gentle compression, provided there is no clotting defect.

1. Primary haemorrhage occurs during operation or injury.
2. Reactionary bleeding results in the postoperative period when the blood pressure recovers, or straining raises venous pressure, dislodging arterial and venous clots, respectively.
3. Secondary haemorrhage is the result of infection, with bacterial dissolution of occluding clots.

Key points

- Uncontrolled bleeding encourages hasty, ill-considered actions that prejudice surgical success.
- Anticipate and prevent bleeding by correcting anaemia and clotting defects. Stopping anticoagulation may require bridging with shorter-acting anticoagulants. Consider stopping antiplatelet agents if appropriate.
- If bleeding is likely, ensure you have ordered adequate volumes of cross-matched blood. Consider ordering other blood products such as platelets, cryoprecipitate and fresh frozen plasma as required.

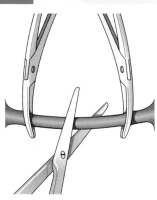

Fig. 10.1 Doubly clamp and divide the vessel. Note that the curved haemostats are placed with their concave surfaces facing each other. This will facilitate the application of the ligatures beneath them.

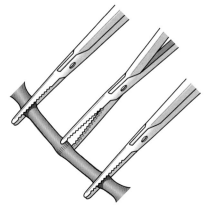

Fig. 10.2 To create sufficient space between the clamps when a short segment only can be exposed, gently apply three clamps side by side and remove the middle one. This ensures that there is a sufficiently long stump presenting beyond the ligatures.

PREVENTION

1. Study the anatomy so you can expose and control major vessels before you cut them.
2. When you encounter an important blood vessel that must be preserved, obtain control by placing across it a noncrushing vascular clamp ready to be closed if necessary, or encircle it with flexible silicone rubber slings or tape (see Ch. 5).
3. If you wish to divide a major vessel, display it, pass two ligatures under it, tie them at a distance from each other and divide the vessel between them. Alternatively, apply haemostats on each side of the point of division, section the vessel, then ligate each cut end (Fig. 10.1). Do not apply the clamps too close together or the ligatures will be too near the cut ends and may slip off. You will find it easier to ligate if you apply each haemostat so that the curve is facing where the cut end will be. Sometimes you can achieve sufficient space by applying three clamps, removing the middle one, and cutting through the space left by it (Fig. 10.2).
4. When tying very large arteries be prepared to place three artery forceps side by side and cut through the vessel leaving two forceps on the proximal stump. Tie a ligature under the deeper of the two forceps and remove it, then tie and tighten a second ligature before removing the second pair of forceps.
5. If an arterial stump continues to pulsate after ligation it may gradually roll off a ligature. The safest method of avoiding this is to apply

a transfixion suture–ligature. Pass a needled thread through the artery and tie it to the short end, encircling half the circumference, then take a full turn around the vessel and tie a triple throw knot. The transfixion prevents the ligature from being displaced.

6. If you are operating on vascular tissues or organs, obtain control of the feeding vessels. You can sometimes apply noncrushing clamps across a soft structure such as a kidney or liver, without damaging it, or encircle a portion with a tape that can be pulled sufficiently tight to constrict the vessels without injuring the organ. The classic method of controlling bleeding from the liver was described by the Australian-born Hogarth Pringle (1863–1941) from Glasgow Royal Infirmary in 1908; he compressed the hepatic artery and portal vein in the free edge of the lesser omentum between his fingers and thumb.
7. Be doubly careful when working in the depths, since any bleeding will rapidly create a pool, hiding the site. Take particular care not to injure large veins at sites where they are held open by surrounding structures, as in the pelvis.
8. Do not open large central veins such as the internal jugular vein unless you have good control. When the patient inspires, air may be sucked into the heart as an air embolus, causing frothing, with immediate circulatory failure.
9. When dissecting in vascular tissues, avoid mass exposure. Prefer to tackle small sections at a

time, gaining complete control before proceeding to the next section.

Pre-empting

1. If you are going to operate on a case where there is a known risk of bleeding it is wise to have a Group and Save or Group and Cross Match available. If your patient has had multiple blood transfusions in the past, they may have formed antibodies, so you may need to request cross-matched blood a few days in advance.
2. In operations where there is the risk of large-volume bleeding, an autologous blood-saving system such as a Cell Saver machine may be used to suction up the blood and process it to be transfused back into the patient by the anaesthetist.
3. If your patient is having an operation where you have given intravenous heparin anticoagulation to prevent intraoperative clotting (such as in cardiovascular surgery) you may ask your anaesthetist to monitor this with regular point of care ACT (activated clotting time) testing and a TEG (thromboelastogram).

ADJUNCTS

Elevation

1. If you can lower venous pressure in the area of operation, the veins and capillaries collapse. When vessels are cut, bleeding is minimal and usually stops without delay. Do not do this with the jugular veins for the reasons noted above.
2. Limbs can often be raised above body level during operations.
3. The whole body may be tilted. Sideways tilt allows the limb on the opposite side to be raised. Head up or down tilt is a standard part of many operations. The distinguished surgeon Friedrich Trendelenburg of Leipzig (1844–1923) placed the patient's head down when operating on varicose veins to avoid venous congestion in the leg veins. It can also be used when operating in the pelvis, allowing the intestines to shift caudally. 'Reverse Trendelenburg', or head up, is a valuable position when operating on the head and neck, or in the upper abdomen.
4. At the end of the operation place the limb or patient into a natural relationship before closing the wound to reveal any bleeding when the usual venous pressure is restored. The part may then be raised in some cases to maintain a lowered venous pressure and avoid congestion during healing.

Fluid infiltration

1. This is an effective and often ignored method of reducing bleeding during operations on vascular tissues. Inject sterile physiological saline as you move the needle point, after initially aspirating the syringe to ensure the needle point is not in a large vessel. The fluid raises the tissue pressure and renders the tissues translucent.
2. In appropriate circumstances, as an extra aid, add adrenaline (epinephrine) 1:200,000 to produce local vasoconstriction.

Transillumination

1. If you are entering an area where there may be large blood vessels. You may be able to raise it and view the light through it, particularly if you have rendered it translucent by fluid infiltration. Alternatively, you may insert a mobile sterile light source behind it. This is useful when viewing the mesentery.
2. Do not forget, though, that if there is a large vein in a part that you have elevated under tension, it will empty and so will not be visible. Gently relax it.

Tourniquet

1. This is a valuable method when carrying out delicate operations on the limbs.
2. It is contraindicated in the presence of ischaemia, venous thrombosis from vascular disease or trauma if the soft tissues are injured or infected, or if there are bony fractures.
3. First empty the limb by elevating it for 2 minutes.
4. Encircle the proximal part with orthopaedic wool and apply a pneumatic tourniquet over this. Secure the tourniquet with a bandage to prevent it from slipping.
5. You may further exsanguinate the limb by applying an Esmarch bandage of thin, flat, elastic rubber, starting at the tips of the digits, with overlapping turns. Run it as a spiral as far as the tourniquet and secure the end (Fig. 10.3). There are also inflatable devices that serve the same purpose.

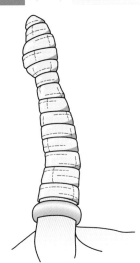

Fig. 10.3 Place a pneumatic cuff proximally around the limb while it is held vertically. Apply an Esmarch bandage from distal to proximal. Inflate the tourniquet and then remove the Esmarch bandage.

6. Inflate the tourniquet quickly to 50 mmHg above systolic blood pressure for the upper limb—but no higher than 250 mmHg—and inflate the tourniquet to 90–100 mmHg above systolic arterial pressure for the lower limb, but no higher than 300 mmHg. Now unwind the Esmarch bandage.
7. Record the time of tourniquet inflation and frequently check the pressure. It is conventional to limit continuous inflation to 1 hour for the arm and 1½ hours for the leg. Release the tourniquet for at least 10 minutes before reinflating it. There is clinical research being undertaken to look at the effectiveness of much lower pressures (e.g. 20 mmHg above systolic pressure) and there are calculation tools for working out recommended pressures based on a series of systolic blood pressure readings.
8. At the end of the procedure release the tourniquet so you can ensure that all the blood vessels are sealed before you close the wound.
9. Remember that prolonged or too-high tourniquet pressures can result in ischaemic nerve injury, muscle necrosis, pain and swelling.

Technical aids (see also Ch. 2)

1. Diathermy is a well-established method of sealing vessels before dividing them, sealing

and dividing them simultaneously, or sealing vessels already cut and bleeding. Bipolar diathermy has additional safety because current passes only between the tips of forceps in which the tissue is grasped, and this is coagulated. LigaSure compresses vessels and electrosurgically obliterates the lumen by melting the collagen and forming a seal so a knife can be triggered to transect the vessel.
2. Ultrasonic vibration produces intracellular cavitation, cellular disruption, tissue heating, coagulation, and tissue welding, depending on the frequency and power. If a vessel up to 2 mm in diameter is gently compressed and low-power ultrasound applied, it reliably welds and occludes the lumen. At higher power, it has a disruptive cutting effect and coagulates the vessels.
3. Laser produces a coherent high-intensity beam that causes vaporization of the tissues. The wavelength and thus the tissue absorption is determined by the medium within which the radiation is generated, such as carbon dioxide, neodymium yttrium aluminium garnet (Nd:YAG), or argon. The heating associated with tissue vaporization produces tissue destruction with coagulation of the small blood vessels.

Drugs

1. Tranexamic acid is now widely used to reduce bleeding in major surgery. It is an antifibrinolytic drug and trials have shown that whilst it reduces bleeding by 25%, there is no significant increase in thrombosis with its use.

Topical haemostatic applications

1. When there is an oozy area in the surgical field a topical agent that promotes clotting may be applied. This does not apply to frank bleeding, which you must address more definitively. Cellulose products are widely used; as they are biodegradable and plant-based, they are thought to act by absorbing blood cells and active clotting components and then forming a framework for clot to form on. Surgicel is one such example and is available in gauze form, a fluffy cotton wool-like form or powdered.
2. Glue-like applications are also available, e.g., Floseal (a combination of gelatine and

thrombin) and Tisseel (based on the antifibrinolytic aprotinin).

3. Alginates, such as Kaltostat or Sorbsan, are topical dressings with haemostatic properties. These cannot be left in a closed wound but can be applied to an oozy wound that you are going to leave to heal by secondary intention.

> **Key points**
>
> - Bleeding is better prevented than arrested.
> - Just before you make a cut into unknown tissue, are you confident there is no blood vessel within it?

CONTROL

1. Control generalised oozing with manual pressure, possibly expanded and extended with a gauze pack, or a metal retractor pressing on a pack. Sometimes you can push a pack under a wound edge to exert pressure. You may be able to control a small area of generalised oozing with the application of an absorbable collagen-based haemostatic agent (see below) or seaweed-based gauze. The former can be left in a wound, but the latter is applied topically to open wounds only and must be removed when the dressing is changed.

2. Once bleeding has occurred, identify and isolate the vessels, pick them up and ligate them or seal them with diathermy current.

3. If your first clip catches the vessel with its tip alone, it may be difficult to apply a ligature that does not fall off. Do not risk it. Hold the first clip vertically while you apply a second clip beneath it across the vessel with its tip projecting. Then remove the first clip (Fig. 10.4). Make sure, though, that you do not tent the surrounding tissue, lifting a deeper structure into the jaws of the second clip and damaging it. Do not pick up surrounding tissue and ligate it together with the vessel. Your ligature does not directly contact and hold the vessel; arteries can retract, escape from the ligature and rebleed.

4. If you inadvertently divide a major vessel, control it initially with direct finger pressure or by compressing the supplying vessel until

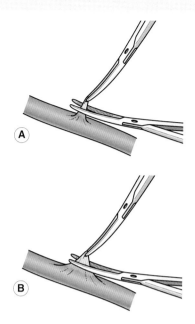

Fig. 10.4 (A) If you have merely captured the tip of a bleeding vessel with your first haemostatic clip, gently lift it up while you place a second clip across it, with the tip projecting. Now remove the first clip and ligate the vessel. (B) Do not clamp and ligate tissue surrounding the vessel, which could then retract out of the ligature.

you have identified it. If you cannot identify the supplying vessel but know it passes through a particular tissue, try applying a noncrushing clamp such as sponge-holding forceps. Do not be hasty; you may wish to repair the vessel. Do not compound the problem by risking injury to other structures. If you can control it with pressure, wait 5 minutes timed by the clock. As you cautiously reduce and eventually release the compression you will be surprised and encouraged at how much less dramatic the bleeding appears. Do not proceed until you have made sure that you have identified the vessel, assessed the likelihood of further bleeding and confirmed that you have not caused any damage. If you are unable to safely apply a vascular clamp to control the bleeding at the cut ends, you will need to dissect proximally along the vessel while your assistant continues to compress the bleeding end. Once you have proximal exposure, you can apply a vascular clamp to this and achieve proximal control. The same would then apply to the distal cut end. This will give you more space to assess the cut ends and deal with them.

5. Prevent calamitous generalised bleeding from happening during a well-conducted operation by proceeding step by step, controlling any bleeding as it occurs. You then have only a single problem on which to concentrate at any time.

6. Tears of vascular organs such as the liver and spleen may sometimes be controlled with sutures, but bleeding may continue behind the stitches. There are a number of haemostatic agents available that may be used. Absorbable collagen-based products are widely used and may be available as a woven fabric, a ball of wool, or a sponge. You can tear the wool into smaller pieces and sprinkle them on the affected area. Massive resection, however, is sometimes indicated, or in the case of the spleen, removal of the whole organ; in this case, it is important to give the patient a polyvalent vaccine (and in the case of children, prophylactic penicillin is usually given). These are problems for specialists since bleeding can often be controlled by interventional radiology.

7. In addition to collagen-based haemostatic agents, there are other products available. Fibrin glues and sealants may be sprinkled onto an oozing area. Likewise, gelatin-based gels can be applied. Fibrinogen and thrombin are often incorporated in these preparations. Biological glues can sometimes be applied to seal an oozing area. Ensure that you read the operating instructions of each before using them.

8. In some cases, simple packing suffices, as in the nose. Use a long pack; start in the depths and lay it back and forth like a jumping-jack cracker (Fig. 10.5). After 24–48 hours, return the patient to the operating theatre and, with the same preparations you used for the initial operation, cautiously remove the pack. Again, you may find that the bleeding has stopped.

9. Consider checking the clotting status and correcting it accordingly.

10. On occasion, if massive bleeding occurs you may have to make the decision to abandon the original procedure to allow the patient to stabilise and come back at a later date.

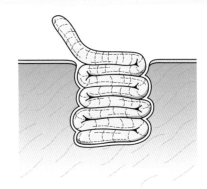

Fig. 10.5 Insert a long pack to control intracavity bleeding. Start in the depths and fold it back and forth like a jumping jack cracker. Either close the wound over the pack or bring out the end through the wound. Plan to remove it after 24–48 hours.

11. Many hospitals have a major haemorrhage protocol. If you are faced with a massive haemorrhage, activate this protocol immediately. This will bring into action a number of hospital personnel including haematology, anaesthetics, and porters, to bring the necessary expertise and blood products to your patient. Ensure you know how to activate your local pathway.

Key points

- When faced with calamitous, life-threatening bleeding, never forget why you are here—to stop the bleeding!
- Do not get carried away and perform any procedure that is not equally and urgently lifesaving.
- Always notify your anaesthetist if you have unexpected bleeding, so that they can ensure adequate fluid filling, ordering of cross-matched blood and, if necessary, inotropic support.

Intracavity bleeding

1. Unfortunately, you do not have control of bleeding when a patient is admitted as having sustained an injury or disease that has resulted in severe, life-threatening bleeding. A typical problem is bleeding within a closed cavity such as the abdomen and chest, since when you enter you may have no idea where the

source lies. Tension builds up and eventually reduces the rate of bleeding. This is called tamponade.

2. When the cavity is opened, tension falls, and bleeding starts with renewed force. Bleeding from a ruptured ectopic pregnancy, treated by open operation, requires prompt control. The introduction of laparoscopic methods allows the intraperitoneal pressure to be maintained and raised by insufflation, reducing the need for urgency.

> **Key points**
>
> - When there is bleeding from an unknown source into a closed cavity, defer opening it until you have everyTHING you need to deal with the problem and have ensured that everything works. This might include having everyONE there that is needed, such as a senior surgical colleague, a vascular surgeon and an experienced anaesthetist.
> - As soon as you release the pressure, bleeding will start with renewed vigour.

3. Your hand may be forced when bleeding in the chest is causing serious cardiorespiratory distress. Have available a generous supply of large packs, two powerful suckers, large dishes in which to collect the large blood clots and long-handled vascular clamps and artery forceps for clamping vessels in the depths. In addition, order vascular surgical instruments and sutures.

4. If you open the cavity and merely suck out the blood, you may exsanguinate the patient. Therefore, in the abdomen, open it swiftly and extensively, insert packs into each quadrant, then pack the central area (Fig. 10.6). If necessary, apply pressure until you have controlled the welling up of blood, but remember that compression squeezes out blood from the packs. Do nothing further except to scoop out loose blood and clots that will obscure your subsequent search for the origin of the bleeding, while the anaesthetist resuscitates the patient, restoring the blood volume, checking clotting and infusing blood products as required.

5. If you have controlled bleeding and the patient's condition is improving, do not rush to 'do something', but carefully consider your options and tactics. Be willing to change your mind from your initial intentions. Ensure that

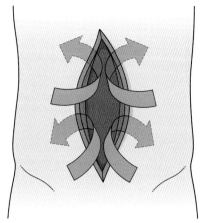

Fig. 10.6 Place large packs into each quadrant of the abdomen to control calamitous bleeding.

you have all the help, equipment and instruments that you are likely to need.

6. Arm your assistant with a sucker from which the guard has been removed. Peel back the edge of the central pack, compressing the part just behind the revealed area. If you see bleeding, isolate the smallest possible area and have your assistant maintain a clear field, using the sucker. Do not automatically clamp a vessel; you may wish to repair it. In many cases apply pressure just sufficient to control it with a finger, a pack or a gently applied noncrushing clamp.

7. If you have an autologous blood recycling system available this can be very useful in massive haemorrhage. A special sucker is used which draws the blood into a machine which filters the blood and prepares it for retransfusion. If this is used, be careful to use it to suction up clean, non-contaminated blood only. Do not use it if there is bleeding in relation to abscess drainage, faecal contamination or bile leakage.

8. As you control each area, continue to peel back the pack until you can remove it and start on the pack in the quadrant least likely to lie over the culprit. When this is finally removed, unpack the next most unlikely quadrant and so on, until, if all goes well, you are left with a final quadrant, having carefully checked and controlled all the others. Try to start at the highest point so that any bleeding will drain elsewhere. You may be pleasantly surprised to find that bleeding has diminished in the interval. Control it while you decide how best to deal with it.

Key points

- When you have stopped the bleeding, do not close up!
- Wait while the anaesthetist restores the blood pressure and improves the patient's general condition.
- Have you removed all the blood that has been collected? Stagnant blood makes an ideal culture medium.
- Have you counted all of the swabs?
- In your efforts to control the bleeding, have you injured or imperilled any other structure?
- Once the bleeding is under control, the situation is no longer urgent.

INTRACRANIAL BLEEDING

1. You may not rotate through a neurosurgical service but note that generalists sometimes see more head injuries than do neurosurgeons. Many of the consequences of head injury result from intracranial bleeding. Extradural haemorrhage may follow fracture of the temporal bone with tearing of the middle meningeal vessels; subdural haemorrhage may result from tearing of cerebral veins passing to the venous sinuses, often in elderly patients taking anticoagulants, following trivial injuries; intracerebral vessels rupture from distortion of the brain. Some patients develop small aneurysms, especially around the circle of Willis, which may rupture, causing a subarachnoid haemorrhage.

2. In addition to the primary brain damage, the patient may deteriorate as a result of secondary damage from ischaemia and oedema. Remember that the brain utilises approximately 20% of the total body oxygen consumption and that ischaemia also produces cerebral oedema. The *basic surgical action* required is to maintain cerebral perfusion and oxygenation.

Key points

- Remember to maintain **A**irway, **B**reathing and **C**irculation.
- Be competent to administer oxygen at 12–15 L/min via a close-fitting face mask.
- Monitor neurological signs closely using a system such as the Glasgow Coma Score.

FURTHER READING

Devereaux PJ, et al. Tranexamic Acid in Patients Undergoing Noncardiac Surgery. *NEJM* 2022;386(21):1986–1997.

Chapter | **11** |

Handling drains

Abnormal accumulation of fluids—liquid, vapour or gas—may have deleterious effects on, for example, the space they occupy, pressure they exert, tracking within the tissues, susceptibility to infection or spread of existing infection, and absorption of toxic substances.

1. The value of most drains is hotly debated. As a trainee, follow the practice of the consultant who is responsible for the patients and watch the outcome so that you can draw your own conclusions about their value.
2. The use of drains can often be avoided by delaying operations if there is swelling that can be allowed to settle, by taking extra care over haemostasis, closure of vessels and ducts, and elevating parts to prevent the build-up of fluid swelling. In some cases, the possible source of a collection can be brought to the surface.
3. In some circumstances, drains are inserted as sentinels to warn of complicating blood or fluid discharge, but they are unreliable.
4. Drains can be used to bring together or keep together surfaces that would be separated by intervening fluids, such as air in the pleural cavity or oozing of blood from apposed raw surfaces.
5. In some cases, the source can be brought to the surface, where it can discharge and—if the fluid to be drained is within a tube—a stoma can be formed.

> **Key points**
>
> - The value of drains is hotly debated.
> - Proponents claim they remove harmful fluids, monitor complications and cause little harm.
> - Opponents claim they cause irritation, perpetuate discharge and offer an inward track for contamination.

CAUTION

1. In the absence of scientific knowledge or extensive personal experience, use drains where orthodox practice favours them.

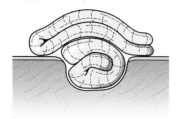

Fig. 11.1 Pack a wound with sterile cotton gauze. Make sure the pack is large enough to absorb the expected discharge. Cover it with dry gauze, which should remain dry and not become soaked.

2. As a trainee, follow the practice of your chief, but observe the results so you can develop your own views.
3. Use the softest and least irritant materials; ensure the drain does not press onto damaged, delicate or vital structures, or suture lines.
4. If there is a main wound, prefer to bring the drain to the surface through a separate wound to avoid prejudicing the healing of the main wound.
5. When possible, make the track lead outwards and downwards to benefit from gravity drainage. When this is not possible and you must lead a drain down to a sump and suck it out, ensure that the drain tip reaches the lowest point, where fluid is likely to collect.
6. Whenever possible, used a closed system to avoid the possibility of inward contamination.

TYPES

Packs and wicks

1. Gauze packs are sheets of sterile cotton gauze (Fig. 11.1) placed on a raw surface where discharge is expected to occur over a wide area, such as an abscess cavity, a laid-open superficial fistulous track, or as the initial treatment of an infected wound. It soaks up fluid most effectively if it is dry, but some surgeons prefer it moistened with sterile isotonic saline solution or antiseptic solution. Unfortunately, it needs to be changed frequently.
2. Gauze in contact with raw tissues soon adheres as it is invaded with fibrin threads. You can avoid this by soaking it in sterile liquid paraffin alone or emulsified with an antiseptic such as proflavine. This destroys its ability to soak

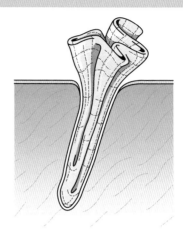

Fig. 11.2 Gauze wick. This is a folded gauze sheet or ribbon, passed down a track to keep the track open.

up fluid, which now tracks between the pack and the raw surface. As an alternative, first lay on a thin nonadherent net of tulle gras (from the French *tulle* = net + *gras* = fat), e.g., Jelonet, or a silicone substitute.
3. The absorbent pack may be overlaid with cotton wool so that it can be compressed with a crepe bandage or by means of elastic adhesive strapping. Compression may reduce oozing and oedema. Since the cotton wool is intended to remain dry and elastic to distribute the pressure evenly, make sure that it does not get soaked or it will form a hard cake; moreover, a completely soaked pack forms a moist channel for microorganisms from the exterior to the raw surface.
4. When the source of discharge cannot be brought to the surface, a wick of folded gauze or a gauze ribbon can be passed down to it (Fig. 11.2). It may block rather than hold open the channel. It is fully effective only until the gauze is soaked; thereafter it lies moist and inert in the channel. To avoid the wick becoming adherent to the tissues, it may be passed through a thin-walled latex tube open at both ends (Fig. 11.3); a so-called 'cigarette drain'. For very small tracks, twisted threads are sometimes inserted.

Sheet drains

1. A track may be kept open by inserting a sheet of latex rubber or plastic material (Fig. 11.4), which is often corrugated to create spaces. Alternatively, a Yeates drain (Fig. 11.5) comprises

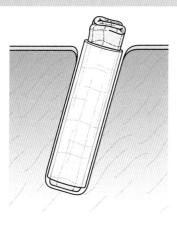

Fig. 11.3 'Cigarette' drain. Pass a folded gauze sheet or ribbon through a thin-walled rubber tube open at both ends, where it acts as a wick.

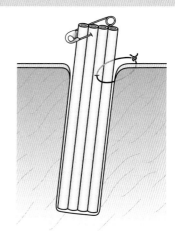

Fig. 11.5 Yeates drain—a sheet formed of parallel tubes of plastic material.

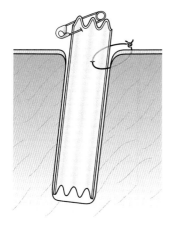

Fig. 11.4 A corrugated sheet drain of latex rubber or plastic material. It has been sutured in place and transfixed by a safety pin in the projecting portion.

> ### Key point
>
> - Packs, wicks and sheets are imperfect forms of drains, but they are simple and usually serve their purpose in localised infections after a track has developed spontaneously or been provided surgically.

parallel plastic tubes. However, these are inert, and fluid reaches the surface by gravity or *vis a tergo* (from Latin, meaning to push from behind), where it must be soaked up by gauze packs. Fix them to prevent them from slipping into the wound by stitching them to the skin and also placing a large safety pin through the projecting portion.

2. Although these are not very effective, they are popular for the drainage of abscess cavities and to provide a track in case there is any subsequent discharge.

Tube drains

1. These have the great advantage that they can lead away any content into a receptacle, such as a bag or other reservoir, thus forming a closed system, reducing the possibility of infection tracking back into the tissues. Tube drains usually have side holes as well as end holes (Fig. 11.6).

2. When fluid has entered the tube, it may stagnate unless the tube is inserted upwards so it can drain by gravity. Fluid will flow only provided it is not viscous and only if the tube is sufficiently wide so that air can displace the fluid. If the tube is too narrow, the force of capillarity tends to retard the flow. However, fluid empties by *vis a tergo* if, for example, it is pushed out by a rise in intraabdominal pressure. A limb may be compressed with a bandage to express any fluid into a drain, but compression of an infected area pushes the causative organisms into the bloodstream.

3. Usually, the most effective method is to apply suction. Insert the tube so the tip lies at the lowest

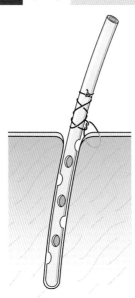

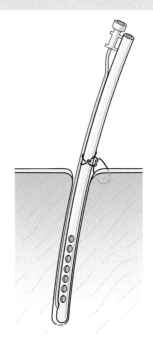

Fig. 11.6 A tube drain of silicone rubber or plastic material with multiple side holes. Note how it is secured by tying the suture thread back and forth around it, then with a stitch through the skin that is loosely tied. The tube has not been transfixed and therefore will not leak.

Fig. 11.7 The Shirley wound drain incorporates a side tube guarded by a bacterial filter so that, when you apply suction to the main tube, sterile air can be drawn down to the drain tip, helping to prevent tissues from being sucked into the side holes and blocking them.

part where fluid is most likely to collect. The tube may be connected to a vacuum-sealed bottle.

4. The most versatile method is to apply suction directly from an electrically driven vacuum pump, incorporating a reservoir to collect any discharge from the drain. The suction tends to drag tissue into the holes of the drain and block them, rendering the system ineffective. This can be partially overcome by using a pump that automatically and intermittently breaks the vacuum, allowing the pressure to rise to atmospheric; however, the tissues may remain trapped in the holes. The Shirley drain (Fig. 11.7) allows air to leak throughout, drawn in by the suction through a side tube protected by a bacterial filter. However, the most effective method is to use a sump drain (Fig. 11.8). Place a large tube with side holes at the bottom of a cavity so that any fluid will collect in it. Lying free within this is a suction tube which can take up the fluid but cannot be blocked by sucking in tissues.

5. The need for surgical creation of a path to the site of drainage has markedly diminished as methods of imaging have improved so that percutaneous aspiration and drainage can be

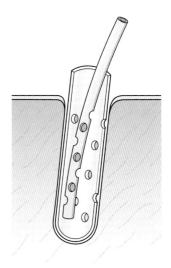

Fig. 11.8 Sump drain. The large outer tube creates a sump in which fluid collects. Lying freely in the bottom of the sump is a smaller tube attached to a sucker. Because the tissues are separated from the holes in the suction tube, they cannot be drawn in to block them.

accomplished, often using the Seldinger technique (Ch. 5). In some cases, a pigtailed catheter can be passed into a cavity and the curl at the inner end acts as a retainer; alternatively, a Foley balloon catheter can be passed.

6. Normal fluids may be drained to monitor them. A classic example is a 'T-tube' inserted into a bile duct that does not necessarily drain bile unless the distal flow is blocked (see Fig. 4.12). When free flow is confirmed, the tube can be gently withdrawn. The hole closes spontaneously unless subsequent distal blockage develops.

SITES

Subcutaneous

1. Subcutaneous tissues vary in depth and vascularity in different individuals and in different parts of the body. Blood and reaction fluid collect, especially when the skin has been extensively undermined. Small collections can be drained using gauze wicks, corrugated sheet drains, or soft tubes with many side holes, connected to a gentle suction pump. They may be preferable to attempting to apply external pressure by means of cotton wool and crepe bandages in the hope of preventing fluid collecting.

2. Following extensive resection of the breast, for example, the large potential space left following skin closure may accumulate oozed blood. Some patients develop a 'seroma', a collection of serum. The best way of avoiding these complications is to encourage the skin to adhere to the base and obliterate the space. Compression is often ineffective and restricts respiration. Some surgeons insert multiple fine tubes with side holes connected to a suction pump or one of the many portable suction devices that are available such as a compressible bulb which exerts suction as it attempts to expand to its spherical shape.

3. In the presence of severe contamination or infection, do not attempt to close the skin with the hope that the drains will provide adequate removal of any discharge.

Subfascial and intramuscular

Do not trust drains in the presence of damaged muscle trapped beneath strong fascial coverings, since fluid collecting here raises the pressure, thus causing ischaemia with the risk of infection from anaerobic organisms.

Extraperitoneal

After removing a source of intraperitoneal infection, there is a risk of infection of the extraperitoneal tissues. Many surgeons close the peritoneum and leave a drain to its external surface, usually through a separate stab incision. An alternative is to leave the skin wound open and carry out delayed primary closure.

Intraperitoneal

1. These are usually made of Silastic.
2. On occasion, intraperitoneal drains continue discharging fluid for prolonged periods if the amount of fluid generated prevents the surfaces from coming together and sealing off. This occurs in ascites.
3. Although drains usually discharge fluid that is already present, the fiercest arguments centre around their ability to channel subsequent fluid collections to the surface and thus to signal a haemorrhage or the breakdown of an anastomosis with subsequent leakage into the peritoneal cavity. Do not assume that there is no fluid collecting in the peritoneal cavity because there is nothing in the drain.

> **Key points**
>
> - Use intraperitoneal drains if it reassures you.
> - However, do not allow the insertion of a drain to replace careful performance of the procedure.

4. Having inserted a drain, do not rely upon it to warn of a leak or a bleed if other features point to a complication.
5. Soft latex drains promote fibrosis and the formation of a track. Today, drains are more likely to be made of silicone elastomer, polyurethane or polyvinyl chloride, which are inert.
6. Insert drains through a small separate stab wound when possible. Take care to avoid major nerves and blood vessels in the abdominal wall. Keep the track straight by grasping the retracted peritoneum and posterior rectus sheath of the main wound on the side of the drain and draw them

towards the opposite side. Now lift the whole abdominal wall upwards, clear of the viscera. Cut straight through the full thickness of the abdominal wall with a scalpel, taking care to cut the peritoneum under vision. Insert straight forceps through the stab wound and grasp the external end of the drain to draw it out through the stab wound.

7. In some cases, it is permissible to bring out the drain at one end of the main wound. If you do so, make sure you use separate stitches to secure the drain from those that close the wound. Eschew this, though, if infected material is likely to be discharged, for fear of contaminating the main wound.

8. Carefully place the inner end of the drain in the most dependent part where fluid is likely to accumulate, but make sure there are no sharp ends pressing upon delicate structures.

9. Now insert a stitch through the skin and the drain and tie it, leaving the ends long. If it is a sheet drain, place a large safety pin through it as an extra safety precaution to prevent it from dropping into the abdomen. If you are using a tube drain, insert the skin stitch, tie it loosely, then take a number of turns around the drain tube, back and forth, tying the ligature onto the drain without puncturing it. The tube drain can be connected to a collecting bag in a closed manner.

10. Plan to remove intraperitoneal drains after 48 hours unless there is copious discharge. When a drain has been placed very deeply, it is sometimes removed by 'shortening it' a little each day.

Pleural cavity

1. Although liquid such as an effusion, pus or blood may be drained, an important function of chest drains is to remove air that has accumulated, has leaked following lung damage or enters through a breach in the thoracic wall. If the pleural space is occupied by air, the lung is compressed and collapses.

2. Introduce a tube through the chest wall, just above the upper border of a rib, in order to leave the neurovascular bundle that runs in a groove beneath the ribs undamaged (Fig. 11.9).

3. If there is a chest X-ray, examine it to determine the level of the diaphragm on each side, whether the lungs are collapsed, and whether there is any liquid in the pleural cavity. From the X-ray and by percussion and

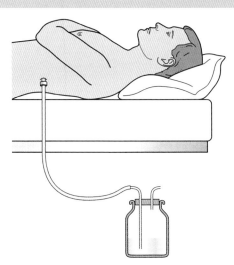

Fig. 11.9 Intrapleural drain with underwater seal. The tubular drain emerges through the chest wall, where it is secured by an encircling but not piercing stitch, which then catches the skin. Connect the tube to the vertical plastic tube passing through the bottle bung, the tip of which lies below the surface of sterile water in the bottom of the bottle. The short, angled tube allows air to escape from the bottle but can be attached to a source of suction.

auscultation, decide where to insert the drain. You may decide the safest place is the fifth or sixth intercostal space in the anterior axillary line, the seventh or eighth space in the posterior axillary line or the second interspace anteriorly 3–5 cm from the lateral edge of the sternum.

4. You may insert the drain at the conclusion of a thoracic operation under general anaesthetic, in which case you can insert it under visual control. You may need to insert it in the ward with strict aseptic precautions after infiltrating the skin and deeper tissues with local anaesthetic.

5. Make a 1–2 cm incision just above and parallel to the chosen rib and gradually deepen it to the pleura. Open the pleura and insert a finger to sweep it round 360° to ensure there is no adherent lung.

6. Clamp the chest drain and then gently insert it (remove the trocar if there is one); there are side holes, so make sure that they are all well inside the pleural cavity.

7. Attach the outer end of the tube to sterile tubing that leads to an underwater seal bottle, then remove the clamp from the drain. The tubing is attached to a vertical plastic tube

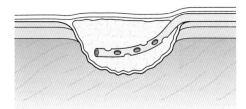

Fig. 11.10 Negative pressure wound healing. The wound is filled with plastic foam shaped to fully occupy it. A tube is buried within the foam. The area is now sealed with plastic film which is stuck to the surrounding skin with adhesive. The tube is connected to a suction pump.

that pierces the bottle stopper and descends almost to the bottom of the bottle, which contains sterile water covering the lower end of the tube. There is another open tube that pierces the stopper and bends at a right angle so that organisms do not fall into it. If necessary, this tube can be connected to a vacuum pump.

8. Place the bottle on the floor. The bottle should remain dependent.
9. Insert strong, deep stitches on either side of, but not through, the tube, including the skin. Tie one loosely, leaving the ends long, then pass it back and forth around the tube, tying it after each encirclement in the fashion of 'English lacing' to grip but not penetrate the tube, preventing it from being pulled out. Leave the other stitch untied and long, to be used to close the wound after withdrawing the tube.
10. Arrange for a check X-ray.
11. In the presence of a pneumothorax, if the intrapleural pressure rises above atmospheric, as the patient exhales, air is forced down the vertical tube and bubbles out through the water. As the patient inhales, a short column of water is temporarily drawn up the vertical tube. During normal breathing, the water level in the vertical tube oscillates, signalling that the tubes are patent and functioning correctly.
12. If liquid drains out of the chest, it may be trapped in a dependent loop of tubing, damping the oscillation of the level in the vertical tube. Doubly clamp the tube emerging from the chest, disconnect the tubing distal to this, elevate the drain tube to allow the liquid to run into the bottle, then reconnect the tubes and take off the double clamps. Check that oscillation is now normal.

13. You can estimate the amount of liquid draining from the chest by marking the initial water level in the bottle and subsequently comparing the mark with the water level. If the bottle fills rapidly with blood, be suspicious that active bleeding continues and call for senior assistance.
14. If air leaks rapidly into the pleural cavity, bubbling will continue in the bottle and the lung cannot reexpand. Check any leakage around the chest drain and correct if necessary. If not, connect the open tube emerging from the bottle to a vacuum pump set to maintain the pressure in the bottle at slightly below atmospheric pressure. This results in an increase in bubbling, but eventually the lung will reexpand before sealing against the parietal pleura, at which time the bubbling will cease. While you are applying suction, do not expect to see any oscillation.
15. To remove the drain, first clamp it. Then, cut the stitch attaching the chest drain and withdraw it; as you do so, tighten the loose stitch to seal off the hole. It is often valuable to apply suction as you gently withdraw the drain so that any last fluid collection is removed. Now tie the loose suture and apply a dressing.

NEGATIVE PRESSURE DRAINS

1. Negative pressure drains can be used to aid wound closure (Fig. 11.10) (see Ch. 16).

ABSCESSES AND CYSTS

These are eminently suitable for drainage (see Ch. 12). The discharge will be small after you have evacuated the contents, but continue drainage to allow the cavity to shrink and become partly or completely obliterated. Depending on the site and size of the cavity, you may use open or closed drainage. Infected wounds should be left open.

EXTERNAL FISTULAS

1. An external fistula opens on the body surface. Some produce little discharge and do not need

to be drained. Others need to be excised or laid open and prevented from bridging over by applying packs.

2. Some fistulas, especially those carrying digestive juices from the gastrointestinal tract, may produce voluminous discharge, which is usually intensely irritating to the skin or excoriating (from the Latin *ex* = off + *corium* = skin). The discharge can often be collected in a stoma bag. Cut an accurate hole in the flange of the stoma bag to fit closely around the discharge site. Clean and dry the skin around the stoma and apply the flange carefully to the skin. The stoma bag ring may have hooks to which you can attach an encircling belt. Clip on the stoma bag. This can be removed as necessary without disturbing the backing ring. In some cases, the bag may be emptied from time to time without removing it through a tap at the bottom or by removing and replacing a clip on a spout.

3. Occasionally, you may be able to pass a Foley-type catheter into the fistulous track, gently inflate the catheter balloon to seal the passage, and allow the catheter to drain into a bag.

Chapter | **12**

Handling infection

Infection (from the Latin *in* = into + *facere* = to make) strictly signifies disease spread through the air, while both contamination and contagion (from the Latin *con* = together + *tangere* = to touch) indicate transmission by direct contact. Sepsis (from Greek, meaning decay) usually implies the invasion of pathogenic bacteria or their toxins into the bloodstream or tissues.

PRINCIPLES

1. The capacity of microorganisms to cause infection depends on the balance between the virulence and numbers of the organisms on the one hand, and the health, vigour and nutritional state of the tissues on the other hand. It is increasingly recognised that local lack of tissue oxygen results in deprived and inactive phagocytes.[1] Another identified influence is the ability of communities of microorganisms to adhere and develop a polymeric matrix biofilm, impairing the efficiency of antibacterial efforts, particularly in elderly and immunocompromised patients.
2. While we should hope to operate on patients who are uninfected and clean, many of our patients require operation specifically because they are already infected.
3. It is essential that we employ our expertise as physicians to keep or raise the patient's condition to the best attainable state before operation, correcting fluid, electrolyte and nutritional status, recognizing and alleviating the effects of old age and obesity, and treating co-morbidity, including organ failure, compromised immunity, diabetes and drug addiction. Expertly performed surgery is useless if it is performed inappropriately, or on an ill-prepared patient.

4. Wounds are often classified in order to help predict the risks of subsequent infection:

   Clean wounds are typically elective, nontraumatic, technically perfect and primarily closed.

   Clean contaminated wounds include emergencies with minimal spillage such as appendicectomy in the absence of perforation.

   Contaminated encompasses nonpurulent inflammation or spillage of gut, biliary, urinary or other fluids. Other conditions are those resulting from a major technical failure, penetrating trauma of less than 4 hours and chronic open wounds.

   Dirty wounds result from pus formation, gross perforation of the gut, biliary or urinary tract and penetrating trauma more than 4 hours old.

INFECTIONS

Skin and soft tissue infections (SSTIs)

Most SSTIs are caused by a limited group of organisms—β-haemolytic Streptoccoci A, C and G and *Staphylococcus aureus*—though less common organisms are also found, such as *Clostridia* and *Klebsiella*. The clinical manifestations range from mild localised symptoms to systemic sepsis.

1. Cellulitis is confined to the skin and may be treated with oral or intravenous antibiotics depending on the severity.

2. Necrotising fasciitis is a bacterial infection of the deeper soft tissues, and the patient may present with symptoms out of keeping with the appearance of the overlying skin and will require surgical debridement in addition to intravenous antibiotics. Fournier's gangrene is a form of necrotising fasciitis confined to the scrotum and perineum.

3. Pyomyositis is a bacterial infection of the muscles and will also require surgical debridement. The presentation is insidious because it is deep-seated, and swelling of the muscle may cause compartment syndrome.

4. Pseudomembranous colitis. Over-use of antibiotics can alter the microflora of the gut. The exotoxins of *Clostridium difficile* (a Gram-positive anaerobic Bacillus) produce inflammation and mucosal cell necrosis in the gut, with severe diarrhoea as a result of changes in intestinal flora usually following prolonged courses of broad-spectrum antibiotics. The patient will have diarrhoea. Send a stool specimen for *Clostridium difficile* toxins. Consider stopping the antibiotic therapy and seek microbiological advice regarding specific antibiotic therapy to treat the *Clostridium difficile*, often oral metronidazole or vancomycin.

Abscess

An abscess (from the Latin *abs* = from + *cedere* = to go) is an enclosed cavity filled with necrotic material and the products of liquefaction, consisting mainly of dead phagocytes, which form pus (from the Greek *pyon* and Latin *pus*).

1. If an abscess forms near a surface, it may 'point', spontaneously rupture, and discharge to the body surface or to an internal space such as the peritoneal cavity, or into a hollow viscus such as the bowel. At first, the swelling becomes reddened, hot and tender (classically described in Latin as *tumor, rubor, calor, dolor*). The rise in pressure empties the overlying blood vessels so that the centre becomes white, then darkens as it undergoes necrosis. At the body surface, you can detect a point of maximal tenderness and softening and elicit fluctuation in a larger abscess.

2. A boil (from the Old English *byl* = an inflamed swelling) is an infection of a hair follicle, usually from *Staphylococcus aureus*, and may develop into a small abscess. It usually discharges or subsides spontaneously (a 'blind' boil).

VIRAL TRANSMISSION

1. Important viruses are the hepatitides A, B, C, D and E, the human immunodeficiency virus (HIV) and SARS CoV-2 (Covid-19).

2. You can protect yourself and your colleagues by ensuring that you do not risk coming into contact with human blood or blood products and human natural secretions. Make sure you do not sustain, or cause anyone in the team to sustain, skin damage. Be especially careful of needle-stick injuries and injuries with other sharp instruments. Never pass them from hand to hand; always place them in a dish whenever they are not being used or when they are being passed from one person to another.

3. Make your precautions universal. It is dangerous to assume that people who do not fall into the so-called high-risk categories are free of infection.

SEPSIS

1. The definition of sepsis seems to vary. However, it is largely a condition where there are clinical signs of an infection somewhere in the body. If that infection is in the bloodstream, it is septicaemia. Severe sepsis is present when there are signs of organ dysfunction, such as hypoxia, oliguria or lactic acidosis as a result of the infection. Septic shock occurs when as a result of the infection the blood pressure remains low despite fluid resuscitation.
2. The Sepsis Six is a bundle derived from a multicentre international set of guidelines that looked at reducing negative outcomes from sepsis. If you have a patient with sepsis you should do the following:
   • Give oxygen.
   • Obtain cultures before giving antibiotics.
   • Give broad-spectrum antibiotics early.
   • Give adequate intravenous fluids early.
   • Measure the lactate and other blood tests (such as white cell count, CRP, platelet count, clotting, renal function tests and liver function tests).
   • Monitor the urine output.
   In addition, you should consider the following:
   • Obtain early imaging to identify the source of sepsis.
   • If you find a source of sepsis, you should deal with it appropriately.
   • If there is no response or a poor response to fluids, give vasopressor agents to maintain blood pressure.
   • Remeasure the lactate within six hours if it was previously elevated.
   • Your patient should be moved to a high-dependency or intensive therapy facility at the earliest opportunity.
3. Remember that a patient with severe sepsis and septic shock may die and you should not work outside your depth of competence. Call for help early as needed.

UNIVERSAL PRECAUTIONS

These rules were developed, in addition to standard precautions, in response to the outbreak of acquired immune deficiency syndrome (AIDS) in the 1980s.
1. The title is often quoted with the assumption that the precautions are well understood. Most rules are discretionary; 'universal' signifies 'without exception'.
2. All patients with whom you come into contact must be assumed to be possible carriers of pathogens in certain body fluids, such as blood, semen and vaginal secretions, and peritoneal, pleural, pericardial, synovial and amniotic fluids.
3. Wash hands before and after each medical procedure or apply nonaqueous cleaner.
4. Wear protective gloves when at risk of coming into contact with body fluids.
5. Wear a protective gown, face mask and eye cover if there is a danger of bodily fluid splashing onto you.
6. Safely dispose of contaminated sharp instruments including needles. There should be a sharps box close to where you are using sharps so that you do not have to walk around carrying them.
7. Safely dispose of contaminated protective equipment.

Key point

• Do not ignore universal precautions in emergency situations.

TRAUMA

Traumatised tissues are often contaminated and resulting loss of vitality means that sepsis may develop. Devitalised tissues should be debrided.
1. Before operation on a patient with an injury, carefully assess and investigate the injuries to soft tissue, skin, bones and joints, blood vessels and nerves and the presence of foreign bodies. This allows you to plan your strategy ahead and to order any equipment and backup that you will need.
2. Every surgical operation is traumatic. Do not compound it by handling the tissues roughly. Injured tissues have increased susceptibility to infection as a result of contamination.
3. Under suitable anaesthetic induction, open and explore the wound one layer at a time. Gently remove all dead tissue, ensuring that all remaining tissue is clean and viable. Viable muscle should bleed when cut, and contract when pinched or touched by diathermy. Dead muscle appears pale, homogeneous, and friable. Seek and remove all fragments.
4. Make use of lavage with sterile physiological saline to wash out fragments of foreign material.

This can be done with a syringe if direction is required.

5. It is particularly dangerous to introduce, or fail to remove, microorganisms that require little or no oxygen for their metabolism within damaged, dead or ischaemic tissues.
6. Battle injuries and traffic accidents cause the risk of severe infections. Penetrating injuries allow organisms to be carried deeply. High-velocity missiles, especially bullets fired from high-velocity rifles and shrapnel scattered from an explosion, are particularly dangerous. They carry in clothing and other foreign material. If the kinetic energy of the missile is rapidly dissipated in the tissues, it acts like an explosive, disrupting the cells. Anaerobic organisms flourish in the resulting dead tissue. For this reason, it is essential to remove all dead tissue and foreign material and expose the retained healthy tissue to the air.

Key points

- Systemically administered antibiotics cannot reach dead or ischaemic tissues.
- Do not close a wound if you are uncertain whether it is recent, healthy, with no foreign material and tension-free.
- In case of doubt employ delayed primary closure (see Ch. 6).

7. Debridement (from the French *débrider* = to unbridle) of devitalised tissues is imperative to prevent the spread of infection. Tissues may have died as a result of infection, ischaemia or both. Surgical debridement involves cutting away the tissue with a scalpel or sharp scissors until healthy, bleeding tissue is reached. Debridement can also be achieved by applying larvae (laboratory-grown maggots) to the wound.
8. Slough, the layer of devitalised cells that adheres to chronic open wounds, and gangrene may also be debrided. Slough can be debrided with a scalpel or with some hydrocolloid dressings which absorb the exudate from the wound to form a gel softening the dead tissue so that it is more easily removed.

PREOPERATIVE

1. We all have microorganisms constantly with us on our skin, in our noses, mouths, and gut and we may become infected as a result of contact with other people or infected material, especially if we have exposed cuts or injuries or have diminished resistance.
2. Many of the operations surgeons perform are for the treatment of existing infection. Patients submitting themselves to operation often carry organisms that could be carried to the site of operation. Many organisms are harmless in one site, as in the gut, but are harmful elsewhere.
3. Hospitals are reservoirs of nosocomial infection (from the Greek *nosos* = sickness + *komeien* = to tend; hospital sickness) from organisms often resistant to antibiotics. Although they may be harboured in instruments, dressings and bedding, many studies have demonstrated that transmission of the majority of infections is by personal contact. This can occur between patients, or via nurses and doctors, especially if effective hand-washing is neglected between encounters.
4. Consider the need for prophylactic or peroperative antibiotics, especially for someone at increased risk, including patients with a prosthesis such as a heart valve replacement.

BLEEDING

Stagnant blood provides an ideal culture medium for microorganisms. The incidence of wound infection is increased after operations in which excessive bleeding has occurred. Make every effort to leave the operative field completely dry, remove all spilt blood, and guard against continuing or recurring bleeding when the procedure is completed.

OPERATING ROUTINES

1. Before 'scrubbing up', check your hands for cuts, abrasions and ulceration. If you find any, apply a waterproof adhesive dressing.
2. During procedures placing you at risk, wear a long apron, an impervious gown, eye shields and double gloves. As a preference, use a dark-coloured glove underneath and a normal cream-coloured glove over the top. Then, if there is a perforation in the outer glove, the darker colour will show through, alerting you to the breach. Most people wear a glove half a size larger than their normal glove underneath,

covered by a glove their normal glove size to allow ease of movement of the fingers. If your gloves are damaged, change them.

3. Keep all sharp instruments in separate dishes. Never pass them by hand.

4. For high-risk infections, use blunt needles rather than sharp, and cutting diathermy instead of a scalpel, where possible.

5. Avoid spilling blood as far as possible by sealing vessels before you divide them.

6. To reduce the risk of spreading infection on surgeons' gloves during the operation, Sir Arbuthnot Lane (1869–1943) successfully popularised 'no touch' techniques. All the procedures were carried out using instruments. A modification of the technique is continued in minimal access procedures.

7. If you sustain a needle-stick injury, encourage bleeding, wash your hands, and put on fresh gloves as soon as you can. Afterwards, report it to the occupational health officer.

8. As a routine, check your hands at the end of every operation for any injuries you may not have noticed while concentrating on the procedure.

Key points

- 'Universal precautions' means employing safe routines as part of your automatic behaviour.
- To repeat, this is particularly true in emergency situations.
- Do not relax them, thinking, 'It will be safe this time'.

OPERATION

1. In the past the skin was assiduously shaved, washed and prepared with sterilizing applications before operation. Close shaving is now avoided because of the resultant damage to the skin; if necessary, the hairs are clipped short, using a clipper with a disposable head.

2. Antibiotic prophylaxis is routine for many operations. You will find that many hospitals have their own regime for different operative scenarios, and you should make yourself familiar with your local protocols.

3. Before making the incision, clean the skin with an antiseptic solution such as 2% iodine in 50% ethanol or 0.5% chlorhexidine in 70% ethanol. Drape the area with sterile towels, usually proprietary disposable sheets, to isolate the operation site. Some towels cover a wide area and have a central hole through which you make the approach. If you apply several towels, fix them together with towel clips. Alternatively, or in addition, you may apply a sterile, transparent, adhesive sheet through which you make the incision. You may prefer an adhesive sheet impregnated with iodine for those procedures where skin contamination could be a disaster.

4. You may be operating to deal with an existing infection, or in an area where there are organisms present that are harmless here but would be dangerous if they spread elsewhere. In both cases take every possible precaution to avoid disseminating the organisms. Pack off tissues outside the immediate area of the operation. Immediately remove or isolate contaminated material. Keep all the instruments used in the contaminated area in a special container, to be discarded as soon as the 'dirty' part of the operation is completed. If it is essential for you to handle contaminated or potentially contaminated material and tissues to assess them, or as part of the procedure, discard your gloves and replace them with sterile ones before completing the operation. Similarly, discard and replace soiled drapes.

5. If you encounter infection, always take a specimen or swab for culture and tests of sensitivity to antibiotics.

6. At the end of the operation the whole area should be clean and viable.

7. Should you close the wound?

8. Be willing to lightly pack the wound and wait until it is clean, healthy, and free of discharge; then close it, if necessary by applying a skin graft.

9. If you have closed the wound, or if you are dealing with a closed injury, frequently and carefully watch to exclude swelling and tissue tension. This may be most obvious in a limb. If necessary carry out debridement (from the French to *unbridle*—the original meaning was to cut away constricting bands; only later was it extended to mean excision of dead tissue). Incise the skin and deep tissues longitudinally to release the tension. Lay in sterile gauze and replace it at intervals until the wound is suitable for closure or grafting.

10. Mesothelial-lined cavities such as the peritoneal space may be contaminated, as when a large bowel is breached surgically, by trauma or disease, releasing organisms within the peritoneum. It may be necessary to create an artificial opening of the colon onto the abdominal wall (a colostomy). Remove every trace of colonic content from the peritoneal cavity with warm, sterile, physiological saline. Once it is free of contamination, the peritoneum is usually well able to resist infection. However, the superficial part of the wound is much more susceptible. You should either drain the superficial layers or leave them open.

11. The precepts of Kocher, Halsted and Cushing of gentleness, haemostasis and perfect tissue apposition did not specifically include oxygenation. Ischaemia (from the Greek *ischein* = to restrain + *haima* = blood) was well recognised but tissue anoxia (from the Greek *an* = not + oxygen + *ia* = indicating a pathological condition) is not always clinically detectable.

12. If you leave the abdomen open as a laparostomy there are a number of ways that you can cover the wound. Gently laying on large saline-moistened swabs will protect the bowel and can then be covered with a large sterile, transparent adhesive sheet. An alternative is to apply a Bogota bag. This is usually a large thick plastic sheet fashioned out of a large sterile irrigation fluid bag, with the fluid discarded; you place the bag, the inside (shiny side) facing the bowel to protect the bowel and place interrupted nonabsorbable sutures to temporarily fix it to the open abdominal wall. If you have available a negative pressure wound system, then you may either use the sponge and plastic sheet system supplied with it or you may take two sheets of sterile transparent adhesive plastic and sandwich a large gauze swab between them (adhesive sides facing the gauze on both sides). Use a scalpel to perforate this (away from the patient), to allow fluid to be withdrawn through it. Place this over the abdominal contents, tucking it under the edges of the abdominal wall. Another large swab can then be placed over this and then the suction mechanism placed over this and sealed with a further sheet of sterile adhesive plastic adherent to the surrounding abdominal wall. A good seal is required for any negative pressure system to work. Remember a negative pressure wound system in contact with bowel requires a non-adherent layer (plastic) in contact with the bowel.

SURGICAL SITE INFECTION

The incidence of infection at the site of operation is related to bacterial factors, surgical technique and the patient.

1. Bacterial factors include the type: *Staphylococcus aureus* and *Escherichia coli* are commonly involved but other organisms including fungi may be causative. Bacteria in one site may be harmless, for example within the gut, but be pathological elsewhere.

2. Surgical factors include whether the wound is clean or dirty, the perfection of the operating technique, operating time, the presence of necrosis and the presence of foreign materials or prostheses.

3. The patient's age, immune status and nutritional state affect resistance and this is reduced in obesity, diabetes, malignancy, comorbidity and as a result of smoking.

4. Common organisms are *Escherichia coli* and *Staphylococcus aureus*.

5. The incidence of surgical site infections is dependent on wound type, operation class, use of drainage, the operating surgeon and American Society for Anesthesiologists (ASA) category: I, healthy; II, mild systemic disease; III, severe systemic disease; IV, severe disease a constant threat to life; V, moribund, unlikely to survive 24 hours. To enable comparison of outcomes, the Health Protection Agency Surgical Site Infection Surveillance Service (SSISS) collects results from mandatory surveillance according to the type of operation and issues comparative tables.[3]

TREATING INFECTIONS

Cellulitis

1. Early, adequate treatment with a well-chosen antibiotic is usually the most important step in the management of many forms of cellulitis.

2. It may not be possible to obtain a specimen for culture, but if there is an adjacent wound, this can be swabbed. Immediately deliver it to the microbiologist, at the same time taking advice on the antibiotic most likely to be effective.

Necrotising fasciitis

1. Operative treatment is urgently required. All the necrotic tissue must be excised, leaving only healthy tissue.

Abscess

1. One of the principal functions of surgeons was traditionally to 'let out the pus'. Access to imaging methods has replaced many operative procedures. Simple ultrasonic viewing of the collection of pus facilitates the insertion of a drain following the injection of local anaesthetic. Small abscesses can be drained through a needle, or catheter carried on a needle or using Seldinger's technique (see Ch. 5). Larger abscesses may demand a small incision to accommodate a formal drain (see Ch. 11).
2. Be sure that there is no continuing cause for the abscess or simple drainage will not suffice.
3. Local anaesthesia is less effective in the presence of inflammation but in many localised situations, it spares the patient the need for a general anaesthetic. If you intend to employ it, raise an intracutaneous bleb in adjacent uninflamed skin and slowly and gently inject ahead of the needle until you have reached the pinnacle of the abscess. If you are impatient and inject under pressure, raising the tissue tension, you will cause pain. If you do not wait long enough for the anaesthetic to take effect, you have wasted your time and will hurt the patient. Never incorporate adrenaline (epinephrine) with the local anaesthetic or you may cause extensive necrosis. In the case of a finger pulp infection, if you create a ring block at the base of the finger, you must avoid at all costs creating a constricting ring of swelling; if you do, the whole finger may undergo necrosis. Inject only within the web space where the volume of fluid will not have any constricting effect.

Key points

- Many abscesses can be drained using a needle and syringe with a three-way tap to empty the syringe.
- Deep abscesses are often best drained using a catheter introduced under imaging control.

---

4. Incise an abscess at the point of greatest tenderness, or on the pinnacle of the swelling. Obtain a swab for culture and determination of antibiotic sensitivity. Clean out the contents, taking a specimen for culture. If you have any doubts about the aetiology, excise a portion of the edge for histological examination.
5. Empty the contents not by squeezing, which will introduce organisms into the bloodstream, but with a scoop, or by washing out with fluid from a syringe. Squeezing of infected lesions is particularly deprecated on the face around the nose and upper lip. Organisms will drain by the anterior facial vein into the cavernous venous sinus and may cause septic thrombosis.
6. Unless this is an obviously small local abscess, insert a finger or an instrument to explore the interior for loculations (from the Latin *loculus* = diminutive of locus = place) or track. The collar-stud abscess is notorious in the neck when a diseased lymph node undergoes necrosis and liquefaction; the resulting pus then tracks through a hole in the deep fascia to form a subcutaneous abscess. A tuberculous cervical lymph node is a well-known cause. An infected branchial cyst may also create a collar-stud abscess.
7. An abscess near the anus may develop from an infected anal gland, presenting close to the anal margin. An ischiorectal abscess, developing higher up, usually presents laterally and further away. You may be able to feel and open up loculi and detect an upward extension with a finger in the abscess cavity. Do not attempt to probe it in search of an internal opening. It is usual to pack the wound to prevent it from healing until the base has filled up. If the skin is allowed to close over, an abscess may reform.
8. An intraabdominal abscess usually results from localised disease that has been limited from spreading by the adhesion of surrounding structures. The primary pathology will need to be addressed. A typical condition is an appendix abscess. When the appendix becomes inflamed, surrounding structures usually adhere and form an appendix mass. If the appendix then ruptures, it does so into a constrained cavity. You need to be very cautious and gentle in approaching the mass for fear of releasing the contents into the general peritoneal cavity, or of damaging any of the inflamed, fragile viscera forming part of the wall of the mass. Be content to drain the abscess unless the appendix is easily found

within the cavity and can be removed without disturbing the other structures.

9. Some other abscesses within the abdomen, which have an underlying cause, may not settle after you drain them. Leakage from a viscus may continue and a track will form to the surface, creating a fistula (see Ch. 4).

10. Having emptied the abscess, you need to maintain drainage. A wick or ribbon of gauze is sometimes inserted into a small abscess. Very often this merely acts as a plug. The drain should keep the wound open until the cavity is completely empty, and in some cases until it has had time to shrink and fill up with granulation tissue. Therefore, prefer soft latex corrugated sheet, usually held by a single stitch. If the cavity is deep, insert a safety pin into the projecting portion as an extra precaution so that it cannot fall into the cavity (see Ch. 11).

11. If possible arrange that the drainage hole will be dependent so that the cavity will drain by gravity. This may be difficult in the breast. It is rarely necessary to make a second incision from the undersurface of the breast to drain a high, deeply placed abscess.

12. If an abscess recollects or has no obvious primary pathology, it may be drained percutaneously with a pigtail catheter under ultrasound guidance. Though it is likely that you will be asking a radiologist to perform this for you, you should be responsible for ensuring that a specimen has been sent to the laboratory for appropriate microscopy and culture.

INFECTED PROSTHESES

When a surgical implant (e.g., a joint replacement or a vascular graft) becomes infected, it is a disaster. Once infective organisms have seeded onto an indwelling foreign body, they are very difficult to eradicate. The basic principle is to remove them, though sometimes removal can be limb- or life-threatening. Management will be via a multidisciplinary approach with senior surgeons and microbiologists or infectious disease physicians.

REFERENCES

1. Allen DB, Maguire JJ, Mahdavian M, et al. Wound hypoxia and acidosis limit neutrophil bacterial killing mechanisms. *Arch Surg.* 1997;132:991–996.

2. WHO. Global Guidelines for the prevention of surgical site infection. ISBN 978 92 4 154988 2 (2016).

FURTHER READING

Dellinger RP, et al. Surviving Sepsis Campaign: International guidelines for management of severe sepsis and septic shock: 2008. Intens *Care Med.* 2008;34:17–60.

Chapter | **13** |

Handling minimal access surgery

Key points

- As new approaches and techniques are developed in one area; they are seised upon and utilised in others; skills are transferable!
- Anticipate soundly based advances and be prepared to acquire new skills that are often needed to exploit demonstrable patient benefits.

EXAMPLES

Minimal access procedures comprise those internal manipulations that can be performed without the need for extensive exposure to reach the target tissue. Patients often refer to these procedures as 'keyhole' surgery, though undoubtedly some keyholes have larger keys than others. Traditionally, surgeons were encouraged to employ generous incisions, allowing careful exploration and ample access, by the adage that 'wounds heal from the sides, not from the ends'. The need for wide exposure has been markedly reduced by the development of improved imaging methods and technical advances; these have often been achieved by incremental improvements in what were originally unpromising innovations. Often this results in the patient recovering and going home quicker.

1. Conventional open procedures performed through the smallest possible incisions, prefixed 'mini-', such as laparotomy, cholecystectomy, and appendicectomy. Special long-handled but conventional instruments may be used.

2. Radiological, magnetic resonance, ultrasound and other methods of imaging allow interventions using needles and cannulas. Many of them depend on developments of Seldinger's technique (see Ch. 5) by means of which access can be gained into blood vessels, ducts, and natural, pathological and created spaces. In neurosurgery, carefully targeted instruments may be passed through burr holes to biopsy, or to destroy special tissues or tumours by ultrasonic, electrosurgical or other means. A frame can be attached to the skull to hold the

instrument, but this has largely been replaced by computer-generated targeting.

3. Endoscopy is generally recognised to have developed from fibreoptics in rigid or flexible guided instruments passed through natural ducts with any procedures performed along the line of sight or aided by imaging techniques. Endoscopic retrograde cholangiopancreatography (ERCP) allows visualization which can be augmented by imaging for diagnostic and therapeutic procedures.

4. 'Minimal access surgery', or so-called 'keyhole surgery', generally implies procedures carried out in the main by surgeons as opposed to radiologists and endoscopists (though many surgeons now undertake both radiological and endoscopic procedures). It depends upon simultaneous developments in illumination, visualization, instruments—and more importantly, the willingness of pioneers to acquire new, complex skills that often require natural movements to be reversed. A major step forward was the realization that instruments that were previously inserted along the line of sight could often be inserted through separate ports allowing them to be viewed with better depth perception. It has succeeded in spite of other deficiencies: two-dimensional viewing on a screen with loss of binocular vision, haptic loss (the sense of touch) with reduced appreciation of force and torque transmitted to the tissues, and reversal of some natural manipulative functions. Wherever a cavity exists, even though it is potential only, it may be possible to expand it with carbon dioxide, saline, or initially with a balloon, to allow the insertion through separate portals of a combined light and camera, and instruments to perform a rapidly increasing variety of surgical procedures. In some centres, space is created within the abdomen by lifting the abdominal wall instead of inflating it with gas.

5. Robotic surgery is a further demonstration that once a technique has been shown to be practicable, small incremental improvements are developed that make it likely to become widely available. It offers the advantage that the operator's surgical movements feel natural, hand tremor is eliminated, binocular vision is available and haptic sensation is promised. Furthermore, the surgeon may be comfortably sitting and thus tire less easily. In the past, the initial high cost of all electronically controlled instruments has rapidly fallen as manufacturers compete for the market and demand increases as users compete to exploit the newly available technical possibilities. Surgical robots are now commonplace in developed countries.

LAPAROSCOPY

Access

This is not a new concept. For many years abdominal surgeons routinely employed a rigid sigmoidoscope inserted through a small stab incision, inflating the abdomen using the hand pump. Limited areas could be visualised, and biopsies removed along the line of sight. The German physician Kalk was the first to use separate access points for needles inserted across the line of sight to obtain liver biopsies. The gynaecologist Kurt Semm of Kiel is considered the father of modern laparoscopy. Laparoscopy (from the Greek *lapara* = flank or loins from *laparos* = soft, loose + *skopein* = to view) is normally carried out under general anaesthesia.

1. Obtain consent for the procedure to be converted to an open operation if necessary.
2. Make sure the bladder is empty; if necessary, pass a catheter.
3. If the stomach is distended, pass a nasogastric tube.
4. Carefully palpate the relaxed abdomen to identify any masses and locate the sacral promontory. Percuss the abdomen to detect the lower level of liver dullness.

Two methods have been developed to allow safe penetration of the abdominal wall without damage to intraabdominal viscera or major blood vessels.

Closed pneumoperitoneum

This was initially popular, but concerns relating to potentially unseen visceral injuries have seen its popularity wane. If you are a new learner, use the open technique.

1. Make a small subumbilical incision down to but not through, the peritoneum. Pick up the abdominal wall and gently insert the Veress needle (Fig. 13.1). As the point penetrates the peritoneum, a spring-loaded, round-ended obturator projects, pushing away any underlying structure.

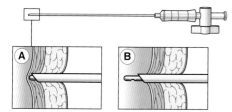

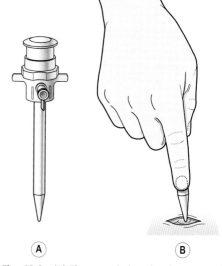

Fig. 13.1 A Veress needle. (A) The needle is just about to pierce the inner lining of the cavity. (B) As soon as the needle has entered the cavity, the round-ended, spring-loaded obturator projects, pushing away any structure that might be punctured by the sharp needle and exposing the gas inlet.

> **Key point**
>
> • Listen for, and feel for, the click as the Veress needle obturator extends.

Fig. 13.2 (A) The cannula has the sharp trocar in place. (B) The head of the trocar sits in the palm of your hand and your index finger extends along the shaft of the cannula to prevent too deep penetration. Aim the trocar towards the anus, i.e., below the previously identified sacral promontory using a gentle twisting motion.

2. Check your confidence in the safety of peritoneal puncture by opening the tap on the Veress needle and placing a drop of sterile saline on the Luer connection. The drop should be drawn into the needle when the patient inhales. Gently inject 10 mL saline through the needle, then try to aspirate it; if you can, the needle tip must be in a closed space. Switch on the insufflator (from the Latin *in + sufflare* = to blow) with a gas flow of 1 litre/min and check the pressure, which should not exceed 8 mmHg. Confirm that liver dullness has been lost.

3. If all is well, cautiously inflate the abdomen with 3–5 litres of carbon dioxide, provided the abdomen is evenly distended and pressure is 10–15 mmHg. Now withdraw the Veress needle and enlarge the incision down to the peritoneum.

4. Insert the cannula (port) with its trocar, which has a flap or trumpet valve to prevent gas leakage (Fig. 13.2). Hold the cannula (port) and trocar in the palm of the hand with the index finger extended to limit the extent of penetration, inserting it with a twisting motion, directing the tip below the previously identified sacral promontory, pointing towards the anus. You can meanwhile distend the lower abdomen by gently compressing the upper abdomen. As the trocar pierces the peritoneum, a spring-loaded collar may project, extending beyond the sharp tip of the trocar. Listen for the click. It may be preferable to do this with a special cannula that has a transparent trocar

within which fits the camera; the cannula is thus placed under direct vision.

5. Withdraw the trocar and replace it with the combined light carrier, telescope and camera, attached to the light source and television monitor. View the interior to check that there has been no damage.

Open pneumoperitoneum

This open Hasson technique is now generally preferred and allows a trocar to be placed under direct vision.

1. Make a 1.5–2 cm incision, either vertical just below the umbilicus, or curved transversely subumbilical. The size of your incision will depend on the size of the cannula that you are going to insert. This, in turn, will depend on the size of the instruments that you will use, in particular the camera. Standard cannulae are 10 mm or 5 mm. Carry it down to the linea alba, identified by the white fibres after which it is named (from the Latin *albus* = white). Other sites may be more appropriate if there are nearby scars on the abdomen. Incise the linea alba and place a stay suture on each side leaving the peritoneum intact, to be tented and incised separately, or grasp and lift the linea

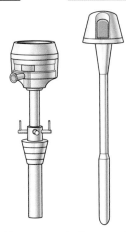

Fig. 13.3 Hassan cannula. The coned neck blocks the entrance hole. The cannula is usually held in place by deep stitches on each side, tied over projecting shoulders to prevent displacement of the cannula. Some models have a screw shape and remain in place even without retaining stitches. The insufflator, camera and lighting systems are connected. Subsequent ports are inserted while you watch their entrance from within, to avoid damage to internal structures.

alba on each side with strong forceps while you cut through it and proceed to open the peritoneum.

2. Insert a finger and sweep it in a full circle to confirm that you have reached the peritoneal cavity and that there are no adherent viscera.

3. Insert a 10 mm diameter Hasson cannula (Fig. 13.3), which has a blunt obturator and a conically shaped neck intended to block the entrance hole and stop leakage. Some Hasson ports have spiral collars that can be rotated through the fascia to provide a snug seal which helps maintain the pneumoperitoneum. Modern-day commercially available disposable Hasson ports (generally referred to as 'balloon ports') consist of a retention disc and balloon which when approximated across a variable width of the abdominal wall can reduce port-site bleeding. They also allow for balloon deflation and port removal to allow periodic specimen retrieval before reinsertion and resumption of laparoscopy.

4. If using a standard reusable Hasson cannula, draw the stitch or stitches tight, tie them around the cannula projections and loop them over the gas inlet. Do not knot the threads

but clip them, so you can use them to close the incision at the end of the procedure.

5. Gently ensure that the cannula moves freely. If all is well, connect the gas inlet to the insufflator, which is set to deliver carbon dioxide at 1 litre/min and against a pressure not exceeding 12–15 mmHg.

6. Insert the camera, attached to the light source and ensure that you can see clearly around the peritoneal cavity and that there is no intraabdominal injury or undue bleeding running directly down from the cannula site. Cameras come with the lens at varying degrees of angle from direct forward view and your choice will depend on the procedure that you are undertaking.

PLACING A SECOND CANNULA (PORT)

1. When placing a second cannula, direct the camera placed in the umbilical cannula towards where you wish to place the new cannula. Ensure there are no adhesions to this area and that intraabdominal contents are sufficiently out of the way; it often helps to tilt the patient into reverse Trendelenburg and sometimes to the contralateral side to achieve this.

2. In a slim patient, the light from the camera transilluminating through the skin can be used to identify where to make the small incision in the skin. Placement of your skin incision will depend on what operation you intend to undertake. Incisions are made away from the site of the procedure to allow for leverage of instruments, and yet not so far that the instruments cannot easily be manipulated at the site of the operation. The skin incision is made in a Langer's line and is just large enough to accept the chosen cannula diameter.

3. The cannula is inserted with its trochar under direct camera vision and pointing away from internal structures. Some surgeons inject a local anaesthetic into the wound and push the needle into the abdominal cavity under direct vision to ensure that the exit site in the abdomen is where they would wish the cannula to be. The trocar is removed to allow insertion of further instrumentation.

TECHNICAL ASPECTS

1. Space has been created with carbon dioxide gas from the insufflator, delivered at a predetermined rate to the required volume, up to a preset pressure, sounding an alarm if this is exceeded. Low-pressure laparoscopy has physiological advantages over prolonged high-pressure laparoscopy but has traditionally been difficult to achieve. Innovative insufflation devices such as the AirSeal system are now widely available and provide for a stable pneumoperitoneum combined with constant smoke extraction and valve-free access to the peritoneum For some procedures, carried out extraperitoneally, such as in a TEPP (totally extraperitoneal preperitoneal) laparoscopic hernia repair and retroperitoneal approach to the kidney, a space can be developed by inserting a balloon without breaching the peritoneum. This technique does not require a pneumoperitoneum, but insufflation of gas may still subsequently be required to maintain a suitable operating space. DD Gaur initially described the use of a sterile glove finger tied by silk over a suction catheter to atraumatically displace fat and peritoneum to create space prior to port placements. A variety of commercially available devices are now available for the development of extraperitoneal spaces but work essentially in the same way as the originally described approach.

2. When introducing additional cannulae, identify and avoid large vessels, particularly the inferior epigastric blood vessels. Because instruments can then be manoeuvred across, rather than along the line of sight, their spatial relationships with the target structure can be accurately judged. Site these ports in order to provide the most advantageous approach and available space for instruments. There are standardised port sites for many operations but take into consideration the patient's build and the presence of scars.

3. A single fixed camera entry point limits the view of structures, usually to one aspect and, at present, a two-dimensional view on the monitor screen. A second monitor provides a view for the assistant controlling the camera and for the scrub nurse.

4. The instruments are long-handled and slide in and out through the fixed entry portal in the abdominal wall, which forms the fulcrum.

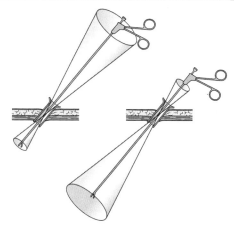

Fig. 13.4 The effect of withdrawing and advancing an instrument through the access port on the volume of accessible space. The effect also alters the inverse relation between hand movements and movements at the instrument tip. If the instrument is almost fully inserted a small hand movement produces an extensive movement of the instrument tip, and vice versa. This demonstrates the importance of carefully placing the entry portal to achieve a correct balance between the internal and external lengths of the operating instrument.

As the instruments are withdrawn and advanced, the relationship changes between the inner and outer portions, thus changing the amount of movement produced at the tip of the instrument resulting from a standard movement of the handle (Fig. 13.4). The tip can be moved anywhere within a cone whose apex is at the body wall.

Key points

- When siting the entrance port, carefully consider the required range of movement of the instrument tips in relation to your hand movements.
- Ports sited too close to the target structure commit you to wide hand movements; sited too far away, they commit you to making very limited hand movements and exaggerated tip movements.

5. Retractors, suckers, irrigators, forceps clip applicators, staple applicators, Lahey-swab-on-a-stick and other instruments are available. It is time consuming to change instruments, so some are designed to be multipurpose;

for example, a combined diathermy hook, irrigator and sucker. Versions of most of the stapling machines available in open surgery can be used laparoscopically (see Ch. 2). Blood vessels can be isolated and ligated; intraperitoneal ligature tying and pretied endoloops have largely superseded extraperitoneal knot-tying. Sutures and suture ligatures are similarly inserted and tied intraperitoneally. Clips can be applied and an intraperitoneal stapling machine, resembling a miniature GIA intestinal stapler, safely inserts lines of staples on each side as it divides larger vessels or ducts.

6. Dissection techniques have been modified from those used in open surgery. Wherever possible the tissues are separated into layers and sequentially identified and sealed. Unipolar diathermy has long been a popular and effective method; small amounts of tissue are separated, hooked up clear of the main mass, identified, coagulated and simultaneously divided. Bipolar diathermy is increasingly popular. Because your view is restricted, you may not notice that tissue outside the intended area has been burned via metal in contact with the diathermy applicator. When two metal instruments are in close proximity and the alternating diathermy current is passed through one, it may induce a current in the other, even though they are insulated from each other, and so the current may reach the patient. Use the lowest power setting, prefer bipolar to monopolar and select cutting in preference to coagulation current. Pulsed pressurised saline may also be used to dissect, as may the harmonic scalpel.

7. Vessels can also be sealed after clamping to appose the walls using electrosurgery, with the LigaSure system which automatically senses the melting of collagen to weld the walls. The harmonic scalpel ultrasonic coagulator and cutting device coapts and seals the tissues with a protein coagulum at a relatively low temperature, compared with electrosurgical instruments, of 50–100°C. In some cases, large masses are disrupted using laser beams. Dissection through solid tissues using simple or sophisticated instruments demands the greatest familiarity and highest skills, but can be achieved by experts. A diathermy probe with a pea-sized metal ball can be used to coagulate an oozy area. However, be careful not to touch any other structures with it.

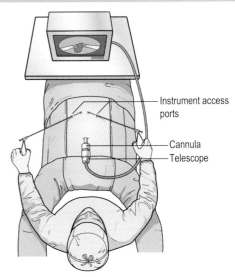

Fig. 13.5 Diagram from above of a surgeon laparotomist manipulating instruments while watching the television monitor connected to the camera inserted into the patient's peritoneal cavity.

8. When using instruments that are either sharp or hot, always withdraw them into the cannula immediately after use to avoid inadvertent damage to other structures.

9. Because your hands may be widely separated (Fig. 13.5), they cannot be held as steadily as they would be during open surgery when the base can usually be brought close to the point of action, and the hands are close together working in practised harmony.

10. The most experienced assistant takes charge of the camera. Since multiple access ports are used, you can delegate to assistants responsibility for some instruments. Some surgeons use voice-directed, body or eye-movement-directed control, in the absence of an experienced assistant. Retraction and steadying of tissues can be delegated to another; a number of versatile retractors and graspers have been designed.

11. Excised tissues can sometimes be withdrawn through the largest or a surgically enlarged port site or fresh incision. A useful method is to place the tissue within a strong, flexible bag, bring out the neck of the bag through a small exit hole and exert traction combined with a side-to-side motion to draw it out. Alternatively, a morcellator (from the French *morceau*, cognate with morsel, from the Latin *mordere* = to bite) can be used to chop up a

large piece of tissue into small particles within the bag for withdrawal through a small exit port. In women, you can create a posterior colpotomy (from the Greek *kolpos* = vagina).

12. A variety of procedures are 'laparoscopy assisted', part open surgery, part laparoscopy. In some cases, dissection is performed laparoscopically, and anastomoses are fashioned at the surface. In low rectal anastomoses, circular staplers can be inserted transanally. Hand assistance can be employed using a special glove sealed to the margins of an incision. Although such procedures may take longer than purely open operations they often cause less disturbance and recovery is quicker.

13. Single-incision laparoscopic surgery (SILS) utilises a camera with a side port so that instruments can be passed alongside it to perform the procedure. Natural orifice transluminal endoscopic surgery (NOTES) is an endoscope used to pass from a natural orifice through to the cavity of choice and the procedure conducted through the endoscope.

14. If you are assisting with a robotic procedure, you will be standing by the patient, manning the ports.

CLOSURE

1. At the end of the procedure, first carefully check that there has been no inadvertent damage, no residual bleeding, and no free bodies left in the peritoneal cavity.

2. Remove each instrument in turn while observing the withdrawal from within, to guard against herniation into the defects.

3. Close each secondary port hole after ensuring that there is no bleeding within the track. Inject local anaesthetic into the surrounding tissues (if not given at the start of the procedure) and close the fascia using interrupted stitches. Insert a single subcuticular synthetic absorbable stitch, then close the skin with adhesive strips. There is still some debate as to which ports should be formally closed. There is general agreement that those ports which are greater than 1 cm in diameter require repair in adults and those over 5 mm require repair in children. The peritoneum should be included in a full-thickness repair. The repair can be undertaken under direct vision before the camera is removed. A number

of laparoscopic instrument devices have been developed to facilitate the process. The Endo Close device consists of a spring-loaded stylet mechanism that retracts as the needle is passed through the abdominal wall and advances automatically once the peritoneum is passed. The stylet tip has a notched end which can be used to capture a suture that has already been passed full-thickness through the abdominal wall and is thus retrieved to complete the surgical knot externally.

4. Finally withdraw the laparoscope under vision.

5. Gently compress the abdomen to expel any residual gas.

6. Elevate the margins of the telescope portal by means of the stay stitches inserted at the beginning of the procedure and tie them after ensuring that no abdominal contents have insinuated themselves into the gap. Close the skin with adhesive tape.

ACQUIRING SKILLS

1. You need new skills for minimal access procedures beyond those you have acquired for open surgery. Some surgeons find it difficult to adapt.

2. On a flat, two-dimensional screen, you can see the tips of the instruments in relation to the tissues from one aspect only. Misperception from the restricted view, added to lack of touch sense, leads to incorrect speculative and occasionally wrong conclusions, particularly noted during cholecystectomy,[1] leading to error.

3. In open surgery your hands are close to the point of action of the instruments and are able to feel and assess the tissues, approaching the target from different angles. Now they are at the ends of long shafts and may be wide apart and well away from the 'business' ends. Coordination of hand movements is difficult to achieve in this unnatural posture and with a limited range of approach to the target. Hand movements do not correspond to those of the instrument tips, being spatially reversed and varying with the relation of the instrument shafts to the abdominal wall, which acts as a fulcrum; novices are found to exert 130–138% greater force and torque than experts to achieve the same result.[2]

4. Minimal access surgery lends itself to material simulation and virtual reality courses more

than almost any other formally taught surgical skill. The reason is that you need to learn and practise using a new set of instruments while seeing your objective on a flat screen. It is remarkable how rapidly some surgeons have adapted to the new circumstances by assiduous practice.

> **Key points**
>
> - Remember that the instruments that you learn to wield skilfully are merely intermediaries between you and the living tissues when you come to apply your training to clinical use.
> - No simulator has yet been invented that challenges you with living, often diseased and displaced tissues—the real target of your skills.

5. Every laparoscopic unit should have simulators where trainees can spend spare time acquiring facility with the techniques. This is not yet provided universally, and the simulator may not be available when you wish to practise. You can provide yourself with a simple simulator, using cleaned, worn-out or disposable instruments (Fig. 13.6). Start by placing objects in an open-topped box with direct viewing and holding the instruments directly, then introduce them through holes in the lid, and finally cover the top to prevent you from seeing the objects directly by using two mirrors or a mobile phone. Practise holding a structure with forceps held in one hand after manipulating it to present it most advantageously and cutting it with scissors held in the other hand (Fig. 13.7). Practise dissection using, for example, a chicken leg or an orange.

6. Suturing is commonly performed in a similar manner to that used in open surgery. In order to facilitate inserting stitches, try to insert them from the dominant to the nondominant side (Fig 13.8) or from far to near. Make use of your ability to pronate and supinate, to drive the curved needle smoothly through the tissues.

7. Initially, many knots were created externally and pushed down with a pusher (Fig. 13.9). Preknotted loops are available which can be tightened using a pusher, or you may create a Roeder knot (Fig. 13.10). Many laparoscopic surgeons now tie intracorporeal (intraperitoneal) knots constructed in a similar manner

to the instrument ties employed in open operations. A simple method is shown step by step in Fig. 13.11 but there are many variations. Initially practise this tie with multifilament threads, using straight forceps, then with laparoscopy instruments under direct vision, and finally by indirect viewing. Remember

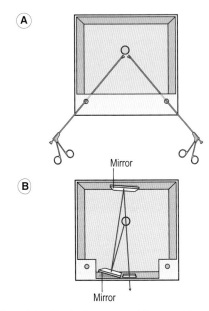

Fig. 13.6 Simple 'homemade' boxes with which to practise minimal access surgery. (A) Remove part of the lid so that you can view the target and instrument tips directly. (B) Place two mirrors so that you can view the target area indirectly. Place a screen so that you cannot see the target directly.

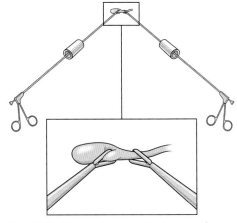

Fig. 13.7 Hold a structure steady using forceps held in one hand while cutting it using scissors held in the other hand.

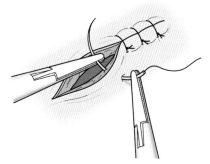

Fig. 13.8 One simple method of intracorporeal suturing. Try to suture from your dominant to nondominant side, exerting counter pressure on the nondominant side and steadying the emerging needle to be recaptured and withdrawn with the needle driver.

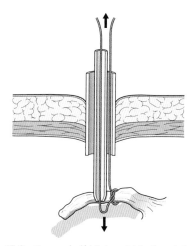

Fig. 13.9 Form a half-hitch outside the abdomen and thread one end through the pusher tube. Tighten the half-hitch by pushing down the pusher tube against counter tension exerted on the other thread. Repeat this for the other half-hitch to form a knot.

that grasping threads with metal instruments severely weakens them, so hold them in parts that will be discarded. Keep a firm hold on the needle before cutting sutures.

8. Thread ligation and suturing have been greatly reduced by the introduction of mechanical staplers and stapling instruments developed as miniaturised open surgery instruments.

9. Dissection techniques have been modified or adapted. Blunt dissection can be performed using retractors to steady the tissues and against which to create mild tension. Sharp dissection requires preliminary exploration

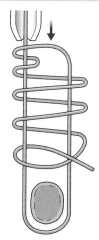

Fig. 13.10 A preformed Roeder knot. The standing part is led to the exterior within a hollow pusher tube. Place the loop over the structure to be ligated. Tighten it by pushing the knot down with the pusher tube against the counter tension on the standing part. The knot will not slip. Cut off the standing part and withdraw it with the pusher tube.

behind the area to exclude vital structures that in open techniques could be palpated or transilluminated from behind. Distension of tissues by injecting saline is an aid to dissection by separating structures. Monopolar diathermy can be applied using a hook to seal, then disrupt flimsy connective tissue, but it can produce smoke that temporarily reduces visibility. Bipolar forceps develop heating only between the tips of the forceps. For piercing and disrupting certain dense tumours, Nd:YAG lasers are sometimes valuable. Ultrasound at a vibration rate of 55,000 cycles/second using a Harmonic scalpel is popular because it causes limited heating and does not produce smoke. Because even a slight amount of bleeding obscures the view through the laparoscope, there is an imperative to seal even small blood vessels before dividing them.

Key points

- Laparoscopic surgery offers a valuable lesson: haemostasis before dissection.
- Transfer the attitude to open surgery by identifying and sealing blood vessels before—not after—dividing them whenever possible.

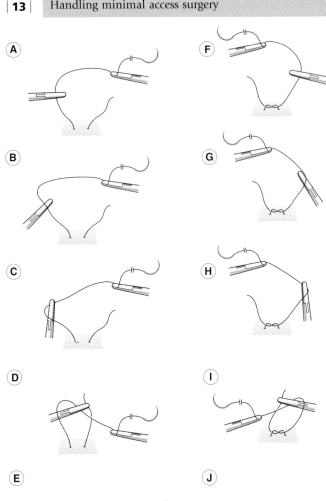

Fig. 13.11 Internal knot-tying resembles the instrument tie described in Chapter 3. (A) The short end is on the right, and the long, needled end is on the left. Slackly raise the left thread with the right forceps and push the thread into a bight with the left forceps. (B) Now pass the left forceps behind the lower part of the bight, (C) in front of the upper part. (D) Draw the right forceps down to keep the thread loop around the left forceps which now grasp the tip of the short thread on the right. (E) Pull the short thread through the looped long thread and tighten the half-hitch by separating the forceps. (F) Tie the second half-hitch by lifting the long thread slackly with the right forceps while forming a bight by pushing the slack thread to the right with the right forceps. (G) Now pass the right forceps behind the lower part of the bight. (H) Push the tip of the right forceps up in front of the upper bight, (I) while drawing the long thread towards you to keep the loop around the right forceps with which you grasp the short thread. (J) Draw the short end through the loop to form the second half-hitch and tighten it onto the first by separating the forceps.

OTHER PROCEDURES

1. Because of the pioneering work of Kurt Semm of Kiel in Germany, gynaecologists utilised minimal access techniques before general and other surgeons and have extended the number of procedures that can be carried out by the technique. Large excised structures are frequently removed through the vagina.

2. Urologists pioneered many single-channel techniques because of the early development of the cystoscope and have adopted minimal access procedures. Although many of them are endoscopic, it is possible to approach the kidney extraperitoneally, first creating a space by inserting and inflating a balloon without transgressing the peritoneum.

3. Orthopaedic surgeons face the problem that joint spaces are difficult to develop although the suprapatellar pouch of the knee forms a capacious space. Joint spaces are distended not with carbon dioxide but with saline. Arthroscopy often needs to be carried out using general anaesthesia because it is usually necessary to manipulate and distract the joint. Many conditions previously treated by open operation can now be treated in part or whole through minimal access procedures. A torn knee cartilage can be repaired, trimmed, smoothed and reattached, avoiding meniscectomy. Arthroscopic assisted repair of a ruptured anterior cruciate ligament is frequently employed.

4. Thoracoscopic access allows diagnostic inspection and a number of procedures to be performed, including sympathectomy. Cardiovascular surgeons employ minimal access techniques including valve repairs. Cardiac valve replacement can be carried out robotically.

5. Otolaryngologists have pioneered many techniques to provide access to small areas difficult to approach. Operations upon the middle ear and the minute ossicles are now commonplace. Cochlear implants for the relief of deafness are constantly improving.

6. The size of corneoscleral incisions in ophthalmology was previously large enough to extract a hard, opaque lens. By liquefying the lens using ultrasound phacoemulsification (from the Greek *phakos* = lens) it can then be aspirated and replaced with a soft plastic lens that is rolled up and spontaneously unrolls within the intraocular capsule. This can be carried out through a very small incision.

7. Neurosurgeons have also embraced minimal access techniques in many areas. Localised lesions may be dealt with using stereotactic procedures (from the Greek *stereos* = solid + *tassein* = to arrange), first used in 1906 by Robert Clarke and Sir Victor Horsley (1857–1916). The original metal helmet frame is mostly replaced now by three-dimensional computing, allowing electrodes to be inserted through burr holes, for electrical stimulation, DC tissue destruction, or AC coagulation, or to obtain biopsies. Cobalt-60 'gamma-knife' irradiation can be accurately targeted from a specialised helmet after obtaining the three-dimensional coordinates.

Robotic surgery

Whilst much emphasis inevitably focuses on the technical challenges facing the primary console surgeon in robotically-assisted laparoscopic procedures; the patient-side assistant plays a pivotal role in the successful implementation of the surgical procedure and has arguably greater technical challenges to overcome. Current robotic systems faithfully and intuitively translate console surgeon hand movements to intracorporeally placed instruments whilst eliminating tremors. Likewise, the primary surgeon is provided with a three-dimensional high-definition image and benefits from the improved dexterity that accompanies instruments with seven degrees of freedom and 90 degrees of articulation. By contrast, the patient-side assistant contends with the traditional two dimensions offered by a standard screen system (and its associated lack of depth perception), poor ergonomics and the restricted degrees of freedom imposed by rigid laparoscopic instruments (albeit with a degree of haptic feedback denied by the console surgeon).

1. Unlike the console surgeon whose hand movements are translated faithfully by the robotic system, the patient-side laparoscopist contends with the counterintuitive instrument movements and a fulcrum effect which enhances the effect of tremor. The patient-side assistant will need to contend with all these whilst delivering sutures to and from the operative field and whilst deploying surgical clips etc. during a procedure.

2. As an assistant in a robotic case you may be involved in insufflation and port placement. Once you have learnt this you will learn how to dock the robot, and then how to exchange the instruments on the robot arms.

3. You may also be assisting through a separate port site (e.g., retraction, lavage or suctioning).

4. Practice standard laparoscopic techniques in order to be a good robotic assistant.

REFERENCES

1. Way L, Stewart L, Gantert W, et al. Causes and prevention of laparoscopic bile duct injuries: analysis of 252 cases from a human factors and cognitive psychology perspective. *Ann Surg.* 2003;237:460–469.
2. Rosen J, MacFarlane M, Richards C, et al. Surgeon-tool force/torque signatures: evaluation of surgical skills in minimally invasive surgery. In: Proceedings of Medicine Meets Virtual Reality (MMVR-7). San Francisco, CA Online. IOS Press; 1999. Available http://bionics.soe.ucsc.edu/publications/CP_03.pdf June 26, 2009.

FURTHER READING

Greaves N, Nicholson J. Single incision laparoscopic surgery in general surgery: a review. *Ann R Coll Surg Eng.* 2011;93:437–440.

Rodriguez-Sanjuan JC, et al. Laparoscopic and robot-assisted digestive surgery: present and future directions. *World Journal of Gastroenterology* 2016;22(6):1975–2004.

Sgarbura O, Vasilescu C. The decisive role of the patient-side surgeon in robotic surgery. *Surg Endosc.* 2010,24(12):3149–3155.

Chapter | **14**

Handling the patient

Remember that the prime reason for performing a procedure or operation is to prolong or improve the quality of life of the patient. Be careful not to focus solely on the pathology; there is a whole patient and their environment to consider. To be a good surgeon, you must also be a good doctor.

PREOPERATIVE FACTORS

The general preparedness of your patient for the intended procedure is a combination of physical and psychological factors. Physical factors to consider include general fitness, whether or not they are on anticoagulation or antiplatelet agents, what allergies they may have, what age they are, whether they have any fixed preferences and whether they have had previous related surgery. The ability for you to prepare your patient may depend on whether they are having an emergency, urgent or elective procedure.

Physical preparedness

General fitness can be quantified in a number of different ways. The American ASA system designed by the American Society of Anesthesiology is widely used:

ASA I: A normal healthy patient with no comorbidities and a nonsmoker.
ASA II: A patient with mild systemic disease but little functional limitation, which may include smoking, pregnancy, obesity, diabetes.
ASA III: A patient with severe systemic disease with functional limitations such as poorly controlled diabetes, ischaemic heart disease, COPD, alcohol dependence.
ASA IV: A patient with severe life-threatening systemic disease such as a recent myocardial infarction or stroke, end-stage renal failure.
ASA V: A patient who is moribund such as in current massive haemorrhage, septicaemia.

P-Possum scoring is another that calculates relative risk from a combination of patient factors such as age, cardiorespiratory dysfunction, vital signs and blood parameters.

What I call the 'end of the bed test', whilst unscientific, should not be dismissed. Despite our ability to measure so many patient parameters, overall clinical impression can be a useful indicator.

There are other considerations that you will need to address when planning a procedure.

Allergy

If your patient has a specific allergy, remember to note this on their records and take heed. Common allergies to consider are iodine (used in both antiseptic skin preparations and in radiological contrast agents), latex (present in some disposable gloves and some tubing), some dressings (often the adhesives that stick to the patient's skin), and antibiotics. Remember that a patient with a fish allergy may be allergic to iodine. Remember, also that there may be cross-reactivity between some antibiotics, such as the ten percent crossover with penicillins and cephalosporins. Use alternatives and ensure the whole team are aware.

Anaesthesia

Whilst the ultimate choice of anaesthesia type might be determined by your anaesthetist and your patient, you should consider the type of anaesthesia that might be best for the type of operation that you will be doing and the overall patient status. For instance, if it is a small, localised and superficial procedure you might elect to do it under local anaesthetic, but if the patient is a child or unduly anxious you might prefer a general anaesthetic, or local anaesthetic under sedation. Regional blocks and other alternatives to a full general anaesthetic are becoming more common for some operations.

Anaesthetic preassessment

If your patient is having sedation or a regional or general anaesthetic it would be wise to send them to see a member of the anaesthetic team to be assessed. However, as a doctor, you should have a good idea of the risks associated with your patient's comorbidities and consider organising relevant workup tests and opinions.

Anticoagulation

If your patient is anticoagulated, this should be stopped before an invasive procedure except in an acute emergency. Some indications, such as noncomplicated atrial fibrillation, may mean you can stop the anticoagulation for the relevant number of days (for instance, 3–4 days for therapeutic warfarin) and simply proceed with your procedure. For other indications, such as recurrent pulmonary embolus or an artificial heart valve, you may need to bridge the decreasing level of anticoagulant with a short-acting low-molecular-weight heparin by injection at therapeutic levels up until you undertake the procedure. Remember to restart the anticoagulation once you are happy that there is no risk of bleeding after the procedure.

Anti-platelet agents

If your patient is to undergo a procedure where it will be difficult to gain haemostasis by direct compression (such as a resectional procedure in a luminal or ductal structure), or where they may be anaesthetised with spinal or epidural anaesthesia, antiplatelet agents, in particular clopidogrel, should be stopped 10 days prior to the procedure.

Age

You should remember that patients at extremes of age have their own considerations. Children are often physically more robust but more likely to be frightened by a surgical procedure. Women of childbearing age may be pregnant; in which case the foetus should also be considered. Where pregnancy status is not known, many offer a routine urinary pregnancy test prior to anaesthesia. The elderly are often frailer, may have greater comorbidity and are more prone to delirium after a general anaesthetic.

Nutritional status

The undernourished may not have satisfactory immunity and may not heal as well as normal. The morbidly obese may present you with difficult surgical access and you should check that your operating table can take their weight and that you have appropriate retractors and long-handled instruments.

Immunosuppression

If your patient is on long-term steroids, has poorly controlled diabetes, is on chemotherapy, has some autoimmune disorders, or is taking other immunosuppressive drugs there may be a degree of immunosuppression. Bear this in mind when handling tissues, as healing will be poor. In these patients, you may need to leave skin sutures in for longer than usual.

Previous surgery

This may render tissue scarred and distorted. The anatomy will be altered, and you should ensure that you have read the previous operation notes so that you know what to expect. Allow yourself more time to undertake surgery in a previously operated area compared with virgin territory. Your patient should also be warned of the greater risk of potential complications.

Optimisation

There may be some comorbidities that require optimisation before embarking on a planned procedure. It may be helpful to discuss cardiac issues with a cardiologist. It may be necessary to prehydrate a patient with chronic kidney disease. It may be necessary to control the heart rate of a patient with a tachyarrhythmia or bradyarrhythmia. Tobacco smokers should be advised to quit. Patients with certain infections may require eradication; a patient with MRSA (methicillin-resistant staphylococcus aureus) will require eradication before placing an implant such as a vascular graft or joint replacement. Consult prevailing guidelines for the recommended interval from infection to operation (for instance, it was 6 weeks for Covid-19 during the 2020–2023 global pandemic). A female patient on the oral contraceptive pill may be required to stop it temporarily for 4–6 weeks prior to surgery if the surgical procedure poses a higher risk of deep venous thrombosis.

Anaemia

Your patient may require a transfusion or iron therapy well in advance of surgery. Jehovah's Witness patients will not accept blood transfusions; you should discuss with your patient whether they will refuse all blood products or only certain components.

Psychological preparedness

Psychological preparedness varies from patient to patient and in the same patient from one procedure to the next and one day to the next. Be prepared to spend the necessary amount of time with your patient to ensure that you have explained what they need to know and managed their expectations as best you can. Many patients will be anxious prior to any procedure, and you must do your best to gain their confidence and allay their fears. It may help to talk to your patient with a relative or friend of their choice present.

Your patient may have preconceived ideas about what to expect. It may be wise for you to gain an understanding of what their expectations are. Occasionally they have been misinformed by a third party, including non-peer-reviewed entries on the internet.

Your patient may have previously expressed a wish to have or not have a particular procedure. In some cases, this is tangible in a legal document called an advanced directive. At other times close family may relay information about previous wishes. At all times you must act in the patient's best interests and within the law.

Informed consent is not just asking your patient to sign a form agreeing to undergo the given procedure. It should be a full explanation of the given procedure, any alternative procedures (including what happens if no procedure is undertaken), the risks, the benefits, the consequences and the expected timescales. In particular, all risks to which you think they will hold relevance should be discussed even if that risk is extremely small.

Types of consent form

For many procedures requiring no or local anaesthetic a consent form is not necessary; for instance, if you are going to take a routine blood test. However, you must still explain what you intend to do and why. If the competent patient offers you their arm and allows you to take the blood test, consent is implied. If you intend to undertake a more involved procedure and certainly those where the patient is not fully conscious, be it under general anaesthetic or sedation, you should take written informed consent. In the UK health system, there are four types of written consent forms, numbered 1–4:

Consent form 1. Where the competent patient over the age of 16 years signs on their own behalf. If an interpreter has been used to translate during the consenting process, there is a place for them additionally to sign.

Consent form 2. Where a parent signs for a child under 18 years. A competent child over 16 may, however, give their own consent and should use consent form 1 for this. If a child under 18 years refuses treatment that would be lifesaving, their parents may sign the consent form, and overrule the child's decision. Where a competent child wishes to sign to have a procedure, the parents are not in a position to overrule it. Alternatively, in the UK, you may apply to the Court of Protection to decide for you.

Consent form 3. Where a patient signs for a procedure where their consciousness is not impaired. For instance, this may be for a local anaesthetic procedure.

Consent form 4. Where a patient is unable to sign for themselves and the clinician believes the procedure will be in their best interests, in particular a lifesaving procedure, the clinician can complete a consent form 4. This is commonly used when a patient is unconscious or lacks capacity through delirium. It should not be used to override an advanced directive, and it is good practice to discuss it with the next of kin even though they are not signing it. It is good practice for two clinicians who have been looking after the patient to sign it.

There are instances when additional consent is also required. This might occur if you wish to get permission from your patient to include them in a research project, to retain tissue for research or a tissue bank, to include them on a database (local, national or international) or to take photographs (stills, video footage or live streaming of their operation). Ensure that you know the consequences of each of these acts and can justify them to your patient. Often, separate consent forms are used.

Ensure that you have afforded your patient opportunities to ask questions and if available give them relevant leaflets about their intended procedure.

PLANNING THE ORDER OF AN OPERATING LIST

When considering the order of a planned operating list you should consider the patients, the operating team and the theatre.

It is unkind to starve paediatric patients for longer than is necessary, so it is better to place them early in a list of patients of mixed age. Likewise, diabetic patients are better placed earlier in the list as diabetic control is easier without prolonged periods of fasting. Diabetics are often placed on an insulin sliding scale on the morning of surgery. A patient with a significant latex allergy may similarly be placed first on the list before materials containing latex are brought into the theatre for subsequent patients.

If there is a particularly long or strenuous operation on the list, most surgeons prefer to undertake this at the start of the list when they are mentally and physically freshest. That is not to say that you should concentrate less when operating on patients at the end of the list. If there is a patient who is having a combined procedure with another team, then the availability of that team may dictate when that case is scheduled.

A patient undergoing an operation involving overt infection or high infective risk (such as abscess drainage or where bowel contamination is likely) should be placed at the end of the list to reduce the risk of cross-infection in the operating theatre. Likewise, a patient having an implant placed should be scheduled earlier, especially before any 'infected' cases, for the same reasons. The theatre is still cleaned between patients.

PERIPROCEDURAL FACTORS

Before undertaking a procedure or list of procedures, consider the following:

Preprocedural marking

You should mark the site of the operation with a skin marker before a patient is given a general anaesthetic or sedation, and indeed before they have reached the anaesthetic room. This is particularly important when differentiating between left and right. In some procedures, you may need to organise preoperative marking by a radiologist (such as guidewire local excision, marking of an impalpable foreign body). Many bedside procedures also need preprocedural marking (such as peritoneocentesis).

Nil by mouth (NBM)

Patients undergoing general anaesthesia or sedation should be starved before the procedure to prevent aspiration of stomach contents. Starvation should be for 6 hours for solid food and drinks and 2 hours for clear water. Patients should not chew chewing gum for 6 hours to prevent stimulation of gastric secretions. Likewise smoking will irritate the airways and should be avoided. In a dire emergency, your anaesthetist will decide if measures such as rapid sequence induction can be undertaken.

Special equipment

If special equipment is required for your procedure, ensure that it is present (and you know how to use it) before you start. This could range from the microscope slides and fixative for an FNA to hired-in equipment for an orthopaedic operation, an ultrasound machine, a particular endoscope, a laparoscopic stack, or use of a hybrid or laser theatre room.

Radiographer

If you are performing a procedure that requires radiological imaging, remember to inform the radiographer in advance. Often in a theatre suite, more than one theatre will require the services of the radiographer, and radiographer availability may impact the timing of your case.

Frozen section

If you will need the services of a pathologist for your procedure, such as for a frozen section, then remember to inform them in advance.

ITU

If your patient is likely to require admission to a high dependency unit (HDU) or intensive therapy unit (ITU) after your procedure then it is wise to inform them beforehand. This allows them to prepare to receive your patient. For an elective case, you may need to book several days in advance.

Prion disease

If your patient is at risk of carrying prion disease then it is customary to use disposable surgical instruments. This should be notified to the theatre staff.

Nonspecimen retention of tissue

If you are providing tissue for research (having gained the patient's consent) or if, as in some faiths, you are retaining a body part for burial, appropriate arrangements should be made before starting your case.

IN THE OPERATING THEATRE

If you are organising a list of procedures in the operating theatre there will be a number of checks that you should make, once there.

It is customary to have a team briefing beforehand. This involves all personnel involved in the operating list such as anaesthetic staff, scrub staff and surgeons, to ensure that everyone knows what to expect in the list. The expected list order (and reasons for the order) is often discussed. Special circumstances such as a significant latex allergy or infection control measures can be planned for.

The WHO checklist was devised by the World Health Organisation and is widely used. You should ensure that the checklist is followed for every patient before starting an operative procedure. It identifies the patient by name and local identifier, confirms the procedure and consent, confirms marking, the presence of appropriate imaging, any pertinent allergies, estimated blood loss and any concerns from the surgeon, anaesthetist and scrub staff.

You should consider if your patient will need a urinary catheter, whether any special monitoring is required and whether to institute any components of the Sepsis Six (see Ch. 12).

DVT prophylaxis

Venous thromboembolism is an unwanted consequence of prolonged immobility, particularly under anaesthesia. Preventative measures should be undertaken. If there is no contraindication, chemical DVT prophylaxis may be given, often as a daily dose of low-molecular-weight heparin. Positioning on the table is an important consideration. The calves should be elevated so as not be compressed against the table using ankle rests. These also take pressure off the heels, preventing pressure sores. Intermittent pneumatic calf compressors can be applied for longer operations to prevent venous pooling. This is particularly important if the patient is in a prolonged reverse Trendelenburg position or if undergoing a laparoscopic procedure where there is an increase in intraabdominal pressure. Where there is no history of lower limb ischaemia, Class I graduated compression hosiery can be used.

Positioning on the table

The patient's position on the table will be determined by the procedure being undertaken. It is important that you discuss this with your anaesthetist, as the anaesthetic may vary; for instance, if the patient is to be turned prone, an endotracheal tube will be used (and not a laryngeal mask), it will be taped to the corner of the mouth and the eyes will be well padded. If access to the perineum is required the legs may be up in Lloyd-Davis or lithotomy, which will require the relevant stirrups. If the patient is to be placed on their side, particular equipment is required to secure the patient on the operating table. If you need access to one of your patient's arms, the anaesthetist will place all monitoring on the contralateral arm. Likewise, a femoral line will be avoided if surgical access is required in that area. A head-ring or other such supports should be requested before you start.

Protection of pressure areas

The anaesthetised patient is prone to pressure sores if vulnerable areas are not protected. Bony prominences should be well padded. The eyes should be covered or shielded from inadvertent injury. Elbows should be padded if the patient has subluxing ulnar nerves.

Diathermy pad

It is routine to remove any external metal adornments from the patient to prevent conduction of electricity. The diathermy pad for monopolar diathermy is positioned away from any internal metalware such as a hip replacement, and out of the way of any potential dripping fluids such as blood. Bipolar diathermy may be a preference in an awake patient and certainly when operating near important nerve structures (such as in the popliteal fossa) and in a patient with a cardiac pacemaker.

Implanted devices

If your patient has a cardiac pacemaker, ICD (implantable cardioverter defibrillator), a cochlear implant, metalwork, ventriculoperitoneal shunt, arteriovenous fistula, or CAPD catheter, there are specific considerations. This would include use of diathermy, avoidance of contamination of indwelling catheters, positioning of the blood pressure monitoring cuff and intraarterial and intravenous cannulae. An ICD may need to be temporarily disabled prior to surgery if monopolar diathermy is to be used, particularly if surgery is in the upper torso, and a cardiologist should be consulted. Bipolar diathermy should be used if the patient has a cochlear implant.

Local anaesthetic infiltration

Always check the permissible dose of local anaesthetic before using it. For 1% lignocaine (lidocaine) the maximum dose is 3 mg/kg and if it contains adrenaline (1:200,000) then this increases to 7 mg/kg. Lignocaine has a fairly rapid onset of action and begins to wear off after a couple of hours. Other local anaesthetics, such as bupivacaine, take longer to take effect but will last for about 4 hours afterwards and would therefore give good postprocedural pain relief.

Warming devices

In a prolonged procedure, your patient may become relatively hypothermic. A mattress warmer may be used, or a warming blanket. The latter is often a disposable quilted paper sheet through which warm air is circulated. When preparing the patient ensure that you have left enough prepared skin to stick down the warmer and then the drapes to cover it.

Wearing appropriate personal protective wear

If you are performing a procedure by the bedside you will use an aseptic no-touch technique, wearing disposable gloves and an apron if necessary. If you are performing a procedure in the operating theatre you will do so using a sterile technique, being properly scrubbed, gowned and masked. In addition, depending on the procedure you may require a lead apron, goggles, visors, or double gloving.

Skin preparation

Be cognizant of any skin allergies when painting on the skin preparation. Do not use alcohol-based preparations in open wounds. Do not allow liquids, especially alcohol-based liquids to pool under the patient. There have been reports of skin burns, particularly of the perineum where the monopolar diathermy current has passed to the liquid pool and caused thermal injury.

Communication

Throughout the operation maintain a line of communication with both your scrub team and your anaesthetist. If you think you may need an instrument that is not on your regular set, or a consumable not usually kept in your theatre, ask for it well in advance, to give the theatre 'runner' time to obtain it. If you are struggling with bleeding, or the operation is taking longer than expected then it is wise to let your anaesthetist know so that they can plan accordingly.

Swab, needle and instrument count

At the end of the operation, this is the responsibility of the first surgeon in the operation. In practice, the scrub nurse will undertake the count on your behalf. Always believe your scrub nurse if they say there is a needle, instrument or swab missing at the final count before closing the wound. Your scrub nurse will traditionally count all swabs in groups of five. All swabs used in an open procedure should have a radio-opaque marker. If the count is not 'correct' an X-ray should be taken before closing the skin to look for the missing object.

Postoperative team briefing

A briefing at the end of a list of procedures is useful to have a team briefing and to summarise any postoperative instructions. If there have been any issues that were detrimental to the running of the list they can be noted and prevented next time. Likewise, any actions that contributed to its smooth running can be reinforced the next time.

Writing the operation note

As the operating surgeon, it is your duty to ensure that the operation note is well written whether it is by hand, dictated or typed, and whether on loose leaf, in a booklet, free typed or uploaded onto a programme or database. It should include the following:

- Patient's name and identifier, surgeon's name, surgical assistant's name, anaesthetists' names, the name of the procedure, the skin preparation used, the volume and type of any local anaesthetic given, any antibiotics or other drugs given (such as heparin), the location and plane of the skin incision, a step by step description of the procedure, details of any significant findings, details of any intraoperative complications, the types of sutures used for the different stages, the type of skin closure. Any blood loss should

be recorded. The swab, needle and instrument count should be noted as correct. The dressing type should be recorded.

In addition, the operation note for specific procedures might include details of any drains used and when to remove them, tourniquet time, details of any prosthetic materials used, when to remove skin sutures or clips, whether antibiotic therapy needs to be continued and for how long, whether anticoagulation should be started or restarted, when a second-look procedure should be scheduled, if the patient is to remain nil by mouth, if the patient is to be transferred to the ITU, if specimens have been sent for histology or microbiology, when the patient can mobilise, and whether the patient can bear weight. If you have done an operation on an arm, you may wish to note that blood samples should not be taken from that arm. It is sometimes helpful to reinforce instructions by writing them on the dressing (e.g., 'no tourniquets or blood samples from this arm' or 'leave this dressing for 5 days from date x').

It is your responsibility to ensure that appropriate labels and request forms have been made for any specimens sent to the laboratory. Indeed, it is also your responsibility to check on the results when they are available. Likewise, if postoperative imaging is required, such as a check X-ray, then you should request and check it.

POSTOPERATIVE CARE

After an operation or procedure, it is good practice to review your patient a short while after. Even in the modern era of nurse-led discharge, it is reassuring for both you and your patient to check that the patient is content and that there are no immediate postoperative complications. If you have been involved in a prolonged or major procedure, it is often kind to speak to the relatives afterwards as well, assuming that you have permission from your patient. You will receive fewer complaints if you maintain lines of communication with the patient and their next of kin. If you are going off duty, you should hand over to your colleagues any specific concerns or instructions. Always document the details of your review in the notes.

If there has been an unfortunate complication or mishap, it is your duty to be open and transparent with your patient. This duty of candour is integral to your professionalism. A carefully worded apology where due, should be made. An apology is not an admission of guilt but of respect.

EMERGENCY PROCEDURES

You should conduct yourself in the same way for emergency procedures as you do for planned procedures. The difference is that you may have less time and will need to be particularly efficient in your organisation. It is easy to panic and cut corners. However, this is not advisable because an important component of the process may be missed; if you must cut corners, at least go through each stage in your mind and make a conscious decision to miss a step rather than going straight to the latter stages of the process without thought.

FURTHER READING

WHO. Implementation manual surgical safety checklist. WHO Press; 2008.

Chapter | **15**

Handling craft skills

Insulted to be referred to as a craftsman? Don't be. In the Middle Ages, surgeons were trained not in universities but as apprentices to masters. Within a craft, a master can *show* you the required skills, whereas a trainer or coach can teach and correct you but does not necessarily have exceptional skills.

The surgical craftsman's material is living human flesh. Never forget that all your skill must be targeted at the correct treatment of the tissues; you acquired skill with the instruments to enable

you to focus on that commitment. This aim was immortalised by the French surgeon Ambroise Paré (1510–1590), who had the humility to state, 'Je le pansai, Dieu le guérit'–'I dressed him, God healed him'. Whatever your philosophical beliefs, we cannot *heal*, but we owe it to the tissues to help them heal.

Always keep in mind the precepts associated with Kocher and Halsted. They promoted the importance of careful, gentle surgery, perfect haemostasis and perfect apposition of the tissues. Notice that speed is not included. These concerns remain unaltered, although they are sometimes forgotten or ignored. Failing to observe can result in remorseful nights lying awake.

> **Key point**
>
> • Techniques advance but the fundamental precepts of good surgery remain.

PHYSICIAN/SURGEON

1. Never forget that you are primarily a physician with an extra practical skill. Superlative technique on its own is useless. It must be applied correctly at the right time on the right patient. Many surgeons are capable of performing a wide variety of operations but not necessarily of selecting and preparing the patients on whom to perform. Read standard operative texts that describe in detail the individual

considerations required for each patient and each procedure. Ensure, for example, that you can justify your decision to recommend the procedure to your patient and that you have taken every necessary step to ensure that the patient is in the best possible condition, that the timing and facilities are correct, the operation site marked if appropriate, the informed consent form is signed, suitable prophylaxis is arranged for bleeding, clotting and infective complications, and universal precautions are observed.

2. Keep up to date. Do not become an expert in outdated treatments. Remember, though, that innovators are biased. Their reported good results may stem in part from the selection of patients, perhaps the closer monitoring and care of the patients, and overoptimistic interpretation of the outcomes. Remember, also, that negative results are less often published than positive results; many are reluctant to publish their complications. Veer towards waiting for reports from surgeons who do not have a personal commitment to the treatment. Take greater heed from meta-analyses and reviews than isolated reports and be cognizant of levels of evidence. Remember that in prospective trials it is often necessary to exclude patients in order to keep the number of variables to a minimum. Our methods of audit do not yet fully include and compare those patients who are treated conservatively or by alternative methods.

3. Before the anaesthetic is administered, make sure that this is the correct patient and reassure yourself that you are operating on the correct side if this is a unilateral lesion. Be sure that you have personally seen and marked the patient if you are to perform a procedure on them.

4. Do not become a skilful operator who lacks judgment. You may become skilled in a particular technique, but others emerge that are shown to produce better results. Be willing to acquire the new skills required rather than continue with an outdated method because you can perform it expertly. The American novelist Mark Twain aptly summed up this attitude with the statement, 'If your only tool is a hammer, every problem begins to look like a nail'. In contrast, if you can produce results at least as good as those obtained by a newer method, you may be wise not to change.

5. There have been remarkable advances in nonsurgical treatment of many conditions

traditionally treated surgically, including medical treatment, endoscopy and interventional radiology. When you are convinced of their effectiveness, relinquish your patients to those who are experts in the alternative treatment. The well-being of your patient should come above your pride.

Key points

- A good surgeon knows how to operate.
- A better surgeon knows when to operate.
- The best surgeon knows when not to operate.

6. You rely upon your colleagues in the operating theatre to help you and also to warn you of impending or actual danger or disaster. Maintain an atmosphere in which all feel able to speak out in such circumstances. In the WHO check, one of the first things to do is introduce all members of the team and ensure that the whole team are engaged. When you are in doubt, explaining the problem to them often clarifies your course of action, or someone will contribute a valuable suggestion.

SKILLS COURSES

1. Quite rightly, trainee surgeons are introduced to operating in courses, with simulations and virtual reality trainers. These allow aspiring operators to familiarise themselves with the procedures and practise using the instruments and equipment. You must acquire familiarity with the instruments so that you can manipulate them skilfully while your primary awareness is directed to the tissues on which you are operating.[1] This applies particularly in minimal access techniques when the movement of the tip is the opposite of handle movement.

2. When you attend a course and are shown how to carry out a procedure, it does not transfer a skill to you. It shows you how to perform, but to do so skilfully demands intelligent, assiduous practice.

3. At the end of the course, when you are assessed, the examiner has a list of objectively assessable actions to mark. If you succeed in passing all the steps, you pass the assessment; it neither makes you an expert nor necessarily

proves your competence. It is a minimum achievement, not a measure of your skill.

4. This is not to decry such courses; they demonstrate many fundamentals, introduce concepts of 'best practice' and identify errors early before they become habits. But there are other contributions to successful performance that are not identifiable within the limits of artificiality, time, facilities and limited observation. Success on a course does not signify surgical competence; it attests to correct performance in a number of formalised steps.

> **Key points**
>
> - The gap between learning to manipulate instruments and simulations on courses, and mastery as a surgeon, is between handling the instruments and operating skilfully on live people.
> - It is a large, extensible gap, not yet amenable to objective analysis.

5. As in every other complex task, you may observe all the instructions but fail to perform successful surgical operations. The reason is that the outcome depends on your ability to assemble the components in the correct sequence and perform each one perfectly for the right indications. This relationship was recognised in the late 19th century by the German Gestalt psychologists (from the German *gestellt* = put together): *'The whole is greater than the sum of the parts'*. You may have every piece of a jigsaw puzzle, but they have to be put together the correct way to form the picture. The purpose of this chapter is to emphasise how you must combine your individual aptitudes to create a fully competent surgeon.

OPERATING PRECEPTS

Gentleness

Living tissues are easily damaged by rough handling. If previously normal tissues are traumatised, they usually survive. The vitality of already traumatised or diseased tissues is already prejudiced.

1. Rough handling may not manifest immediately, but healing will be delayed or fail, and resistance to infection is lowered. Gentle handling has to be a 100% habit. Never grasp tissue with a metal instrument to displace it when it can be gently manipulated with a finger, swab, encircling thread or tube, retractor or closed forceps.

2. If you crush tissue and release it, within a few moments the vessels will fill with blood, and it will look normal, but it is not normal. It will die in part or whole. If it survives, healing will be delayed, dead or dying cells will be replaced by scar tissue, and if the scar is subjected to tension, it will become stretched. When incisions have been closed with stitches that are too tight, they produce wound scars showing a ladder pattern of white scars resulting from the death of tissue strangled within the stitches.

3. Overdistension of closed spaces and vessels is a frequently overlooked form of trauma. Muscular walls are overstretched and temporarily paralysed or torn and will give way. The delicate cellular lining of overfilled vessels is disrupted, exposing the basement membrane. If such a vessel is united to another, the integrity of the union is prejudiced. In the case of blood vessels, platelets adhere to the bared subintima as a basis for clots that may block the lumen. When mobilizing structures, beware of forcefully stripping them. Veins mobilised for arterial bypass undergo spasm if the adventitia is stripped off.[2]

'Setting up'

This aspect of operating is not well recognised but is in fact vitally important. Watch an expert craftsman in any occupation and you will notice how slowly and carefully the preliminaries are carried out, the problem examined and assessed, the equipment assembled, checked and laid out, and the planning of the approach. When the procedure is finally undertaken, it proceeds smoothly and faultlessly.

1. In the past, when surgeons worked with relatively stable teams, they could rely with confidence on preparedness and checks, even though they knew that the ultimate responsibility was theirs.

2. You may not work in an established, stable team. Ensure that you personally check the full list of requirements or are assured by someone in whom you have complete trust.

3. Do not start until you have personally checked that everything you need is available and

working, and, if it is something likely to fail, make sure you have a functional backup.

4. As you start the operation, if there is anything that could possibly complicate the operation or make it more difficult, correct it now.

5. If you are carrying out a manoeuvre that feels unnatural, stop and consider approaching it from another aspect, perhaps by changing your approach or moving to the other side of the operating table.

> **Key points**
>
> - When you are delegated a task, do not rush to 'get on with it'.
> - Carefully assess what needs to be done, identify what you need and how you should carry it out.
> - Start cautiously. Make all your movements carefully and slowly.
> - Nothing makes the person who delegated the task more apprehensive than watching you rush headlong into the risk of a disaster.

Speed

Obsession with speed is one of the most dangerous and damaging characteristics. It is often driven by the unintelligent belief that by completing an operation at breakneck speed the operator is demonstrating their expertise. William, one of the famous Mayo brothers of Rochester, is reported to have left an operation being performed by William Halsted after 3 hours, muttering sarcastically, 'That's the first time I have seen the top end of the wound healing while the bottom end is still being operated on'. Time has proved Halsted right.

1. Before you enter the operating theatre, you should understand that when you acquire a skill in performing a particular procedure, you must perform it at a natural pace; otherwise, what is ideally accomplished automatically and perfectly is raised to conscious focus and is thus performed clumsily.

2. Hand speed and operating speed are different. Performing an action in a hurry very often fails, requiring it to be repeated, so that the total time taken is the same as if it were performed at a natural speed. What is wasteful of time is unnecessary and ineffectual actions, often due to lack of certainty regarding the correct next step.

> **Key point**
>
> - Next time you are uncertain, stop moving and devote your energy to making the correct decision.

Sequence

1. Unless there are special circumstances, employ the standard sequences that have been developed over many years. If you do not, you may discover that you have prejudiced your access to an important area, inadvertently damaged an important structure or prejudiced local function.

2. Operate deliberately and naturally.

3. As a rule, complete and check each step of the operation before proceeding to the next.

Strategy/tactics

1. These terms, which are often confused, are important concepts if you wish to be a successful surgeon.

2. Strategy (from the Greek *stratos* = an army + *agein* = to lead: generalship). Your planning and preparation of yourself, your patient, your team, equipment and backup are essential. Consider what you will do if there are unexpected findings or complications; these are often called 'what ifs'.

3. Tactics (from the Greek *tassein* = to arrange; was applied to manoeuvring in the presence of the enemy). It refers to how you react to what happens during the operation and how you identify, interpret, avoid and respond to unforeseen problems. For many circumstances, guidelines are laid down and usually, you should adhere to them but exceptionally you recognise that the problem does not conform to that described in the guidelines.

> **Key points**
>
> - Do not dismiss an unusual finding. Investigate and interpret it.
> - Do not rigidly continue the intended actions if the new finding makes them inappropriate.
> - Carefully assess your competence to deal with the new situation and react accordingly.

Tissue oxygenation

1. Kocher and Halsted did not have access to methods of determining tissue oxygenation. They, and many of their successors, could determine vitality only by arterial pulsation and colour. Pulse oximeters are now commonplace, and infrared spectroscopy use is becoming more widespread.
2. We now have methods of determining the oxygen concentration. An important contribution was made by Tom Hunt of San Francisco, who measured the concentration of interstitial oxygen concentration in closed wounds and found that it is severely reduced, especially immediately after operation, and this is often not clinically evident.[3] In contrast, when the method of delayed primary closure is employed, the wound tissues are in contact with atmospheric oxygen concentrations.
3. Hypoxic tissues are particularly susceptible to infection with anaerobic or microaerophilic organisms. In case of doubt, delayed primary closure of wounds ensures that tissues are in contact with oxygen at atmospheric pressure.

EMERGENCIES

'Emergency' (from 'emerge', via the Latin e = out of + *mergere* = to plunge; to arise out of) suggests an unexpected occurrence requiring immediate action. What is often left out is the importance of recognizing exactly what has happened, what it means and what is the best way of dealing with it. Unintelligent action often makes matters worse.

1. If something unexpected happens during an operation, *assess it*. Do nothing until you have done so. Panic will delay the situation further.
2. For many emergency situations, studies have produced guidelines that are suitable for most circumstances. Learn them. Practise the prescribed actions.
3. *Bleeding* is a common emergency. Very often, simple finger pressure is the best immediate action and rushing to apply metal haemostats may be a disaster.
4. *Overreaction* often extends to performing unnecessary procedures as a guard against possible complications.
5. Once you have dealt with the emergency, check that you have not caused or missed further damage.

6. Check that you have achieved your objective and then close.

> **Key points**
>
> - Do not lightly abandon safe routines in an emergency.
> - Perform the simplest procedure that corrects the emergency situation—nothing more.

ERROR AVOIDANCE

You are in a high-risk profession. You will make misjudgements and technical errors.

> **Key points**
>
> - If you embark on an operation without first acquiring or revising the anatomy, you are inviting disaster.
> - Missiles, spreading infections and malignant tumours are not respecters of tissue planes or anatomical boundaries.

1. Many surgical errors occur before the patient reaches the operating theatre, in the selection and preparation of patients, operations and numerous requirements of equipment, backup and technical support. Further errors occur following operation as a result of inadequate monitoring and failure to respond effectively to deterioration.
2. Accept that we are all fallible. Any surgeon who claims not to have made any mistakes is either inexperienced, economical with the truth or lacks insight. You should use mistakes to reflect and build on learning, both self-learning and shared learning. French vascular surgeon Renee Leriche (1879–1955) wrote, 'Every surgeon carries within himself a small cemetery, where from time to time he goes to pray – a place of bitterness and regret, where he must look for an explanation for his failures' (La Philosophie de la Chirurgie, 1951).
3. Those who are concerned with organisations requiring high reliability try to identify changes to the system incorporating safeguards. Procedural rules and guidelines incorporate a practice that has been shown to be safest

overall. Remember, though, that when planning an investigation, in order to reduce the number of variables, some combinations are excluded from the trials. You may in clinical practice encounter such circumstances where the guidelines do not apply. You must recognise this and ask for advice and help.

4. Whereas it is traditional to try to eliminate human variability, it is now recognised that human compensatory and adaptive responses to changing events represent an important safeguard. It is this variability and adaptability of humans' dynamic reactions to rare but dangerous events that can be drawn upon.[4]

5. As a trainee, if you encounter an unusual situation that seems to require exceptional management, do not implement your intentions before discussing it with a senior colleague. Often, what is new to you is well known to experienced colleagues who are also aware of the risks.

6. Errors at operation may be the result of a lack of skilful performance such as overuse of force, coincident damage to nearby structures and clumsily performed procedures. However, it is far more likely that you make an error of judgement.

7. Do not be misguided enough to believe that since it is your error, you are honour-bound to repair it. As a trainee, be humble enough to recognise that recovering the situation is best carried out by an expert.

> **Key points**
>
> - If you damage an important structure, the most crucial actions are to recognise it and react accordingly.
> - Such damage is best dealt with immediately.
> - Ask yourself, 'Am I competent to deal with it or should I call for help?'

8. A much more frequent cause of error, especially in minimal-access operations but also in open operations, is *misperception*. Once a mistaken assumption is made about the nature of a structure, it is likely to persist, and you may accommodate subsequent findings around it. A notorious mistake when operating on an infantile inguinal hernia is to mistake the thickened (Scarpa's) deep fascia for the external oblique aponeurosis. As a result of the misperception, you may not identify the external inguinal ring.

9. In open operations, you run doubtful structures between your fingers to trace them, feeling the texture and mobility. During a minimal-access procedure, you are deprived of haptic input; the sensation of touch, to note the surface and temperature, consistency and kinaesthetic (from the Greek *kinein* = to move + *aisthesis* = perception) appreciation of contours and attachments. This is particularly true of robotic surgery. As a result, serious ductal injuries occur more frequently than during open operations.[5]

> **Key points**
>
> - If you have limited access to confirm your first impression, do not proceed.
> - Doubly check it; trace the limits of an identified structure to confirm its nature.

ASSISTING AT OPERATIONS

1. Do not spurn the opportunity to assist. You will learn how to do it—and sometimes, how not to do it. It is also your opportunity to demonstrate your assiduous attention and trustworthiness that encourages the surgeon to delegate part or all of the procedure to you, under expert guidance, and encouragement.

2. Do not look upon assisting as a necessary boring prelude to carrying out the procedure yourself. The privilege of assisting a skilled operator allows you to acquire judgement and technique both consciously and unconsciously so that when you come to perform the procedure yourself, you will automatically adopt safe and effective techniques. You will notice that the best scrub nurses will hand you the correct instrument before you ask for it. Likewise, the best assistant will anticipate what the next stage of the procedure will be and assist accordingly. This is because you have learnt the sequence of the procedure and understand the variances.

3. Read up on the anatomy and pathology that will be important the night before. This will enormously increase the value you will gain from assisting in the operation.

4. Observe every manoeuvre and, at opportune moments, enquire if you do not understand the reason for it.

5. Note that the surgeon performs some manoeuvres in a routine, relaxed fashion while taking extreme care over other parts. Make sure you know why.

6. Notice that good surgeons keep the operative field tidy.

7. As you are asked to assist, try to anticipate what is required without seeming to try and take over the operation. If you are asked your opinion, give it quietly and honestly. If you think you have seen something the surgeon has missed or you think a mistake is about to be made, say so. If your warning has been heard but there is no change in action, recognise that it is the surgeon's responsibility. Afterwards, at an opportune moment, discuss the matter to improve your understanding.

8. Do not be dazzled by technical brilliance while being, as yet, unaware of the more important judgements that have to be made. They are rarely black and white—more usually they are shades of grey—and the particular shade is contentious.

9. If you are fortunate enough to be delegated part of the operation, concentrate on being calm, careful and receptive to guidance.

10. As you become more competent and are given more personal responsibility you will learn even more from assisting than formerly, since you are then more aware of the problems. You may then be awarded the privileged relationship with the surgeon of being treated on equal terms while you both discuss and demonstrate the finer points of operative surgery.

11. Later in your career you may be privileged to assist your own trainees. It is not a one-way teaching experience. My own career has been nourished and made enjoyable, by a series of outstanding, expert, assiduous, supportive and trustworthy junior colleagues.

MENTORING

1. In the past it was an accepted, informal practice for surgeons at all stages of their careers to attend operations carried out by recognised experts, and they were frequently invited to 'scrub up' and assist, in some cases, even having parts of the operation delegated to them. It was possible to watch many senior colleagues and pick up a great deal of knowledge both consciously and by unconscious 'osmosis'. This valuable facility is no longer possible.

2. Modern surgeons are able to apply for consultant posts when they have much less experience than their predecessors. Many acknowledge this and avoid taking on difficult procedures that are at the limit of their competence. As always happens in progressive societies, surgeons have adapted by seeking further training in their deficient areas.

3. In many specialties the system of mentoring is already in place. A surgeon wishing to take on a new procedure attends formal courses and then joins an experienced surgeon as an assistant, then a monitored operator until the senior surgeon is able to declare the trainee as competent. When the competent but still inexperienced surgeon is authorised to perform unsupervised, the outcomes are carefully audited to ensure that the results are satisfactory.

4. Do not ever fail to accept assistance from a more experienced colleague, even though you may feel fully competent and experienced. It is a two-way learning experience.

Ten reminders

- Operative skill alone does not guarantee surgical success. It is one component, albeit vital, of your general care of the patient as a medical practitioner.

- Do not try to be a skilful surgeon only when you are in the operating theatre. Make it part of your normal behaviour to perform everyday practical tasks neatly, smoothly and with minimal force (see Chapter 1).

- Resist the temptation to 'get on with it'. Double check that you have tested equipment and instruments within reach, and that the field is otherwise clear of unnecessary—and especially loose—objects. Are you approaching the task in the most natural relationship?

- As a craftsman whose material is living tissue, never turn aside from an opportunity to examine it, study its anatomical relationships and assess its physical properties. Remember that diseases and missiles are not respecters of anatomical boundaries.

- Because you use instruments as intermediaries, practise using them in simulators, virtual reality trainers, skills courses and on simple homemade mockups until you do not have to think about them and can concentrate on what is happening at the real target of your skill: human flesh.

- Watch experts. You acquire knowledge consciously by noting how they tackle problems, and you will acquire knowledge unconsciously; the type of knowledge that is not easy to put into words.

- Prepare for and react to unexpected findings. Do not insist on pursuing your original intention but reassess them.
- Do not try to hurry. Your concentration switches from the overall objective to the activities that are normally performed with your subsidiary awareness.
- Do not forget the vital factor of tissue oxygenation. Phagocytes deprived of it are inactivated, making the tissues susceptible to infection and prejudicing healing.
- A major operation is merely a series of minor procedures, but for success, every small step must be perfect.

COMMON SENSE

With the intention of preventing people from making stupid errors, experts are from time to time asked to draw up guidelines. These cannot cover every eventuality but are intended to give the greatest protection to the majority of people at risk. Use them but be aware of exceptional circumstances where they do not apply. This common-sense attitude was exemplified by the famous legless British fighter pilot ace, Sir Douglas Bader (1910–1982), who said, 'Rules are for the guidance of wise men and the blind obedience of fools'.

REFERENCES

1. Polanyi M. *Personal knowledge of Prof Kirk.* London: Routledge and Kegan Paul; 1973.
2. Loesch A, Dashwood MR, Souza DSR. Does the method of harvesting the saphenous vein for coronary artery bypass surgery affect venous smooth muscle cells? iNOS immunolabelling and ultrastructural findings. *Int J Surg.* 2006;4:20–29.
3. Chang N, Goodson III WH, Gottrup F, Hunt TK. Direct measurement of wound and tissue oxygen tension in postoperative patients. *Ann Surg.* 1983;197:470–478.
4. Reason J. Human error: models and management. *BMJ* 2008;320:768–770.
5. Way L, Stewart L, Gantert W, et al. Causes and prevention of laparoscopic bile duct injuries: analysis of 252 cases from a human factors and cognitive psychology perspective. *Ann Surg.* 2003;237:450–469.

Chapter | **16** |

Handling dressings

There are many different wound dressings available, with a multitude of variations on theme. The breadth of dressings available will not be detailed here, but commonly used dressing types will be considered.

1. Dressings are placed on a wound to protect it from external abrasion or trauma and to provide an optimum environment to allow natural wound healing. Our skin is our integument (from the Latin *integer* = to cover) and a breach in this covering results in an entry portal for infection or loss of function of underling structures. Wounds may be acute or chronic, intentional (e.g., surgical incision) or accidental. The wound healing process is touched on in Chapter 6.

2. A healthy wound will heal by itself in the correct environment. Furthermore, wound dressings do not 'make' a wound heal. Appropriate dressings may, however, contribute to improving the environment for a given wound to facilitate the natural healing process. Your patient's wound healing may be delayed in the presence of infection, immunocompromise, diabetes, foreign bodies in the wound, poor nutritional status, poor circulation, excessive oedema or anaemia. Similarly, if a wound is too wet, too dry, too contaminated, actively bleeding or under tension, healing will be delayed. Thus, choosing your dressing will depend on the status of the wound. Also bear in mind that patients with chronic ulcers sometimes develop sensitivities to certain dressings.

3. If a wound is sloughy or has overlying necrotic tissue, it is preferable to debride it before applying a dressing. Totally dry eschar is sometimes left alone pending revascularization of the affected limb (usually on the leg). Debridement may be via the topical application of a dressing or by sharp debridement with surgical instruments. Wounds should be cleaned of any debris, dead tissue or foreign bodies. Patients with infected wounds should have cultures taken and be started on antibiotics. Patients with neuropathic ulceration should have pressure relief. Patients with ischaemic ulceration should be revascularised. Patients with suspicious-looking ulcers should have biopsies. If necessary, a dermatological opinion may be sought.

WOUND CLEANSING

Prior to procedures and surgery, intact skin may be cleansed. Alcohol wipes are commonly used prior to insertion of cannulae. You should allow the skin to dry before inserting the needle.

1. In the operating theatre, you might use a chlorhexidine preparation or an iodine-based preparation. The latter might be aqueous-based or alcohol-based. It is advisable not to use alcohol-based solutions where the skin is not intact.
2. Dry, nonexudative wounds may not need deliberate cleansing. A slightly soiled wound may be cleansed with normal saline. Generally, clean wounds with normal saline. There are also solutions available to clean chronic wounds (e.g., Prontosan, which contains a mild surfactant and an antimicrobial which is said to reduce the biofilm present on the ulcer).

TYPES OF DRESSING

There are many dressings available, but it is worth knowing the basic types. Often, more than one layer of dressing is required, and you should consider the order of laying them on the wound.

1. **Simple** dry covering dressings. This would include a simple dressing plaster with fabric (e.g., Elastoplast), plastic (e.g., Airstrip), paper (e.g., Mepore) or film (e.g., Opsite, Tegaderm) backing. They usually consist of a dry gauze-like centre with a nonadherent layer and an adhesive edge. They are used on freshly made surgical wounds that have been primarily apposed or fresh traumatic cuts with no tissue loss.
2. **Skin closure dressings**. If your patient has a skin wound that would come together without tension, you may not need to suture it. Skin closure dressings may be used. The most commonly used is a simple sticky strip that lies across the wound, such as a Steristrip. Most are white, but beige ones are available that do not appear so prominent on many skin types. When you apply this, the skin edges must be dry. It is best to stick one side down first then pull the free end of the strip firmly over to the opposite skin edge and secure it, thus apposing the skin edges without a gap. Skin glue could also be used for small wounds. Likewise, small apposed wounds could be dressed with a dressing spray (e.g., Opsite spray), particularly in an area that is uneven or difficult to access, such as in the hairline.
3. **Semipermeable film** dressings (e.g., Opsite, Tegaderm) are useful for split skin graft donor sites or affixing intravenous access catheters. They are also useful for affixing plain gauze onto a wound, particularly in uneven areas or over a stoma when preparing a patient for a laparotomy and the stoma bag is removed. Be sure to only use this dressing on clean wounds that do not have much exudate.
4. **Nonadherent** dressings. These are underdressings used for clean, healing wounds which are granulating well. The nonadherent nature of the dressing prevents the granulation tissue from being traumatised when you take the dressing off due to the tissue becoming adherent to the dressing. Simple versions of this include Atrauman, a knitted polyester dressing, or 3M N-A Ultra Dressing or Tricotex, which are knitted viscose dressings.
5. **Silicone** dressings are highly nonadherent and useful if your patient finds dressing changes very painful, or if the granulation tissue is rather tenuous (e.g., Silflex). They are generally porous, allowing exudate to pass out to the next layer of dressings. They are more expensive than simple nonadherent dressings.
6. **Tulle**. When your patient has a wound that is dry but granulating, you can use a paraffin impregnated dressing such as Jelonet or an iodine-impregnated paraffin tulle dressing such as Inadine. The latter also has antiseptic properties.
7. **Foam** dressings are absorbent and used for exudative wounds. Remember that if you leave a dressing on an exudative wound once it has soaked through the moisture will remain in contact with the wound and make the surrounding skin macerated. You might also use a foam dressing as a protective dressing for a recently healed wound or a delicate area of skin. Foam dressings may come with or without an adhesive border (e.g., Allevyn, Allevyn Border). They are generally quite flexible and can be placed on curved areas of the body, such as on the lower leg or on sacral sores. As they are soft, they are also quite comfortable for the patient.
8. **Hydrocolloid** dressings are absorbent with a debriding action (e.g., Granuflex, Duoderm).
9. **Alginate** dressings are derived from seaweed and are very absorbent. They tend to form

a gel as they absorb fluid. They are useful in two particular types of wound. If you are dealing with a wound that is oozy, then application of an alginate with a bit of finger pressure can be haemostatic. It should not be used to stop frank bleeding, which will require definitive surgical management by ligation or with a diathermy. Alginates are also useful to debride lightly sloughy wounds. Examples of alginates are Kaltostat and Sorbsan. Do not use alginates on dry wounds or you will have to pick fragments of dressing off the wound at the next dressing change, which will be painful for your patient.

10. **Hydrofibre** dressings are even more absorbent than alginate dressings and can be available with silver impregnation, also serving as an antimicrobial. An example would be Aquacel or Aquacel Ag. They do tend to be a bit more expensive. They are useful for highly exudative wounds.

11. **Capillary action** dressings are highly absorbent and useful for small cavity wounds, as the dressing can be cut into strips or spirals and packed into the wound. An example of this dressing is Vacutex.

12. **Dressing pads** can be applied over the underdressings for very exudative wounds. Simple dressing pads contain wool wrapped in a less adherent wrapper (a bit like a flattened teabag with a sheet of cotton wool inside). Alternatively, superabsorbent dressing pads (e.g., Zetuvit, Zetuvit Plus) can be applied.

13. **Antimicrobial** dressings can be used to reduce local wound infection. They are not a substitute for systemic antibiotics. Iodine impregnated dressings and silver dressings have already been mentioned. In addition, honey impregnated dressings are both antimicrobial and antiinflammatory (e.g., Activon Tulle, Iodoflex).

14. **Zinc Oxide impregnated** bandages are sometimes used in chronic venous ulcers particularly where there is surrounding venous eczema. They are soothing to the dry skin and do not become adherent. Examples are Viscopaste and Icthopaste. They are usually applied as the first layer under compression bandaging.

15. **Bandaging**. When applying a dressing without an adhesive edge to a wound, particularly if the wound is not on a flat body surface, such as the lower leg, the dressing may be secured with a bandage. It is common to place an underlying layer of wool bandage beneath a crepe bandage for comfort. Thus, a patient may have an absorbent dressing covered with a wool bandage which is then covered with a crepe bandage and secured with a piece of tape. When applying a long stretch of bandage around a limb, ensure that your next wrap of the bandage covers at least half of the underlying wrap, or you will cause a multiple tourniquet effect along the limb. For a limb, a tubular bandage may then be applied over the top of this like a toeless sock; to keep the bandage clean, this may be either elasticated (e.g., Comfifast) or stretchable (e.g., Tubifast), and they come in different diameters. The 7.5-cm width bandage has a blue line along its length and is often referred to as a 'Blue Line Bandage'. Likewise, the 10.75-cm width one is referred to as a 'Yellow Line Bandage'.

16. **Compression** bandaging should only be recommended by someone with experience in wound care and will not be discussed in detail here. It is usually used for venous ulcers, and only in the absence of peripheral arterial disease. Compression is commonly in three or four layers. It is worth noting that if you have a patient who is in compression bandaging, they are probably having it changed once a week by an experienced nurse or doctor. You should not recommend compression dressings or bandages to a patient with significant peripheral arterial disease. As a rule of thumb, you should consider that a patient with a resting ankle brachial pressure index (ABPI) of less than 0.8 should not be placed in compression.

17. **Foam wound fillers**. Some cavity wounds, such as an excised pilonidal sinus, are left to close by secondary intention. You can fill these with an expanding foam dressing that fills the cavity and takes on its shape (e.g., Cavi-Care). This is then fixed in place with a simple dressing. The dressing can easily be removed for wound cleaning and its presence prevents the wound closing over before the base has filled in.

HYPERGRANULATION

If your patient's ulcer has overgranulated and the granulation tissue lies proud of the wound, you can touch it on the hypergranulated areas with a silver nitrate stick. This will shrink the granulation by cauterisation. Be careful not to let the stick or the treated tissue touch normal skin; that will be painful and potentially destructive. Do not use silver nitrate on normal granulation tissue, as it will impair healing. There is a suggestion that topical steroids may prove to be a better treatment than silver nitrate for hypergranulation.

GELS AND CREAMS

There are a number of topical gels and creams that may be applied to open wounds or ulcers.

1. Silver sulfadiazine (Flamazine) is commonly applied to burns and some leg ulcers. The silver is an antiseptic. Beware of using it on a patient with a silver allergy.
2. Iodosorb is an iodine-containing ointment which can be applied to small cavity wounds. It is both antiseptic and absorbent.
3. Mupirocin (Bactroban) is an antimicrobial ointment used in some infected wounds and also to eradicate MRSA in preoperative patients.
4. There are a number of hydrogel gels in use (e.g., Intrasite, Nu-gel). They moisten dry wounds, allowing slough to soften and lift. Be careful not to allow these gels to extrude onto the surrounding normal skin, or they will cause maceration—use them sparingly.

LARVAE

Larvae are essentially laboratory-grown maggots that are applied to wound cavities to 'surgically' debride devitalised tissue and thick slough. They do this by secreting enzymes that break down the tissues which they then consume. They do not consume healthy, living tissue. We used to tip them out into the wound. But now they come in small 'teabags' (without the tea!) that can be applied directly to the wound and left for a few days. They do need to have water applied every couple of days, in order to keep the larvae alive. The patient will not be able to weight bear if the wound is on the plantar surface of the foot or else the larvae will be killed.

STOMA BAGS

These are applied to stomas to collect the effluent.

1. It is important that, when cutting the hole for the stomal opening, it is the correct size for the stoma. It should be a snug fit so that effluent does not spill over onto the normal surrounding skin.
2. The rim that sticks to the patient is fairly firm but warming it slightly in your hands before applying it can render it more pliable and it will stick better. If it does not stick well, a stomas glue such as Stomahesive paste can be applied.
3. The surrounding skin can be protected with a dedicated barrier cream such as Cavilon. When applying a stoma bag, ensure the stoma is definitely inside the opening that you have cut and that the bag is closed.
4. If your patient is immediately postoperative, they will be supine for the next day or so; angle the bag to the patient's lateral side. If your patient is going to mobilise almost immediately, angle the bag caudally. In this way, the bag can fill by gravity. Stoma bags are also sometimes used to cover leaking wounds such as a discharging seroma, or to cover the end of an external open drain.

DRESSINGS FOR DRAINS

If your patient has a drain after surgery it is kind to place a dressing around the base of a drain so that the drain does not lie directly on the skin as it exits. Most people achieve this by making a cut halfway across a simple adhesive dressing and snugging the cut part around the base of the drain.

'Mesentery' dressings for drains. Sometimes it helps to secure a drain to the patient not only close to the skin (with a drain stitch) but also a little further away to stop it catching as the patient moves around. This can be achieved by taking a rectangular piece of sticky dressing, e.g., Mefix, wrapping its middle around the drain a short distance from where it comes out through the skin, sticking it to itself for half its length from the drain and using the two free ends to stick to the patient. This is akin to a mesentery.

PRESSURE DRESSINGS

Where you have an oozy, apposed wound, it is sometimes necessary to apply pressure over the wound to reduce the ooze and stop the bleeding. This is best achieved by placing a roll of gauze along the length of the wound, then stretching an adhesive dressing across it. This can be placed directly in the wound or over a simple dressing. If the latter, then the pressure dressing can be removed later without disturbing the wound.

NEGATIVE-PRESSURE WOUND THERAPY (NPWT)

Negative pressure dressings. Negative-pressure wound therapy (NPWT) varies from a localised portable dressing to a larger dressing that is connected to a vacuum pump connected to mains electricity.

1. There is some evidence that NPWT applied to postsurgical apposed wounds may reduce surgical site infection and possibly wound dehiscence. The dressings come as a complete unit.
2. For open wounds, NPWT is supplied as component parts which you will have to apply yourself (or ask an experienced tissue viability nurse). It is said to work by reducing oedema, promoting granulation tissue, and drawing the edges of the wound inwards. The surrounding skin must be dry, intact, and preferably hairless. First, cut the sponge to fit the exact shape of the wound. Apply the sponge to the wound and stick it down with a layer of adhesive dressing to ensure there is no possibility of an air leak. Cut a small hole in the middle of the adhesive dressing in the middle of the sponge. Stick the head of the collecting device over the small hole so that it is in line to collect any exudate (it will have an adhesive rim). Seal this with a further layer of adhesive dressing. Connect the other end of the collecting device to the vacuum pump and turn it on. A standard negative pressure is 125 mmHg. You will see the sponge withdraw into the wound. Check there are no air leaks. If there is an air leak, place another layer of adhesive dressing over it. Most NPWT dressings are changed twice weekly but frequency may depend on how much exudate builds up in the collecting chamber.

3. NPWT can work well to close laparostomies. Do not apply the sponge directly onto bowel.
4. Irrigation dressings. There are NPWT systems that slowly irrigate the wound with saline (at a rate of 15 mls/hour) whilst the vacuum dressing draws up the excess fluid from the wound. This serves as continuous irrigation. Some systems have a dwell time that allows the wound to be bathed in the fluid for a period of time before being drawn off by the vacuum pump; so-called NPWTi-d (negative-pressure wound therapy instillation and dwell). This is used in diabetic foot ulcers and it is thought that this system reduces infection and softens slough, so debriding the wound. Some centres include additives in the irrigation such as povidone-iodine.

Key Points

- Choose your dressings according to the status of the wound. You may start off with one type of dressing, and as the wound environment changes, change to another.
- Do not apply negative-pressure wound dressings onto a bleeding wound.

WHEN TO CHANGE DRESSINGS

If a dressing is applied in a sterile environment, such as the operating theatre, it is preferable to leave that dressing clean unless the wound needs to be inspected. Change dressings when you need to inspect a wound for strike-through, bleeding, an increase in inflammatory markers and when sutures need to be removed. Change dressings with an aseptic technique. If the dressing change is likely to be painful, or if you are expecting to debride a wound at a dressing change, remember to give the patient adequate analgesia appropriately in advance.

Chapter | **17**

Handling your team

As a surgeon, you are always part of a team. You are part of a large multidisciplinary team, which could be viewed as those on a ward round with you, those in theatre with you, the whole hospital, the whole medical profession, etc. Your immediate team includes your assistant and more senior and junior surgical team members. It also includes your anaesthetists, your scrub nurse, your circulating nurse and the anaesthetic team assistants. You would do well to communicate regularly with your theatre sister. Your team also extends to the teams on the wards, the outpatient clinics and your administrative staff. In some ways, every member of staff with whom you have regular contact—and many with whom you may only communicate remotely—are part of your wider team. Ultimately, all are there to provide good care to the patient.

Being part of a team requires you to be aware of the perspectives of others. Encourage and facilitate team members to do the best job they can. The effectiveness of your team is greater than the sum of its parts. The happier your team, the better care will your patient receive.

COMMUNICATION

Communication is key to a well-functioning team. If your team members are well-informed they will have a sense of inclusion and belonging and will have less fear of missing out (FOMO). In the operating theatre, utilise the 'Time Out' of the WHO check to ensure that all feel involved.

If a team member does not seem to be engaged, rather than admonish them or think unkindly of them, consider that there may be something else going on in their life that is distracting or distressing them.

If your aims as a team are aligned, you will be more productive, produce better results and be happier with yourselves.

DISABILITY AND DIFFERENCE

Be aware of potential disability or unnoticed difference in your colleagues. There may be obvious physical disability, but there may also be less obvious disability. Your colleague that you accuse of not being able to spell may actually have dyslexia or may not have your native language as their first language. Your left-handed assistant may be struggling with the right-handed instruments. If you can facilitate an adjustment to support a colleague who is different or has a disability your working relationship with them will be mutually respectful.

SUPERVISORY ROLES

Preceptors, proctors, mentors and coaches

As you surgeon, you may be, or have a preceptor, proctor, mentor or coach. There may be overlap or transition between these roles.

A preceptor helps their preceptee gain new skills or knowledge by defining specific aims. The preceptor will scrub in for an operative case, gradually decreasing their active involvement as the preceptee improves over time.

A proctor will work with a proctee who already has some skill, observe their performance, provide some guidance for improvement, and assess them on their competence and provide constructive feedback. A proctor does not usually scrub in in an operative case.

A mentor provides holistic support and guidance, usually with some specific goals or aims in mind. This may be to provide guidance for a particular part of the mentee's career. The mentor may work collaboratively with the mentee and provide them with feedback.

A coach generally has a one-to-one relationship with the coachee, supporting them to reflect and self-assess in order to seek their own solutions, improve and advance.

Teaching and training are an integral part of being a surgeon. In a craft specialty, the skills you can pass on to others is of benefit to the profession. You do not have to be a formal teacher. Not everyone either enjoys or is effective at formal teaching. However, even leading by example can help to educate the surgeons of the future.

HUMAN FACTORS—BE AWARE AND CARE

There is much in the literature about human factors and patient and team safety. Attention to human factors will reduce errors, improve patient outcomes and result in a happier team.

It is important to take into account everyone's perspective particularly when there is an ongoing incident or emergency; this has been termed situational awareness. The team should work together and feel that they can speak and be heard—there should be a safe team culture. If one person has been doggedly performing one component of the process, they may be tired and hoping someone else will take over. There should be a team leader for any significant event to direct the process and coordinate team changeovers and the acquisition of any necessary equipment. Who the leader is should be clear to everyone, and if there is an established protocol it should be followed. Any distractions from the emergency in hand should be removed if possible.

Even when there is not a crisis, if one of your colleagues is clearly tired or overwhelmed, facilitate them taking a break. If they are unwell, ensure that have adequate support and encourage them to go home and rest. Treat your colleagues fairly and compassionately.

WHEN THINGS DON'T GO TO PLAN

Doctors, in general, often hold their disappointment inside when things don't go to plan. These instances can include when a patient on whom you have operated suffers a complication or you are involved with a patient that dies. Sometimes, in these heightened times of emotion, there is a grey area between the feeling of responsibility and the feeling of guilt, both in our own minds and the perception of others. It is normal to have a sense of responsibility. If you have done your best and followed normal practice within the confines of your own ability, you should not feel guilt. Likewise, do not make comments that suggest that a colleague is guilty of a misdemeanour when they are in the same shoes. In particular, do not do so to deflect any suggestion of blame from yourself.

Help your team to learn from mishaps and mistakes. A negative culture will suppress any urge to improve and foster resentment. This reduces future prospects of openness and transparency. On the other hand, a listening and sharing culture is inclusive and constructive. If the foundation trainee/intern has forgotten to cross-match some blood for a patient, instead of chiding them, find out if they are overwhelmed with work or if they need educational support to fulfil their role. You could use the situation to encourage them to make a checklist with you of what is needed for a particular case. This will not only make them feel valued but will also improve patient care.

After a major mishap or after a patient has died unexpectedly, a team debrief can be both instructive and supportive. Such a debrief is usually led by the most senior person on the team but does not have to be. Sometimes a person who was involved more peripherally is in a better position to lead and support the team because they can be more objective and are not wrestling with their own inner feelings of responsibility.

Key point

- Your behaviour towards your team will be reflected back on you. In the same way as the reaction to a smile is to smile back, if you are kind and considerate to others, they will return the favour.

FURTHER READING

Sachdeva AK. Preceptoring, proctoring, mentoring and coaching in surgery. *J Surg Oncol.* 2021;124: 711–721.

Index

Note: Page numbers followed by "*f*" indicate figures, "*t*" indicate tables, and "*b*" indicate boxes.

Index

Index

Index